Health Reference Series

Volume Twenty-seven

WOMEN'S
Health Concerns
SOURCEBOOK

*Basic Information about Health Issues that
Affect Women, Featuring Facts about
Menstruation and other Gynecological
Concerns Including Endometriosis,
Fibroids, Menopause, and Vaginitis;
Reproductive Concerns Including Birth
Control, Infertility, and Abortion; and
Facts about Additional Physical Emotional,
and Mental Health Concerns Prevalent
Among Women such as Osteoporosis,
Urinary Tract Disorders, Eating Disorders,
and Depression; Along with Tips for
Maintaining a Healthy Lifestyle*

Edited by
Heather E. Aldred

Omnigraphics, Inc.

Penobscot Building / Detroit, MI 48226

BIBLIOGRAPHIC NOTE

This volume contains individual publications and excerpts from documents produced by the National Institutes of Health (NIH), its sister agencies and subagencies. Numbered publications are: 357-505, 89-2893, 90-8416, 91-502, 91-2097, 91-2151, 91-2413, 92-1191, 92-3193, 92-2720, 93-3219, 94-1181, 94-1556, 94-3220, 94-3589, 94-3677, 94-3700, 95-3871, 95-3894, and 95-3901; unnumbered publications include: "Anorexia and Oral Contraceptives," "Facts about Dysmenorrhea and PMS," "General Information on Pelvic Inflammatory Disease," "What Is a Pap Smear?" and "Women and HIV Infection." Selected articles from *FDA Consumer*, *Age Page*, and *National Center for Research Resources Reporter* are also included. Other documents produced by The President's Council on Physical Fitness and Sports and The New York Department of Health. Copyrighted articles from the Atlanta Reproductive Health Centre, and the American Social Health Association, and Planned Parenthood, Inc., are also included. Copyrighted articles are used by permission. Full citation information is located on the first page of each article.

Edited by Heather E. Aldred
Karen Bellenir, Series Editor, *Health Reference Series*
Peter D. Dresser, *Managing Editor, Health Reference Series*

Omnigraphics, Inc.

Matthew P. Barbour, *Production Manager*
Laurie Lanzen Harris, *Vice President, Editorial*
Peter E. Ruffner, *Vice President, Administration*
James A. Sellgren, *Vice President, Operations and Finance*
Jane J. Steele, *Marketing Consultant*

Frederick G. Ruffner, Jr., *Publisher*

© 1997, Omnigraphics, Inc.

Library of Congress Cataloging-in-Publication Data

Women's health concerns sourcebook : basic information about
     health issues that affect women, featuring facts about men-
     struation and other gynecological concerns . . . / edited by
     Heather E. Aldred.
          p. cm. -- (Health reference series ; v. 27)
     Includes bibliographical references and index.
     ISBN 0-7808-0219-5
     1. Women--Health and hygiene.   2 . Women--Diseases.
I. Aldred, Heather E.   II. Series.
RA778.W7543 1997   97-17093
613'.04244--dc21   CIP

∞

This book is printed on acid-free paper meeting the ANSI Z39.48 Standard. The infinity symbol that appears above indicates that the paper in this book meets that standard.
Printed in the United States

Contents

Part III: Family Planning Decisions

Part IV: Other Common Physical Health Concerns Prevalent in Women

Part V: Emotional and Mental Health Concerns

Part VI: Tips for Maintaining a Healthy Lifestyle

Preface

About This Book

Many of the health issues that concern women differ significantly
from those faced by men. Although gynecological and reproductive
issues are perhaps the most obvious, there are many others. These
include osteoporosis, urinary tract disorders, lupus, eating disorders,
and depression, all of which affect a larger percentage of the female
population than the male population in the United States. In addition to gender-specific diseases and disorders, this book also includes
information for maintaining a healthy lifestyle.

Women's Health Concerns Sourcebook contains numerous publications produced by a wide variety of government and private agencies
including the National Institutes of Health (NIH), the Department
of Health and Human Services (DHHS), the Food and Drug Administration, the Federal Trade Commission, the New York Department
of Health, Planned Parenthood of America, Inc., the Atlanta Reproductive Health Centre, and the American Social Health Association.
The documents were chosen to present basic medical information for
the interested layperson—both for the woman herself and for those
who care about her. Several important subjects pertinent to women
are not covered in great depth here, however, because they are addressed in other volumes of the *Health Reference Series*. For example,
obstetrical information will be covered in *Pregnancy and Birth
Sourcebook*, a forthcoming volume. To help the reader locate additional

sources of information, the final paragraph of this Preface includes references to other pertinent books in the *Health Reference Series*.

How to Use This Book

This book is divided into six parts covering broad areas of interest. Within each part individual chapters discuss individual subjects. To help pinpoint specific topics, some chapters are further divided into sections.

Part I: Menstruation and Related Concerns provides information about menstruation and the associated problems women sometimes face. These include menstrual cramps, premenstrual syndrome, and toxic shock syndrome. One chapter focuses exclusively on menopause.

Part II: Other Gynecological Concerns offers information on other medical issues relating to the reproductive tract, including endometriosis, uterine fibroids, ovarian cysts, and vaginitis along with important facts about sexually transmitted diseases in women. Common symptoms, causes and risk factors, diagnostic tools, and treatments are discussed.

Part III: Family Planning Decisions includes three chapters that provide answers to a wide variety of some of the most commonly asked questions about family planning. These include birth control methods, infertility treatments, and abortion.

Part IV: Other Common Physical Health Concerns Prevalent in Women offers information about many disorders that affect both women and men but which are more prevalent in women. These include breast cancer, osteoporosis, lupus, and urinary tract disorders.

Part V: Emotional and Mental Health Concerns presents information about three common problems: eating disorders, estimated to impact three or four percent of young women between the ages of 12 and 18; depression, a disorder affecting as many as one in ten adults in the U.S. including a disproportionate number of women; and stress, a seemingly ubiquitous feature of modern life that can lead to both mental and physical illnesses.

Part VI: Tips for Maintaining a Healthy Lifestyle supplies practical help for women who want to adopt sound cardiovascular and nutritional habits.

Acknowledgements

The editor wishes to thank the Atlanta Reproductive Health Centre, and the American Social Health Association, and Planned Parenthood, Inc., for granting permission to reprint their useful and important articles; researcher Mary Margaret Missar for locating the documents included in this volume; and Karen Bellenir and Peter Dresser for their technical assistance and advice.

Note from the Editor

This book is part of Omnigraphics' Health Reference Series. The series provides basic information about a broad range of medical concerns. It is not intended to serve as a tool for diagnosing illness, in prescribing treatments, or as a substitute for the physician/patient relationship. All persons concerned about medical symptoms or the possibility of disease are encouraged to seek professional care from an appropriate health care provider.

Note on the Health Reference Series

Further information on a variety of diseases and disorders can be found in the following *Health Reference Series* volumes:

- *Diabetes Sourcebook* (Volume 3)—comprehensive disease and statistical information about diabetes, a disorder that affects a disproportionate number of women.

- *AIDS Sourcebook* (Volume 4)—symptoms, treatments, and preventative measures along with statistics covering the female population.

- *Cardiovascular Diseases and Disorders Sourcebook* (Volume 5)—in-depth information about the number one killer of American women: coronary heart disease.

- *Respiratory Diseases and Disorders Sourcebook* (Volume 6)—more help with smoking cessation along with specific disease information.

- *Mental Health Sourcebook* (Volume 9)—information on other mental health subjects of interest to women including panic disorder and agoraphobia.

- *Cancer Sourcebook for Women* (Volume 10)—important information about gynecological cancers and additional details about breast cancer.

- *Genetic Disorders Sourcebook* (Volume 13)—information and resource listings for a female sex-linked genetic disorders.

- *Substance Abuse Sourcebook* (Volume 14)—answers to questions about substance abuse in women and help related to intervention and prevention.

- *Diet and Nutrition Sourcebook* (Volume 15)—additional information on nutrition, healthy eating habits, and weight management.

- *Immune Disorders Sourcebook* (Volume 17)—further information about lupus and other disorders of the immune system.

- *Fitness and Exercise Sourcebook* (Volume 20)—detailed information on exercise and fitness along with data about specific activities and recent research efforts.

- *Kidney and Urinary Tract Disorders Sourcebook* (Volume 21)—discussions of urinary tract disorders including bladder and kidney cancer.

- *Sexually Transmitted Diseases Sourcebook* (Volume 26)—information on a wide variety of sexually transmitted diseases including a chapter focused exclusively on women's concerns.

Part One

Menstruation
and Related Concerns

Chapter 1

Menstruation and Menstrual Cramps

Chapter Contents

Section 1.1

Facts about Dysmenorrhea

Excerpts from NIH publication, Facts about Dysmenorrhea and
Premenstrual Syndrome, 1983.

Dysmenorrhea (painful menstruation) can disable a woman for a
few hours before or at the onset of her menstrual period and last for
several hours or as long as two days. Pain may be severe and daily
activities may have to be modified.

Hormones and the Normal Menstrual Cycle

Hormones play an important role in the proper functioning of the
menstrual cycle. In studying menstrual disorders, scientists have tried
to determine how menstruation occurs normally.

The onset of menstruation (menarche) is the dramatic marker of
the change from girl to woman. Usually occurring between ages of ten
and sixteen, the beginning of menstruation means that a young girl
is developing the ability to bear children. At first the cycle may be
irregular. Usually, a regular menstrual cycle is established by the end
of the first year after menarche. Interrupted only for pregnancies or
specific health problems, it continues month after month until a
woman is in her forties or fifties when menstruation ceases (menopause). A typical cycle is about 28 days, but cycles varying from 24 to
30 days are not uncommon. Generally, a woman keeps to the established pattern although stress, illness or the use of oral contraceptives may alter her cycle temporarily.

During each cycle, the inner wall or lining (endometrium) of the
uterus thickens to provide a suitable environment for a pregnancy. A
mature egg (ovum) is released from one of the two ovaries in mid-cycle
(ovulation) and remains in the reproductive tract for about three days.
For a pregnancy to occur, the ovum must be fertilized by a sperm. If
there is no pregnancy, the lining of the uterus breaks down and is

discharged as the menstrual flow (menses) over the course of three to eight days.

Although the reproductive organs are located in the body's pelvic area, the reproductive cycle is controlled by an area at the base of the brain containing the hypothalamus and the pituitary gland. The hypothalamus and the pituitary gland orchestrate menstrual cycle activities, sending "start" and "stop" signals each month to the ovaries and uterus.

On the first day of menstruation, hormone levels are low. But after one week and for most of the remaining cycle, *estrogens* are produced to promote ovulation and stimulate the development of the endometrium. During this time estrogens contribute to producing an appropriate environment in the reproductive organs for fertilization, implantation and nurturing of the early embryo. Estrogen production drops off a few days before the next cycle begins.

Progesterone, a hormone produced in large amounts during the latter half of the cycle, stimulates the development of the endometrium in preparation for a pregnancy. If there is no pregnancy, progesterone levels decrease and menstruation begins. If pregnancy occurs, production of progesterone continues throughout the nine months to help maintain the pregnancy.

Other hormone-like substances, prostaglandins, are also produced during the latter half of the cycle. Although the role of prostaglandins is not completely understood, they are believed to stimulate uterine contractions which are recognized as cramps during the menstrual period. The prostaglandins may be one of the possible factors that start labor.

Dysmenorrhea Explained

Many women experience some discomfort when a menstrual period begins. Most can manage daily routines and responsibilities because the discomfort is mild and brief in duration. For others, the discomfort is severe, lasts for hours, and is disabling. In a recent health survey of adolescent women, more than half reported pain during menstruation.

Dysmenorrhea is the medical term for painful menstruation. It is primarily caused by moderate to severe cramping of the uterus. Headache, backache, diarrhea and nausea are associated symptoms.

Dysmenorrhea usually does not begin until six to twelve months following menarche, when a woman's system has developed fully and ovulation occurs regularly. The disorder appears to affect young women and women who have not borne children more so than older women who have had children.

In the past, the young woman's complaints of pain were dismissed with the advice, "It's just part of being a woman. You'll get over it after you have a baby." There is a measure of truth in that latter statement because dysmenorrhea diminishes in many women after a full-term pregnancy. This may occur because uterine muscles are stretched during pregnancy. Another possible explanation is that uterine blood supply and muscle activity may be improved by the process of having a child.

Research Findings

Noting the similarity between menstrual cramps and mild labor pains, scientific investigation in the past had focused on the basic workings of uterine contractions. Prostaglandins were identified as one of the factors involved in causing contractions. These substances are secreted by the uterine lining and affect the smooth muscles of the uterus, thus assisting in the sloughing off of the lining during menstruation.

While attention was directed to this area of research, reports began to appear that oral contraceptive users seemed to have less menstrual problems than nonusers. One explanation given was that the decrease in menstrual flow associated with oral contraceptive use resulted in a reduction of prostaglandin concentration.

Other researchers, however, observed that oral contraceptives suppress ovulation, and in the absence of ovulation uterine production of prostaglandins is diminished. This observation, combined with the knowledge that prostaglandins stimulate uterine contractions, led researchers to conclude that an oversupply of prostaglandins is a likely cause of painful contractions of the uterus.

Although oral contraceptives seem effective in relieving dysmenorrhea, their side effects have prevented many women from using them. As a result, other substances were sought to lessen or inhibit prostaglandin production. Now, through research and careful testing, such products are available. These agents, previously developed for the treatment of arthritis, are similar to aspirin, but many times more potent.

Treatment Options

The first step in arriving at treatment for dysmenorrhea is a thorough pelvic examination. This can rule out certain medical conditions other than dysmenorrhea that can cause pelvic pain. At the time of the examination, other health factors and practices can also be discussed with the physician. For example, for some women reducing the amount of salt, caffeine and sugar in the diet, especially in the week before a period is due, often provides relief, as does moderate exercise and sufficient rest.

For a few women, menstrual disorders may stem from psychological problems and worries. Treating the psychological problems of these women often alleviates their menstrual problems. For most others who suffer dysmenorrhea, the source of their pain is the uterus, contracting too hard or too fast. Traditionally, analgesics and sedatives have been used to treat menstrual pain, although these drugs may affect a patient's normal activities, such as driving a car or taking an exam in school.

As a result of scientific research, new types of medication are available. For moderate to severe dysmenorrhea, drugs that prevent or lessen the production of prostaglandins in the first hours or day of the menstrual period have proved effective without serious side effects in about 75 percent of the patients. The drugs provide relief from pain by reducing the level of prostaglandins which in turn moderates the uterine contractions. Not all women can tolerate these drugs, however, especially those who have gastrointestinal problems.

Researchers continue to search for other possible causes of dysmenorrhea and to develop modes of treatment for women who are not helped by the present array of medications.

Section 1.2

Taming Menstrual Cramps

FDA Consumer, June 1991.

For many women "that time of the month" is one they'd rather forgo. More than half routinely experience some form of pain associated with menstruation, say doctors at the Mayo Clinic in Minnesota, and 1 in 10 suffers such severe dysmenorrhea—menstrual pain—she cannot function normally without taking medication.

Throughout history, women have tried to alleviate these menstrual discomforts themselves. But home remedies—teas, hot baths, heating pads, and such—offered only limited help. As recently as a decade ago, when there were far fewer products readily available for menstrual cramps than now, some doctors prescribed powerful prescription painkillers. Others, many women recall, told patients their problems would disappear as they grew older or after they had children.

But today, the pain associated with menstruation is taken more seriously, and there are new, highly effective treatments for it.

"Nearly all women—I would say 99.9 percent—should be able to function quite well during their periods with the menstrual treatments available now," says Charles H. Debrovner, M.D., a gynecologist in private practice and on the faculty of the New York University School of Medicine in New York City.

What's Causing the Pain?

There are two kinds of painful menses—primary and secondary dysmenorrhea—and it is very important to distinguish between them so both are treated properly, Debrovner stresses.

Primary dysmenorrhea usually starts within three years of the onset of menstruation and lasts one or two days each month. While this type of menstrual pain may lessen for some women as they grow older or after the birth of children, it also can continue until menopause.

Secondary dysmenorrhea is menstrual pain caused by disease such as pelvic inflammatory disease, endometriosis (abnormalities in the lining of the uterus), or uterine fibroids (nonmalignant growths). Endometriosis is a major cause of secondary dysmenorrhea. Pain from it usually starts later in life and worsens with time, according to Debrovner. Another hint that disease might be the cause of menstrual pain is if pain also occurs during intercourse or other parts of the cycle.

Primary dysmenorrhea is a result of the normal production of prostaglandins—chemical substances that are made by cells in the lining of the uterus. (Prostaglandins are also produced elsewhere throughout the body.) The lining of the uterus—which has built up and thickened during the early stages of the menstrual cycle—breaks up and is sloughed off at the end of the cycle and releases prostaglandins, explains Lisa Rarick, M.D., medical officer in FDA's division of metabolism and endocrine drug products.

The prostaglandins, in turn, make the uterus contract more strongly than at any other time of the cycle. They can even cause it to contract so much that the blood supply is cut off temporarily, depriving the uterine muscle of oxygen and thus causing pain. Women who suffer painful contractions may be producing excessive amounts of prostaglandins. Or, it may be that some women are just more sensitive to them, says Rarick.

The cramps themselves help push out the menstrual discharge. Because the cervical opening is often widened after childbirth or years of menstruation, cramps may lessen in severity later in life.

Most women describe their menstrual cramps as a dull aching or a pressure low in the abdomen. The pains may wax and wane, remain constant, or be so severe that they cause nausea, vomiting, diarrhea, backache, sweating, and an achiness that spreads to the hips, lower back, and thighs.

Inhibiting Prostaglandins

For many years, women had little help for these symptoms. Doctors recommended aspirin, heating pads, and hot baths. When those failed, they often prescribed painkillers such as Demerol or Tylenol with Codeine. These treatments were all aimed at the perception of pain rather than the cause of it. Even tranquilizers were sometimes used, according to Debrovner.

But the advent of pain relievers that impede the production of prostaglandins has made it possible to directly treat the cause of the cramps. Called NSAIDs, for nonsteroidal anti-inflammatory drugs, these medications have proven remarkably effective for many women.

Because NSAIDS inhibit synthesis of prostaglandins, and thereby the contractions of the uterus, they may actually reduce menstrual flow. Many of Debrovner's patients report shorter periods when they take the drugs at the first sign of pain. He recommends taking them as early as possible after the menstrual flow starts. Waiting too long may mean they won't be as effective.

The prostaglandin inhibitors can cause gastrointestinal distress, so most doctors also recommend they be taken with milk and food. Labeling on the OTC products contains this information.

While there are about a dozen prescription NSAIDs, three— ibuprofen (Motrin, Rufen, etc.), naproxen (Naprosyn), and mefenamic acid (Ponstel)—are now approved to treat menstrual cramps.

Over-the-Counter Products

FDA approved ibuprofen for over-the-counter use in 1984. It now can be found as the active ingredient in several OTC medications, such as Advil, Nuprin, and Motrin IB. The OTC dose per pill is 200 milligrams. The recommended dose is one tablet every four to six hours (or two, if one does not work), not to exceed six in a 24-hour period. Prescription formulations come in dosages of 400 to 800 milligrams.

Aspirin—long a standard over-the-counter treatment for cramps— works as a prostaglandin inhibitor, although probably not so powerfully as the specific inhibitors such as ibuprofen. While aspirin is known to thin the blood and increase bleeding, it does not appear to have this effect on menstrual flow, according to Rarick.

Researchers are not sure if acetaminophen, an analgesic found in drugs such as Tylenol and Datril, works to prevent prostaglandin production. If it does, its effect appears to be milder than that of aspirin or other NSAIDs. Doctors say, however, that it can successfully treat the headache and backache that often accompany menstrual cramps.

Some OTC menstrual pain medications, such as Midol and Pamprin, contain a mix of ingredients that include an analgesic such as acetaminophen, a diuretic such as pamabrom, and an antihistamine such as pyrilamine maleate. Some newer formulations now use ibuprofen in place of more classic analgesics such as aspirin or acetaminophen. Midol 200 Advanced Cramp Formula, for example, contains ibuprofen as its active ingredient. Maximum Strength Midol Multi-Symptom Formula, however, contains acetaminophen as an analgesic. With the variety of ingredients now available, it's wise to read the label to make sure the product is the best one to treat your symptoms. If in doubt, consult your doctor.

Other Treatments

Women who use oral contraceptives rarely suffer menstrual cramps, so some doctors prescribe them for women whose cramps are unrelieved by other treatments. Contraceptive pills disrupt the normal hormonal changes of the menstrual cycle, resulting in a thinner uterine lining and a decrease in production of prostaglandins. However, menstrual cramp relief is not considered by FDA to be a primary reason to use oral contraceptives; rather, it is included in the labeling as a secondary benefit.

Exercise, too, may be of some benefit, possibly because it raises levels of beta endorphins, chemicals in the brain associated with pain relief. With new knowledge, such as the possible roles of exercise and of prostaglandins in preventing cramps, most women can avoid suffering the monthly anguish of severe menstrual pain.

— by Ellen Hale

Chapter 2

Premenstrual Syndrome

Premenstrual syndrome (PMS) is the term given to the group of physical and behavioral changes that may affect some women in the week or so just before a menstrual period. For unexplained reasons, these women suffer moderate to severe distress and tension during that time. They may experience abdominal bloating, fatigue, irritability, or moodiness. Often they may do and say things that alienate friends and family. Negative self-images may develop as these women attempt to cope with severe PMS symptoms.

In the past, women suffered menstrual discomfort in embarrassed, even guilty silence. Menstruating women were thought to be under a curse, unclean, or at the very least, unwell. The subject was not a topic for public discussion. Similar attitudes persist in certain cultures today. There is, however, an increasing awareness in most modern societies that menstruation is not an illness, but a normal and necessary function that is part of the process enabling women to bear children.

Dysmenorrhea and PMS have been the focus of recent public attention. Reports about both conditions in popular publications have suggested that effective treatment is readily available for menstrual cramps (the cause of pain during menstruation) and imminent for PMS. Scientific reports, however, are more conservative. They show that some medications for dysmenorrhea may help some women, but not all. Relief for PMS, however, is still largely a matter of treating symptoms in the absence of a known cause. Researchers first need to

Excerpts from NIH document entitled Facts about Dysmenorrhea and Premenstrual Syndrome and *FDA Consumer*, June 1991 by Ellen Hale.

understand the precise workings of the menstrual cycle before they can know how and why hormonal imbalances occur.

While dysmenorrhea is a disorder more frequently reported by women in their teens and early twenties, premenstrual syndrome (PMS) is reported more often by women in their late twenties and thirties. Interestingly, PMS patients who have had hysterectomies (surgical removal of the uterus) may continue to have PMS symptoms. This observation has led researchers to conclude that the uterus appears not to be a significant factor in causing PMS.

Based on reviews of health surveys, it has been estimated that four out of five women surveyed experience varying degrees of premenstrual symptoms. Of these, one out of four suffer temporarily disabling symptoms. Behavioral symptoms range from depression, aggression, irritability and anxiety to mood swings, nervous tension, and food cravings. Physical symptoms include fluid retention, headache, acne, fatigue and exhaustion.

Most women can cope with the mild form of PMS, but for others with moderate or severe PMS, the physical discomfort can be stressful. Because of fluid retention, a woman may feel bloated, with swelling in her ankles, abdomen and breasts. The enlargement of her breast can cause tenderness and discomfort. She may feel emotionally unstable and behave in seemingly odd and erratic ways.

As with dysmenorrhea, the traditional approach viewed premenstrual distress as "just part of being a woman." Until recently, the distress had been written off as something a woman could control if she would put her mind to it. The association of the various symptoms with menstruation was difficult to recognize because symptoms occur before a woman's period begins. The very nature of the syndrome often made objective reporting difficult. Only recently have the medical and scientific communities become sensitive to the possibility of physiological causes of the various symptoms.

When the symptoms were finally related to the premenstrual period, hormonal imbalance was suggested as a possible cause of the disorder. Other theories advanced included those linking PMS to nutritional or chemical deficiencies in a woman's body chemistry.

With the advent of oral contraceptives (usually a combination of estrogen and progestin, a synthetic progesterone) reports appeared that women on oral contraceptives experienced less premenstrual depression than nonusers. This observation led some investigators to theorize that progesterone deficiency in the last phase of the menstrual cycle might be involved in PMS.

Although hormone levels in a woman can be ascertained at a particular moment in time, these levels vary throughout the month and from woman to woman. Scientists do not fully understand what amount of progesterone is normal or adequate.

Nevertheless, for a number of years a few physicians in England have been prescribing progesterone to PMS sufferers, specifying only natural progesterone, a scarce, expensive drug that is difficult to administer. One has reported marked improvement in up to 95 percent of his PMS patients using progesterone therapy. Side effects of taking progesterone are rare, but headache, exhaustion, feelings of lightheadedness and uterine bleeding may be experienced.

Relieving PMS

PMS occurs in the last 7 to 10 days of the menstrual cycle—called the luteal phase. The time at which these symptoms occur is very important because it's what allows doctors to track their cyclic nature and make a diagnosis.

While premenstrual syndrome remains a mysterious malady, there is growing recognition that it is a true physical syndrome, and there are a number of new treatments to help lessen its symptoms.

The American College of Obstetrics and Gynecology (ACOG) says from 20 to 40 percent of all women suffer some symptoms of PMS, which it defines as "a recurring cycle of symptoms that are so severe as to affect lifestyle or work." ACOG estimates that 5 percent of women have severely disabling PMS.

The variety and combinations of symptoms are usually divided into four major groups, according to Lisa Rarick, M.D., medical officer in FDA's division of metabolism and endocrine drug products. Breast tenderness, swelling, weight gains and bloating comprise one group of symptoms. A second group includes emotional changes such as depression, forgetfulness, crying, insomnia, and confusion. A third group involves headaches, food cravings (especially sweets), increased appetite, fatigue, and dizziness. The fourth group includes anxiety, nervous tension, mood swings, and irritability.

For the most part, PMS is alleviated by treating its symptoms. For example, for those who suffer from symptoms of water retention, diuretics may help. They are a component of many OTC medications for PMS. In 1988, FDA tentatively proposed that three OTC diuretics could be used in menstrual drug products (including those that treat PMS): caffeine, ammonium chloride, and pamabrom.

It is believed that caffeine may help relieve bloating and water retention because it acts as a mild diuretic, and that it also may help relieve the fatigue many women complain of in the premenstrual period. On the other hand, excessive amounts of caffeine may aggravate anxiety and tension, and some doctors think it may be associated with increased breast tenderness. Some over-the-counter medications for PMS combine several ingredients. One product, for example, contains pyrilamine maleate (an antihistamine approved for OTC use but not specifically for PMS), pamabrom and acetaminophen. Women should read the labels of OTC products and check with their doctors for advice on the best treatments for the specific PMS symptoms they have.

Some doctors believe women may be able to help themselves through the discomfort of PMS without pills by exercising, eliminating or cutting down on smoking, and changing their diets.

"I recommend eating small frequent meals because a lot of food causes blood sugar to swing up and down, and that may effect premenstrual problems," says M. Yusoff Dawood, M.D., director of the Division of Reproductive Endocrinology at the University of Texas Medical School in Houston.

To stem water retention, many doctors recommend reducing salt intake, and to reduce headaches, avoiding liquor. No scientific studies have proven that exercise can reduce PMS, but there is much anecdotal and indirect evidence that it does, doctors say.

"The idea is that exercise raises levels of beta endorphins, [which] have a positive effect on mood and behavior," says Michelle Warren, M.D., co-director of the Division of Reproductive Endocrinology at St. Luke's-Roosevelt Hospital in New York City. Moreover, she believes exercise may reduce water retention.

Vitamin B6, known as pyridoxine, is recommended by some doctors to relieve PMS, but studies on its effectiveness have been inconclusive, according to Dawood. Use of extreme doses of it have been associated with neurological problems.

For those whose PMS is unrelieved by most common treatments, more help is available. While not approved for these uses by FDA, some doctors prescribe birth control pills and use of progesterone suppositories (during the premenstrual phase) for PMS. Oral contraceptives prevent ovulation and therefore prevent the luteal phase from occurring. Although progesterone suppositories have proven no more successful than a placebo in controlled studies, because they seem to help some women, Warren believes they are worthwhile. Prescription painkillers, diuretics, tranquilizers, and antidepressants are also prescribed by physicians in severe cases.

Research Findings

Although success with progesterone treatment has been reported, carefully controlled studies have failed to substantiate either the claim that progesterone deficiency is the cause of PMS or that progesterone therapy is beneficial. Currently, the U.S. Food and Drug Administration considers that progesterone treatment of PMS is not indicated.

A variety of other theories about the causes of PMS and methods of treatment for the disorder have been offered. Nutritional deficiencies, such as the lack of vitamin B6, have been reported among women with PMS. As with progesterone therapy, replacement of the lacking nutrient has relieved PMS symptoms in some women although it is not certain that this is other than a placebo effect.

Most research projects are concerned with understanding the basic mechanisms of menstrual cycle activities. There are a few experimental treatment programs for PMS, usually associated with university medical schools or colleges. Limited success has been reported, such as in a research project using bromocriptine (a drug that suppresses lactation after childbirth) to treat PMS. In this study breast engorgement and tenderness were significantly reduced for some women, but other symptoms were not relieved.

The causes of premenstrual syndrome remain elusive. The subjective nature of the disorder contributes to the problem, as does the wide range of reactions to hormone activities that women can have. Some women react to the smallest shifts in body chemistry or functions, while others do not.

Researchers agree that this and other problems in studying PMS need clarification and further study. For example, one problem that both researchers and clinicians wish to clarify is the method of diagnosing PMS. Usually, when a patient tells a physician about symptoms of a medical problem, the physician can confirm the diagnosis with blood or urine analyses, X-rays or with some other technology. But for PMS, no such tests are yet available. Scientists are looking for a way to assess the severity or occurrence of PMS. One recent project found lower levels of magnesium in the blood of women with PMS than in normal women. This observation may be useful in the future as a marker in diagnosing PMS. A federally funded study at the National Institutes of Health in Bethesda, Maryland, is attempting to document the relationship between the menstrual cycle and mood and behavior disorders.

A comprehensive study of the complex inter-relationships of hypothalamic, pituitary and ovarian function is currently supported by the NICHD. A new theory has emerged from this study indicating certain messenger chemicals from the pituitary (neuropeptides) as the possible source of mood and behavior symptoms reported in PMS. By blocking action of the neuropeptides with other chemicals, researchers hope to control the symptoms. To date, there has been wide variation in reaction to neuropeptide activity among the subjects in the study.

Scientists are just beginning to learn about neuropeptides and the effects the blocking agents may have. This research is expected to continue for the next several years as investigators search for a better understanding of hormones, neuropeptides, and the basic workings of the normal menstrual cycle. The nature of the research means, however, that studies often take months and sometimes years to collect data, perform analyses and reach conclusions.

Treatment Options for PMS

Treatment for this disorder presents a challenge because of the many variables involved. To rule out any other medical or psychological problems that may be causing symptoms, a thorough physical examination by a gynecologist is the first step. Following this, a physician may treat the symptoms, recommending diuretics, special diets or medication. Some women may be referred to a university medical school department of gynecology or possibly to a PMS research program.

For help with the severe psychological aspects of PMS, physicians may recommend that women join behavior modification programs or support groups. Support groups can be valuable therapy for a PMS patient, particularly while attempting behavior modification such as changing diet or other health habits. Meeting other women who share the disorder and having access to current PMS information are important benefits of support groups,

Keeping Informed

Professional, scientific and voluntary organizations interested in women's health can provide information on new developments in menstrual cycle research and in the diagnosis, treatment and possible prevention of dysmenorrhea and premenstrual syndrome.

Another way to keep informed is by reading research reports published in scientific journals. Although generally very technical, the reports offer the reader an opportunity to learn first-hand what is new in scientific research. The journals can be found at medical school libraries or other medical libraries. The facilities of the National Library of Medicine are available for obtaining specific references and articles.

Some sources of information on dysmenorrhea and PMS are:

American College of Obstetricians and Gynecologists
409 12th Street, S.W.
Washington, D.C. 20024
Telephone: 202-638-5577

The Premenstrual Syndrome Program
108 Halket Street
Pittsburgh, PA 15213
Telephone: 412-647-1650

National Women's Health Network
1325 G Street, N.W.
Washington, D.C. 20005
Telephone: 202-347-1140

FDA estimates that 1 to 17 per 100,000 menstruating women develop TSS each year.

Since CDRH's Medical Device Reporting Program began in 1984, FDA has received 76 reports of death related to tampon use. Scientific evaluation showed that all but three of the deaths resulted from TSS.

The exact link between TSS and tampon use is not completely known. Scientists believe it requires the presence of *Staphylococcus aureus*, a bacterium that releases one or more toxins into the bloodstream. *S. aureus* commonly exists on the body in areas such as the nose, skin or vagina, and often causes no problem. But it also can lead to serious infection after a deep wound or surgery or, for reasons not fully understood, during tampon use.

About 4 percent of TSS cases are fatal. Risk of death is higher in cases not related to menstruation, says Anne Schuchat, M.D., an epidemiologist with the national Centers for Disease Control and Prevention. "This may be because of the different toxins involved," she says. "In one study looking for TSST-1 [toxic shock syndrome toxin-1], about 90 percent of isolates of *S. aureus* from menstrual TSS patients produced the toxin, but only about 60 percent of isolates from non-menstrual TSS cases did. At least one other *S. aureus* toxin has been identified in TSS cases, and we think there may be more."

In 1980, an increase in TSS appeared in previously healthy young women who had become ill during or just after menstruation. Studies showed an association with tampon use. Then, in 1981, a three-state study reported an even greater risk with high-absorbency tampons. The National Academy of Sciences' Institute of Medicine supported this finding and recommended in 1982 that women minimize their use of high-absorbency tampons. As a result, FDA issued a regulation on June 22, 1982, to require warning information on tampon labeling, including a list of TSS symptoms and advice to choose the lowest needed absorbency.

Because of concern over tampon safety, FDA's division of mechanics and materials science laboratory began testing the absorbency of all types of tampons. "We found unusual absorbency differences between brands," says laboratory director Donald Marlowe, "especially in 'super' varieties. Only through trial and error could a woman select the least absorbency needed."

Standards Sought

A major problem revealed by this early testing was that industry had no standard tampon absorbency test. To look into this and other

TSS issues, a tampon task force representing consumer groups, industry, and FDA was formed under the auspices of the American Society for Testing and Materials. Marlowe's group worked with the society to modify and make uniform a test that was being used by some manufacturers. The "syngyna test," as it's called, simulates normal tampon use conditions. It is this test that has been adopted as the industry standard under the new tampon rule.

The society's task force sought industry's cooperation to voluntarily standardize tampon labeling terms. For indeed, the absorbency of "regular" in one brand could very well be higher than "super" in another brand.

"The voluntary effort almost worked, but the task force couldn't agree on how to describe absorbency in the labeling," says F. Alan Andersen, Ph.D., acting director of CDRH's office of device evaluation. The group was disbanded in 1984, and FDA announced that summer that it would require standard absorbency disclosure and standard testing through regulation.

The need for regulation gained further momentum in 1987 when a CDC study found that TSS risk increases with each one-gram increase in tampon absorbency. An intensive case-finding study reported in 1989 by FDA, CDC, and the National Institutes of Health showed that the TSS risk is 19 to 48 times greater for women who use tampons than for those who don't, and that tampon users face a 34 percent greater TSS risk for each one-gram increase in tampon absorbency.

While FDA was finishing work on the regulation, the U.S. District Court for the District of Columbia ordered on Aug. 29, 1989, that a final rule amending the 1982 tampon labeling regulation be issued by Oct.30. Under the agency's final rule, manufacturers must comply with a number of requirements.

Labeling Requirements

The package insert or outer package must display prominently, legibly, and in easily understood terms information about:

- the risk of TSS to all women using tampons during their menstrual periods, especially the reported higher risks to women under 30

- the estimated incidence of TSS of 1 to 17 per 100,000 menstruating women per year

23

- the risk of death from TSS

- the reduction of the risk of TSS by using tampons with the minimum absorbency needed to control menstrual flow

- the reduction of the risk of TSS by alternating tampon use with sanitary napkin use during menstrual periods

- the avoidance of the risk of tampon associated TSS by not using tampons. The outer package must display one of the following terms representing the corresponding absorbency range of the tampons in the package:

Table 3.1. Absorbency Range of Tampons and the Corresponding Term Used

Term Used	Absorbency Range (grams)
Junior absorbency	6 and under
Regular absorbency	6 to 9
Super absorbency	9 to 12
Super plus absorbency	12 to 15

FDA requires that the word "absorbency" accompany each of the terms. Tampons sold in vending machines are exempt from absorbency labeling because machines typically offer no choice of brands or absorbencies from which a consumer may choose.

The regulation listed two other absorbency ranges—"15 to 18" and "above 18"—but did not designate absorbency terms for these ranges. Any firm that wants to sell tampons with absorbencies in either of these two ranges must submit a request for FDA's approval of the labeling.

In addition to specifying absorbency, the outer package must give an explanation of the ranges and a description of how consumers can use range descriptions to compare absorbencies among brands. The labeling must continue to advise women to select tampons with the least absorbency needed so they can reduce their TSS risk.

The regulation requires that manufacturers use the syngyna test to measure the absorbency of each run, lot or batch of tampons. Their sampling plan must ensure a 90 percent probability that at least 90 percent of the individual tampons are within the absorbency range stated on the package. The test uses a saline solution to simulate menstrual fluid. The tampon is placed inside a condom on the test apparatus, and external pressure is applied. Fluid is pumped into the tampon. After the tampon is saturated, it is removed and weighed to the nearest 0.01 gram. The absorbency is determined by subtracting the tampon's dry weight from this value. The test is terminated as soon as tampon saturation causes a single drop of fluid to exit the apparatus. A firm wanting to use a different test may submit a petition proving the alternative method will yield equivalent results.

Whether the benefits of tampon use, particularly high-absorbency tampon use, are worth the increased risk of TSS is an individual decision. The labeling regulation helps equip women with the information they need to minimize their risk.

Symptoms of Toxic Shock Syndrome (TSS)

- sudden high fever—102 degrees Fahrenheit or higher
- vomiting
- diarrhea
- dizziness, fainting, or near fainting when standing up
- a rash that looks like a sunburn

If symptoms appear during your menstrual period, **remove your tampon if you're using one and seek medical attention right away.** Symptoms may not appear until the first few days after the end of your period. If you have had toxic shock, seek medical advice before using tampons.

Toxic shock syndrome (TSS) is rare, but it can be fatal. If you have symptoms, call your doctor and ask about the possibility of TSS. Explain what your symptoms are, when your period began, and whether you've ever had TSS. If you use tampons, mention what absorbency you use.

TSS symptoms appear quickly and are often severe. All cases are not exactly alike, and all symptoms may not be present or readily apparent. Some patients have aching muscles, bloodshot eyes, or a sore throat, making it seem like the flu. The sunburn-like rash may not develop until a person is very ill or may go unnoticed if it affects only a small area. Later on, some patients have flaking or peeling of the skin on the palms and soles. An initial episode may be so mild as to go undiagnosed, while a recurrent case may be severe. Once you've had TSS, you are more likely to get it than someone who never has had it. You can reduce your risk if you stop using tampons.

People who get proper treatment usually recover within three weeks. Deaths from TSS are now unusual, generally occurring during the first week of illness. The danger lies in a sudden drop in blood pressure, which could lead to shock if not treated in time. Treatment usually involves large amounts of fluids and drugs to raise blood pressure and lower temperature, and specific antibiotics to reduce the risk of recurrence. Body specimens are cultured to determine whether bacteria are present. Patients are often hospitalized, and severe cases require intensive care.

Women who choose to use tampons should use the lowest absorbency product that is effective for them. It's also sensible to:

- Follow the manufacturer's instructions.
- Store tampons in a clean, dry place.
- Wash hands with soap and water before and after inserting or removing a tampon.
- Try a less absorbent variety if a tampon is irritating or difficult to remove.

Non-Menstrual TSS

Today, only 56 percent of cases of toxic shock syndrome (TSS) are associated with menstruation. This is in stark contrast to the epidemic of 1980, when 90 percent of cases were menstrual TSS, the vast majority linked to tampon use.

Non-menstrual TSS can occur after such medical situations as surgery or a deep wound.

These figures are the result of intense TSS case-finding projects in 1980 and 1986 by the national Centers for Disease Control (now the Centers for Disease Control and Prevention). In 1986, for instance, CDC representatives in six regions across the country contacted hospitals every two weeks to find out whether anyone had been admitted with symptoms remotely resembling TSS. They then followed up to confirm cases.

Since 1980, CDC has operated its national TSS surveillance system. Hospitals and physicians report cases to the local state health departments, who collect the report forms and send them to CDC for tabulation. The number of definite cases—patients who display five clinical symptoms—reported from national surveillance dropped from 892 in 1980 to 55 in 1991. "If you add the probable cases of people with four of the symptoms, you'd likely have twice those totals," says

Anne Schuchat, M.D., an epidemiologist at CDC. But this is *passive* reporting in that CDC does not *actively* search out TSS cases, unlike the intense efforts in 1980 and 1986.

"Our passive surveillance detects only about a fifth as many TSS cases as actually occur, but we think it's a pretty good estimate of trends," says Schuchat. Occurrence of non-menstrual TSS has remained fairly constant, while menstrual cases have declined drastically, she says, attributing the decrease not only to a better informed public but also to changes in tampons themselves. "A super plus tampon in 1980 was a lot more absorbent than those sold in the following years. Absorbency of tampons has been lowered several times since 1980".

— by Dixie Farley

Chapter 4

Menopause

Chapter Contents

Section 4.1

Overview of the Menopause

NIH Publication No. 94-3886, 1994.

What Is Menopause?

"I wasn't sure what to expect with menopause, although I certainly looked forward to not having my period anymore. I have to admit, I'm concerned about how my body will change. My mother never talked about menopause. She says her mother never did either, probably because then it was linked to old age and poor health. Now, you hear about it all the time. The "baby boom" generation is making menopause a big issue because of their sheer numbers, and because they'll live with it much longer than their grandmothers did. Back then, menopause did come near the end of life. Now I'm going through it, but feel like I still have my whole life ahead of me."

More than one third of the women in the United States, about 36 million, have been through menopause. With a life expectancy of about 81 years, a 50 year old woman can expect to live more than one-third of her life after menopause. Scientific research is just beginning to address some of the unanswered questions about these years and about the poorly understood biology of menopause.

Menopause is the point in a woman's life when menstruation stops permanently, signifying the end of her ability to have children. Known as the "change of life," menopause is the last stage of a gradual biological process in which the ovaries reduce their production of female sex hormones—a process which begins about 3 to 5 years before the final menstrual period. This transitional phase is called the climacteric, or peri-menopause. Menopause is considered complete when a woman has been without periods for 1 year. On average, this occurs at about age 50. But like the beginning of menstruation in adolescence, timing varies from person to person. Cigarette smokers tend to reach menopause earlier than nonsmokers.

How Does It Happen?

The ovaries contain structures called follicles that hold the egg cells. You are born with about 2 million egg cells and by puberty there are about 300,000 left. Only about 400 to 500 ever mature fully to be released during the menstrual cycle. The rest degenerate over the years. During the reproductive years, the pituitary gland in the brain generates hormones that cause a new egg to be released from its follicle each month. The follicle also increases production of the sex hormones estrogen and progesterone, which thicken the lining of the uterus. This enriched lining is prepared to receive and nourish a fertilized egg following conception. If fertilization does not occur, estrogen and progesterone levels drop, the lining of the uterus breaks down, and menstruation occurs.

For unknown reasons, the ovaries begin to decline in hormone production during the mid-thirties. In the late forties, the process accelerates and hormones fluctuate more, causing irregular menstrual cycles and unpredictable episodes of heavy bleeding. By the early to mid fifties, periods finally end altogether. However, estrogen production does not completely stop. The ovaries decrease their output significantly, but still may produce a small amount. Also, another form of estrogen is produced in fat tissue with help from the adrenal glands (near the kidney). Although this form of estrogen is weaker than that produced by the ovaries, it increases with age and with the amount of fat tissue.

Progesterone, the other female hormone, works during the second half of the menstrual cycle to create a lining in the uterus as a viable home for an egg, and to shed the lining if the egg is not fertilized. If you skip a period, your body may not be making enough progesterone to break down the uterine lining. However, your estrogen levels may remain high even though you are not menstruating.

At menopause, hormone levels don't always decline uniformly. They alternately rise and fall again. Changing ovarian hormone levels affect the other glands in the body, which together make up the endocrine system. The endocrine system controls growth, metabolism and reproduction. This system must constantly readjust itself to work effectively. Ovarian hormones also affect all other tissues, including the breasts, vagina, bones, blood vessels, gastrointestinal tract, urinary tract, and skin.

Surgical Menopause

Premenopausal women who have both their ovaries removed surgically experience an abrupt menopause. They may be hit harder by menopausal symptoms than are those who experience it naturally. Their hot flashes may be more severe, more frequent, and last longer. They may have a greater risk of heart disease and osteoporosis, and may be more likely to become depressed. The reasons for this are unknown. When only one ovary is removed, menopause usually occurs naturally. When the uterus is removed (hysterectomy) and the ovaries remain, menstrual periods stop but other menopausal symptoms (if any) usually occur at the same age that they would naturally. However, some women who have a hysterectomy may experience menopausal symptoms at a younger age.

"I had hot flashes, but they were fairly mild. Sometimes at night I'd suddenly start to sweat and have to throw all my covers off. But they never lasted long and I could usually get right back to sleep. During the day I noticed they tended to come whenever I had big decision to make or when I felt a little tense. But they only lasted about 2 years. I feel blessed. I've had no other problems."

What to Expect

Menopause is an individualized experience. Some women notice little difference in their bodies or moods, while others find the change extremely bothersome and disruptive. Estrogen and progesterone affect virtually all tissues in the body, but everyone is influenced by them differently.

Hot Flashes

Hot flashes, or flushes, are the most common symptom of menopause, affecting more than 60 percent of menopausal women in the U.S. A hot flash is a sudden sensation of intense heat in the upper part or all of the body. The face and neck may become flushed, with red blotches appearing on the chest, back, and arms. This is often followed by profuse sweating and then cold shivering as body temperature readjusts. A hot flash can last a few moments or 30 minutes or longer.

Hot flashes occur sporadically and often start several years before other signs of menopause. They gradually decline in frequency and intensity as you age. Eighty percent of all women with hot flashes have them for 2 years or less, while a small percentage have them for more than 5 years. Hot flashes can happen at any time. They can be as mild as a light blush, or severe enough to wake you from a deep sleep. Some women even develop insomnia. Others have experienced that caffeine, alcohol, hot drinks, spicy foods, and stressful or frightening events can sometimes trigger a hot flash. However, avoiding these triggers will not necessarily prevent all episodes.

Hot flashes appear to be a direct result of decreasing estrogen levels. In response to falling estrogen levels, your glands release higher amounts of other hormones that affect the brain's thermostat, causing body temperatures to fluctuate. Hormone therapy relieves the discomfort of hot flashes in most cases. Some women claim that vitamin E offers minor relief, although there has never been a study to confirm it. Aside from hormone therapy, which is not for everyone, here are some suggestions for coping with hot flashes:

- Dress in layers so you can remove them at the first sign of a flash.
- Drink a glass of cold water or juice at the onset of a flash.
- At night keep a thermos of ice water or an ice pack by your bed.
- Use cotton sheets, lingerie and clothing to let your skin "breathe."

Vaginal/Urinary Tract Changes

With advancing age, the walls of the vagina become thinner, dryer, less elastic and more vulnerable to infection. These changes can make sexual intercourse uncomfortable or painful. Most women find it helpful to lubricate the vagina. Water-soluble lubricants are preferable, as they help reduce the chance of infection. Try to avoid petroleum jelly; many women are allergic, and it damages condoms. Be sure to see your gynecologist if problems persist.

Tissues in the urinary tract also change with age, sometimes leaving women more susceptible to involuntary loss of urine (incontinence), particularly if certain chronic illnesses or urinary infections are also present. Exercise, coughing, laughing, lifting heavy objects or similar movements that put pressure on the bladder may cause small amounts of urine to leak. Lack of regular physical exercise may contribute to this condition. It's important to know, however, that incontinence is not a normal part of aging, to be masked by using adult diapers. Rather, it is usually a treatable condition that warrants medical evaluation. Recent research has shown that bladder training is a simple and effective treatment for most cases of incontinence and is less expensive and safer than medication or surgery.

Within 4 or 5 years after the final menstrual period, there is an increased chance of vaginal and urinary tract infections. If symptoms such as painful or overly frequent urination occur, consult your doctor. Infections are easily treated with antibiotics, but often tend to recur. To help prevent these infections, urinate before and after intercourse, be sure your bladder is not full for long periods, drink plenty of fluids, and keep your genital area clean. Douching is not thought to be effective in preventing infection.

Menopause and Mental Health

A popular myth pictures the menopausal woman shifting from raging, angry moods into depressive, doleful slumps with no apparent reason or warning. However, a study by psychologists at the University of Pittsburgh suggests that menopause does not cause unpredictable mood swings, depression, or even stress in most women.

In fact, it may even improve mental health for some. This gives further support to the idea that menopause is not necessarily a negative experience. The Pittsburgh study looked at three different groups of women: menstruating, menopausal with no treatment, and menopausal on hormone therapy. The study showed that the menopausal women suffered no more anxiety, depression, anger, nervousness or feelings of stress than the group of menstruating women in the same age range. In addition, although more hot flashes were reported by the menopausal women not taking hormones, surprisingly they had better overall mental health than the other two groups. The women taking hormones worried more about their bodies and were somewhat more depressed.

However, this could be caused by the hormones themselves. It's also possible that women who voluntarily take hormones tend to be more conscious of their bodies in the first place. The researchers caution that their study includes only healthy women, so results may apply only to them. Other studies show that women already taking hormones who are experiencing mood or behavioral problems sometimes respond well to a change in dosage or type of estrogen.

The Pittsburgh findings are supported by a New England Research Institute study which found that menopausal women were no more depressed than the general population: about 10 percent are occasionally depressed and 5 percent are persistently depressed. The exception is women who undergo surgical menopause. Their depression rate is reportedly double that of women who have a natural menopause.

Studies also have indicated that many cases of depression relate more to life stresses or "mid-life crises" than to menopause. Such stresses include: an alteration in family roles, as when your children are grown and move out of the house, no longer "needing" mom; a changing social support network, which may happen after a divorce if you no longer socialize with friends you met through your husband; interpersonal losses, as when a parent, spouse or other close relative dies; and your own aging and the beginning of physical illness. People have very different responses to stress and crisis. Your best friend's response may be negative, leaving her open to emotional distress and depression, while yours is positive, resulting in achievement of your goals. For many women, this stage of life can actually be a period of enormous freedom.

What about Sex?

For some women, but by no means all, menopause brings a decrease in sexual activity. Reduced hormone levels cause subtle changes in the genital tissues and are thought to be linked also to a decline in sexual interest. Lower estrogen levels decrease the blood supply to the vagina and the nerves and glands surrounding it. This makes delicate tissues thinner, drier, and less able to produce secretions to comfortably lubricate before and during intercourse. Avoiding sex is not necessary, however. Estrogen creams and oral estrogen can restore secretions and tissue elasticity. Water-soluble lubricants can also help.

While changes in hormone production are cited as the major reason for changes in sexual behavior, many other interpersonal, psychological, and cultural factors can come into play. For instance, a Swedish study found that many women use menopause as an excuse to stop sex completely after years of disinterest. Many physicians, however, question if declining interest is the cause or the result of less frequent intercourse. Some women actually feel liberated after menopause and report an increased interest in sex. They say they feel relieved that pregnancy is no longer a worry.

For women in peri-menopause, birth control is a confusing issue. Doctors advise all women who have menstruated, even if irregularly, within the past year to continue using birth control. Unfortunately, contraceptive options are limited. Hormone-based oral and implantable contraceptives are risky in older women who smoke. Only a few brands of IUD are on the market. The other options are barrier methods—diaphragms, condoms, and sponges—or methods requiring surgery such as tubal ligation.

Is My Partner Still Interested?

Some men go through their own set of doubts in middle age. They too, often report a decline in sexual activity after age 50. It may take more time to reach ejaculation, or they may not be able to reach it at all. Many fear they will fail sexually as they get older. Remember, at any age sexual problems can arise if there are doubts about performance. If both partners are well informed about normal genital changes, each can be more understanding and make allowances rather than unmeetable demands. Open, candid communication between partners is important to ensure a successful sex life well into your seventies and eighties.

For most women, natural menopause is not a major crisis and does not influence their opinion of their general health.

"In a society that places so much value on youth and beauty, it's not much fun to think about menopause. But when you get there, you find it doesn't really make that much difference; you concentrate on how you feel about yourself; not on how you think others see you. I continue trying to improve myself to keep learning and keep active. It's not your age that counts, it's how you handle it."

Long Term Effects of Menopause

Osteoporosis

One of the most important health issues for middle-aged women is the threat of osteoporosis. It is a condition in which bones become thin, fragile, and highly prone to fracture. Numerous studies over the past 10 years have linked estrogen insufficiency to this gradual, yet debilitating disease. In fact, osteoporosis is more closely related to menopause than to a woman's chronological age.

Bones are not inert. They are made up of healthy, living tissue which continuously performs two processes: breakdown and formation of new bone tissue. The two are closely linked. If breakdown exceeds formation, bone tissue is lost and bones become thin and brittle. Gradually and without discomfort bone loss leads to a weakened skeleton incapable of supporting normal daily activities.

Each year about 500,000 American women will fracture a vertebrae, the bones that make up the spine, and about 300,000 will fracture a hip. Nationwide, treatment for osteoporotic fractures costs up to $10 billion per year, with hip fractures the most expensive. Vertebral fractures lead to curvature of the spine, loss of height, and pain. A severe hip fracture is painful and recovery may involve a long period of bed rest. Between 12 and 20 percent of those who suffer a hip fracture do not survive the 6 months after the fracture. At least half of those who do survive require help in performing daily living activities, and 15 to 25 percent will need to enter a long-term care facility. Older patients are rarely given the chance for full rehabilitation after a fall. However, with adequate time and care provided in rehabilitation, many people can regain their independence and return to their previous activities.

For osteoporosis, researchers believe that an ounce of prevention is worth a pound of cure. The condition of an older woman's skeleton depends on two things: the peak amount of bone attained before menopause and the rate of the bone loss thereafter. Hereditary factors are important in determining peak bone mass. For instance, studies show that black women attain a greater spinal mass and therefore have fewer osteoporotic fractures than white women. Other factors that help increase bone mass include:

- adequate intake of dietary calcium and vitamin D, particularly in young children prior to puberty
- exposure to sunlight
- physical exercise.

These elements also help slow the rate of bone loss. Certain other physiological stresses can quicken bone loss, such as pregnancy, nursing, and immobility. The biggest culprit in the process of bone loss is estrogen deficiency. Bone loss quickens during peri-menopause, the transitional phase when estrogen levels drop significantly.

Doctors believe the best strategy for osteoporosis is prevention because currently available treatments only halt bone loss–they don't rebuild the bone. However, researchers are hopeful that in the future, bone loss will be reversible. Building up your reserves of bone before you start to lose it during peri-menopause helps bank against future losses. The most effective therapy against osteoporosis available today for postmenopausal women is estrogen. Remarkably, estrogen saves more bone tissue than even very large daily doses of calcium. Estrogen is not a panacea, however. While it is a boon for the bones, it also affects all other tissues and organs in the body, and not always positively. Its impact on the other areas of the body must be considered.

Influences on Bone Development

Increases Bone Formation

- Dietary calcium
- Vitamin D
- Exposure to sunlight
- Exercise

Speeds Bone Loss

- Estrogen deficiency
- Pregnancy
- Nursing
- Lack of Exercise

Cardiovascular Disease

Most people picture an older, overweight man when they think of a likely candidate for cardiovascular disease (CVD). But men are only half the story. Heart disease is the number one killer of American women and is responsible for half of all the deaths of women over age 50. Ironically, in past years women were rarely included in clinical heart studies, but finally physicians have realized that it is as much a woman's disease as a man's.

CVDs are disorders of the heart and circulatory system. They include thickening of the arteries (atherosclerosis) that serve the heart and limbs, high blood pressure, angina, and stroke. For reasons unknown, estrogen helps protect women against CVD during the childbearing years. This is true even when they have the same risk factors as men, including smoking, high blood cholesterol levels, and a family history of heart disease. But the protection is temporary. After menopause, the incidence of CVD increases, with each passing year posing a greater risk. The good news, though, is that CVD can be prevented or at least reduced by early recognition, lifestyle changes and, many physicians believe, hormone replacement therapy.

Menopause brings changes in the level of fats in a woman's blood. These fats, called lipids, are used as a source of fuel for all cells. The amount of lipids per unit of blood determines a person's cholesterol count. There are two components of cholesterol: high density lipoprotein (HDL) cholesterol, which is associated with a beneficial,

38

cleansing effect in the bloodstream, and low density lipoprotein (LDL) cholesterol, which encourages fat to accumulate on the walls of arteries and eventually clog them. To remember the difference, think of the H in HDL as the healthy cholesterol, and the L in LDL as lethal. LDL cholesterol appears to increase while HDL decreases in post-menopausal women as a direct result of estrogen deficiency. Elevated LDL and total cholesterol can lead to stroke, heart attack, and death.

Managing Menopause

Hormone Replacement Therapy

"I started taking estrogen for my hot flashes. They went away immediately. I've felt no side effects, which I'm thankful for. I don't think I'll stay on it forever, though—no one seems to know how long it's safe! My mother has never taken hormones and she's in great shape at 87. I hope I'm as lucky!"

To combat the symptoms associated with falling estrogen levels, doctors have turned to hormone replacement therapy (HRT). HRT is the administration of the female hormones estrogen and progesterone. Estrogen replacement therapy (ERT) refers to administration of estrogen alone. The hormones are usually given in pill form, though sometimes skin patches and vaginal creams (just estrogen) are used. ERT is thought to help prevent the devastating effects of heart disease and osteoporosis, conditions that are often difficult and expensive to treat once they appear. The cardiovascular effects of progesterone, however, are still unknown. Hormone treatment for menopause is still quite controversial. Its long-term safety and efficacy remain matters of great concern. There is not enough existing data for physicians to suggest that HRT is the right choice for *all* women. Several large studies are currently attempting to resolve the questions, though it will take several more years to reach any definitive answers.

In the 1940's when estrogen was first offered to menopausal women, it was given alone and in high doses. Today, after 50 years of trial and error, it is well known that estrogen stimulates growth of the inner lining of the uterus (endometrium) that sheds during menstruation. This growth may continue uncontrollably, resulting in cancer. Today, doctors typically prescribe a lower dose of estrogen. However, few doctors still prescribe estrogen alone to women who have a uterus. Most now prefer to add a synthetic form of progesterone called progestin to counteract estrogen's dangerous effect on the uterus. Progestin reduces the risk of cancer by causing monthly shedding of the endometrium. The obvious drawback to this approach is that menopausal women resume monthly bleeding. Once menopause arrives, most women enjoy the freedom of life without a period. Many are reluctant to begin their cycles again. In addition, there are other unpleasant side effects of progestin which often discourage women from continuing HRT. These include breast tenderness, bloating, abdominal cramping, anxiety, irritability, and depression.

Only about 15 percent of women who are eligible for hormone replacement therapy are now receiving it. This leaves 85 percent who either do not want or need it, or do not know about it.

The good news is that researchers are evaluating different schedules of low-dose estrogen and progestin to completely eliminate monthly bleeding. Currently most women receive what is called *cyclic* HRT. They may take estrogen continually and progestin for the first 12 days of each month. The use of a *continuous* combined dose, where estrogen and smaller amounts of progestin are taken every day is also being studied. In theory, this use of progestin stems endometrial growth so no bleeding will occur. Unfortunately, it may take 6 months or more until bleeding finally stops. In many cases, monthly bleeding has been replaced by more bothersome irregular bleeding patterns. Obviously, further research is needed to evaluate and perfect this treatment. Various types of progestins in different dosages, preparations, and schedules are being studied in hopes of reducing its other unpleasant side effects while retaining the known advantages of estrogen.

Estrogen and Your Bones

HRT and ERT are successful methods of combatting osteoporosis. As previously discussed, estrogen halts bone loss but cannot necessarily rebuild bone. Long-term estrogen use (10 or more years) may be required to prevent postmenopausal bone loss. Why estrogen helps protect the skeleton is still unclear. We do know that estrogen helps bones absorb the calcium they need to stay strong. It also helps conserve the calcium stored in the bones by encouraging other cells to use dietary calcium more efficiently. For instance, muscles require calcium to contract. If there is not enough calcium circulating in the blood for muscles to use, calcium is "borrowed" from the bone. Calcium is also needed for blood clotting, sending nerve impulses, and secreting various hormones. Prolonged borrowing from bone calcium for these processes speeds bone loss. That's why it's important to consume adequate amounts of calcium in your diet.

Estrogen's Effect on Your Heart

The majority of past clinical studies have shown that women who use ERT substantially reduce their risk of developing and dying from heart disease. One or two studies demonstrate conflicting evidence, but they are far outnumbered by the positive reports. Results from a 1991 study showed that after 15 years of estrogen replacement, risk of death by CVD was reduced by almost 50 percent and overall deaths were reduced by 40 percent. Some researchers credit this reduction to oral estrogen's ability to maintain HDL and LDL at their healthier, premenopausal levels, through its interaction with proteins in the liver. Others believe it is estrogen's direct effect on the blood vessels themselves (through receptors on the vessel walls) which creates this benefit. In the latter case, both oral estrogen and the skin patch would be effective. Studies are underway to determine which mechanism contributes most to a healthy heart.

Many doctors now believe that estrogen replacement benefits women at risk for heart disease (but not those with blood clots). Risk factors for heart disease include a strong family history of CVD, high blood pressure, obesity, and smoking.

At any time of life, women who smoke are much more likely to develop heart disease or have a stroke than women who do not smoke. But after menopause, a smoker's risk climbs dramatically. Low estrogen levels and smoking are separate risk factors for CVD. When the two are combined, the risk is much higher than either one alone. Smoking also raises your risks for some types of cancer and for chronic lung disease, such as emphysema. Fortunately, quitting smoking—at any age—can cut the risk of disease almost immediately. Studies have shown that when older people quit, they increase their life expectancy. Their risk of heart disease goes down, their lungs function better, and blood circulation improves. So quitting smoking, whether before, during or after menopause, can have a definite impact on both the length and quality of your life.

Many women who have quit smoking say they found support in group counseling sessions. Local chapters of the American Cancer Society and the American Heart Association are good places to start looking for a smoking cessation group. Nicotine gum and nicotine patches prescribed by a doctor may also help.

While we know that estrogen users have a decreased risk of CVD, women with certain pre-existing heart conditions are usually advised not to take HRT or ERT. These conditions include blood clots and recent heart attacks. Researchers hope to further investigate non-hormonal methods of preventing heart disease such as weight reduction or control, exercise, smoking cessation, and dietary modification.

According to a 5-year study reported in 1988, weight gain (a common occurrence among many menopausal women) significantly raises blood pressure, total and LDL cholesterol, and fat levels. Together, these make up a dangerous recipe for heart disease. Several other studies also noted that having about one drink per day had a protective effect on the heart. Physicians advise caution in this area, however, as excess alcohol can increase risks for other serious problems.

While cardiovascular benefits associated with oral estrogen are fairly well-known, there is surprisingly little information on the cardiovascular effects of progestin combined with estrogen. Some studies suggest that progestins counteract the favorable effects of estrogen alone, while other studies show no such effect. This remains just one more gray area where questions outnumber reliable answers.

Should women be treated with a drug to prevent a disease they might never get (osteoporosis, heart disease)? Some people will be placed at higher risk, while others will benefit. Each woman should make a decision about HRT based on her own family history and life experiences.

Drawbacks of HRT: The Cancer Risk

A major issue surrounding HRT and ERT is the influence of estrogen on breast cancer. Researchers believe that the longer your lifetime exposure to naturally occurring estrogen, the greater your risk of breast cancer. It has not been proven, however, that estrogen administered at menopause has the same effect. There is disagreement on the many trials conducted to date because of wide variations in the populations studied and the doses, timing, and types of estrogen used. A recent analysis of previous studies suggests that low-dose estrogen taken on a short-term basis (10 years or less) does not pose an increased risk of breast cancer. Long-term use (more than 10 years) at a high dose may significantly increase the risk. By how much is still a matter of heated debate. *At the very most*, researchers think *long-term* use could possibly increase the risk of getting breast cancer by 30 percent. This means that incidence would rise from 10 women per 10,000 each year to 13 women per 10,000 each year. To reach any consensus, however, more women need to be monitored for an extended period of time. The fear of cancer is one of the most common reasons that women are unwilling to use HRT. Interestingly, actual death rates for breast cancer have not risen at all. This may be because estrogen users have more frequent medical visits and obtain more preventive care including yearly mammograms.

While no one can determine who will eventually develop breast cancer, there are certain risk factors you should be aware of when considering HRT. A family history of breast cancer (sister or mother) is probably the most important risk factor of all. You may also be at an increased risk if: you menstruated before age 12; delayed motherhood until later in life; or have a late menopause (after age 50). Also, the older you are, the higher the risk. Most doctors believe that if you are not in a high risk category for breast or endometrial cancer, the benefits of HRT far outweigh the risks. However, for some women, the side effects of therapy make it impossible to use. This is a personal decision to be made by each woman with help from her doctor.

Other Risks

Physicians usually caution women not to use HRT if they are already at high risk for developing blood clots. Obesity, severe varicose veins, smoking, and a history of blood clots put you in this category. A history of gall bladder disease could also be cause to avoid HRT, as women taking estrogen may have a greater chance of developing gallstones.

In Summary

Cautions to Estrogen Use

Serious Risk

- Stroke
- Recent heart attack
- Breast cancer (current or family history)
- Uterine cancer
- Acute liver disease
- Gall bladder disease
- Pancreatic disease
- Recent blood clot
- Undiagnosed vaginal bleeding

Relative Risk

- Cigarette smoking
- Hypertension
- Benign breast disease
- Benign uterine disease
- Endometriosis
- Pancreatitis
- Epilepsy
- Migraine headaches

Subjective Complaints

- Nausea
- Headaches
- Breakthrough bleeding
- Depression
- Fluid retention

(Source: R.L. Young, N.S. Kumar, and J.W. Coldzieher, *Management of Menopause When Estrogen Cannot Be Used*, Drugs, 40(2):220-230,1990)

Advantages and Disadvantages of Hormonal Therapy

Here is what scientists can say so far about the advantages and disadvantages of hormone replacement therapy (HRT–estrogen and progesterone) and estrogen replacement therapy (ERT–estrogen alone). More research is underway.

Advantages

- HRT and ERT reduce the risk of osteoporosis.
- HRT and ERT relieve hot flashes.
- HRT and ERT reduce the risk of heart disease.
- HRT and ERT may improve mood and psychological well-being.

Disadvantages

- ERT increases the risk of cancer of the uterus (endometrial cancer).
- HRT can have unpleasant side effects, such as bloating or irritability.

- HRT and ERT *may* increase risk of breast cancer; long-term use may pose the greatest risk.
- In women with blood clots, HRT and ERT *may* be dangerous.

However, there is no consensus within the medical community about the risks and benefits associated with hormone therapy. There is also no agreement on normal hormonal changes associated with aging. As one women says, "happiness is when the last tuition is paid for; the youngest moves out and the dog dies. Now I can concentrate on what I want to do. My doctor puts everyone on estrogen, so I tried it for a while but it brought my menstrual flow back just as heavy as before. Who needs that mess again? So now I just exercise, try to eat well, and generally, I feel pretty good."

Keeping Healthy

Good nutrition and regular physical exercise are thought to improve overall health. Some doctors feel these factors can also affect menopause. Although these areas have not been well studied in women, anecdotal evidence is strongly in favor of eating well and exercising to help lower risks for CVD and osteoporosis.

Nutrition

While everyone agrees that a well-balanced diet is important for good health, there is still much to be learned about what constitutes "well-balanced." We do know that variety in the diet helps ensure a better mix of essential nutrients.

Nutritional requirements vary from person to person and change with age. A healthy premenopausal woman should have about 1,000 mgs of calcium per day. A 1994 Consensus Conference at the National Institutes of Health recommended that women after menopause consume 1,500 mgs per day if they are not using hormonal replacement or 1000 mgs per day in conjunction with hormonal replacement. Foods high in calcium include milk, yogurt, cheese and other dairy products; oysters, sardines and canned salmon with bones; and dark-green leafy vegetables like spinach and broccoli. In calcium tablets, calcium carbonate is most easily absorbed by the body. If you are lactose intolerant, acidophilus milk is more digestible. Vitamin D is also very important for calcium absorption and bone formation. A 1992 study showed that women with postmenopausal osteoporosis who took vitamin D for 3 years significantly reduced the occurrence of new spinal fractures. However, the issue is still controversial. High doses of vitamin D can cause kidney stones, constipation, or abdominal pain, particularly in women with existing kidney problems. Other nutritional guidelines by the National Research Council include:

- Choose foods low in fat, saturated fat, and cholesterol. Fats contain more calories (9 calories per gram) than either carbohydrates or protein (each have only 4 calories per gram). Fat intake should be less than 30 percent of daily calories.

- Eat fruits, vegetables, and whole grain cereal products, especially those high in vitamin C and carotene. These include oranges, grapefruit, carrots, winter squash, tomatoes, broccoli, cauliflower, and green leafy vegetables These foods are good sources of vitamins and minerals and the major sources of dietary fiber. Fiber helps maintain bowel mobility and may reduce the risk of colon cancer. Young and older people alike are encouraged to consume 20 to 30 grams of fiber per day.

- Eat very little salt-cured and smoked foods such as sausages, smoked fish and ham, bacon, bologna, and hot dogs. High blood pressure, which may become more serious with heavy salt intake, is more of a risk as you age.

- Avoid food and drinks containing processed sugar. Sugar contains empty calories which may substitute for nutritious food and can add excess body weight.

For people who can't eat an adequate diet, supplements may be necessary. A dietician should tailor these to meet your individual nutritional needs. Using supplements without supervision can be risky because large doses of some vitamins may have serious side effects. Vitamins A and D in large doses can be particularly dangerous.

As you age, your body requires less energy because of a decline in physical activity and a loss of lean body mass. Raising your activity level will increase your need for energy and help you avoid gaining weight. Weight gain often occurs in menopausal women, possibly due in part to declining estrogen. In animal studies, scientists found that estrogen is important in regulating weight gain. Animals with their ovaries surgically removed gained weight, even if they were fed the same diet as the animals with intact ovaries. They also found that progesterone counteracts the effect of estrogen. The higher their progesterone levels, the more the animals ate.

Exercise

"To me, exercise is the key to staying healthy. Some of these ladies have been coming to this class for 10 years. I think that really says a lot. Do you think they'd get up at 7:00 a.m. to jump around if it didn't make them feel better?"

Exercise is extremely important throughout a woman's lifetime and particularly as she gets older. Regular exercise benefits the heart and bones, helps regulate weight, and contributes to a sense of overall well-being and improvement in mood. If you are physically inactive you are far more prone to coronary heart disease, obesity, high blood pressure, diabetes, and osteoporosis. Sedentary women may also suffer more from chronic back pain, stiffness, insomnia, and irregularity. They often have poor circulation, weak muscles, shortness of breath, and loss of bone mass. Depression can also be a problem. Women who regularly walk, jog, swim, bike, dance, or perform some other aerobic activity can more easily circumvent these problems and also achieve higher HDL cholesterol levels. Studies show that women performing aerobic activity or muscle-strength training reduced mortality from CVD and cancer.

Just like muscles, bones adhere to the "use it or lose it" rule; they diminish in size and strength with disuse. It has been known for more than 100 years that weight-bearing exercise (walking, running) will help increase bone mass. Exercise stimulates the cells responsible for generating new bone to work overtime. In the past 20 years, studies have shown that bone tissue lost from lack of use can be rebuilt with weight-bearing activity. Studies of athletes show they have greater bone mass compared to non-athletes at the sites related to their sport. In post menopausal women, moderate exercise preserves bone mass in the spine helping reduce the risk of fractures.

Exercise is also thought to have a positive effect on mood. During exercise, hormones called endorphins are released in the brain. They are 'feel good' hormones involved in the body's positive response to stress. The mood-heightening effect can last for several hours, according to some endocrinologists. Consult your doctor before starting a rigorous exercise program. He or she will help you decide which types of exercises are best for you. An exercise program should start slowly and build up to more strenuous activities. Women who already have osteoporosis of the spine should be careful about exercise that jolts or puts weight on the back, as it could cause a fracture.

Ongoing/Future Research

To gather more data to help women make a well-informed decision regarding hormone therapy, researchers at the National Institutes of Health (NIH) launched the Postmenopausal Estrogen/Progestin Interventions Trial (PEPI) in 1989. With 127 women enrolled at each of seven medical centers, PEPI will address the short-term safety and efficacy of various methods of HRT. The study will compare women who take estrogen by itself to those who take it with different types of progestin. It will also examine the effects of both cyclical and continuous progestin on cardiovascular risk factors, blood clotting factors, metabolism, uterine changes, bone mass, and general quality of life.

Several new studies are now looking at normal body changes as women move from pre- to post-menopause. Up to now, the lack of such data has been one problem in assessing the value of HRT. Without knowing what "normal" is, scientists have difficulty judging the effect of a particular treatment. Another problem with past studies is the "healthy user effect." In many trials preceding PEPI, the HRT users studied had freely chosen to begin treatment, with advice from their doctors. In general, most physicians discourage women with a pre-existing illness or long family history of breast cancer from taking HRT. This factor could skew study results to appear that non-users became ill or died more frequently simply because they failed to take estrogen. Only by randomly assigning study participants to the treatment can this bias be overcome. Until more random trials are completed, the jury is still out on HRT.

Another NIH study is the Women's Health Initiative, a multi-center trial involving 70,000 postmenopausal women ages 50 to 79. The study will assess the long-term benefits and risk of hormone therapy as it relates to cardiovascular disease, osteoporosis and breast and uterine cancer. It will also help determine the effects of calcium supplementation, dietary changes, and exercise on women in this age group. Some of the specific questions to be addressed by the Women's Health Initiative include:

- How long is estrogen effective for each system of the body (skeletal, cardiovascular, nervous, endocrine)?

- What is the best dose and route of administration of estrogen and progestin to prevent side effects yet maintain efficacy?
- How long is estrogen safe to take?
- Does estrogen act the same way in older women as in younger women?
- Are there effective alternatives to HRT?

Clearly, no one has all the answers about menopause. Medical research is beginning to give us more accurate information, but some myths and negative attitudes persist. Women are challenging old stereotypes, learning about what's happening in their bodies, and taking responsibility for their health. The important thing to remember as you go through menopause is to be good to yourself. Take time to pursue your hobbies, be they gardening, painting or socializing with friends. Have a positive attitude toward life. Sharing concerns with friends, a spouse, relatives or a support group can help. Don't fight your body—allow the changes that are happening to become a part of you, a part that is natural and that you accept.

Glossary

Angina. A disease marked by brief attacks of chest pain.

Arthralgia. Pain in a joint; experienced by some women during climacteric.

Biopsy. Removal and examination of living cells from the body.

Breakthrough bleeding. Any visible blood when not expected.

Cardiovascular Disease (CVD). Disorders of the heart and circulatory system.

Climacteric. The years leading up and following the last menstrual period. Also called "peri-menopause".

DUB. Dysfuctional uterine bleeding; excessive and/or unpredictable bleeding from the womb, not due to any abnormality, that frequently occurs in the few years before menopause.

Dyspareunia. Difficult or painful sexual intercourse.

Endometrium. Lining of the uterus (womb).

ERT. Estrogen replacement therapy; the use of estrogen alone for the treatment of menopausal symptoms and the prevention of some long-term effects of menopause.

Estrogen. One of the female sex hormones produced by the ovaries before menopause and by fat tissues after menopause.

FSH. Follicle-stimulating hormone; stimulates development of sacs that hold the eggs.

GnRH. Gonadotrophin-releasing hormone; stimulates the release of FSH and LH.

HDL. High density lipoprotein cholesterol, the "good" cholesterol thought to have a cleansing effect in the bloodstream.

HRT. Hormone replacement therapy; the use of estrogen combined with progestin for the treatment of menopausal symptoms and the prevention of some long-term effects of menopause.

Hysterectomy. Surgical removal of the uterus.

IUD. Intrauterine birth control device, which prevents implantation of an embryo into the uterus should fertilization occur.

LDL. Low density lipoprotein cholesterol, the "bad" cholesterol believed to be linked to fat accumulation in the arteries.

LH. Luteinizing hormone; stimulates the release of the egg from the sac.

Leiomyoma. Also called a fibroid; a non-cancerous growth in the womb that occurs in 20 percent to 25 percent of women before menopause and causes no symptoms in most women.

Menorrhagia. Heavy menstrual bleeding and excessively long periods.

Menopause. The point when menstruation stops permanently.

Myomectomy. Surgical removal of fibroids from the uterus.

Oligomenorrhea. Infrequent menstruation with diminished flow.

Oophorectomy. Surgical removal of the ovaries, sometimes called castration.

Oral contraceptives. Pills which usually consist of synthetic estrogen and progesterone that are taken for three weeks after the last day of a menstrual period. They inhibit ovulation, thereby preventing pregnancy.

Osteoporosis. A disease in which bones become thin, weak and are easily fractured.

Paresthesia. Sensation of tingling, prickling or creeping of the skin; experienced by some women during climacteric.

Peri-menopause. The time around menopause, usually beginning 3 to 5 years before the final period.

Progesterone. One of the female sex hormones produced by the ovaries.

Progestin. The synthetic form of progesterone.

Tubal Ligation. A surgical procedure in which the uterine tubes are cut and tied to prevent pregnancy.

Urinary incontinence. Loss of bladder control.

Vasectomy. In males, the surgical removal of part of the sperm duct (vas deferens) to induce infertility.

Withdrawal bleeding. "Planned" bleeding while on a medication that occurs during the hormone-free period of a cycle or after progestin has been added to a continuous estrogen cycle.

Organizations Providing Further Information

National Institute on Aging (NIA)
9000 Rockville Pike
Bethesda, MD 20892
800-222-2225

North American Menopause Society (NAMS)
University Hospitals Department of OB/GYN
2074 Abington Road
Cleveland, OH 44106
fax: 216-844-3348 (written requests)

National Women's Health Network
1325 G Street, NW
Washington, DC 20005
202-347-1140

American College of Obstetrics and Gynecologists (ACOG)
409 12th Street, SW
Washington, DC 20024
202-638-5577

Alliance for Aging Research
2021 K Street, NW, Suite 305
Washington, DC 20006
202-293-2856

Older Women's League (OWL)
666 11th Street, NW
Suite 700
Washington, DC 20001
202-783-6686

National Women's Health Resource Center (NWHRC)
2440 M Street, NW
Suite 201
Washington, DC 20037
202-293-6045

Wider Opportunities for Women (WOW)
National Commission on Working Women
1325 G Street, NW
Lower Level
Washington, DC 20005
202-638-3143

American Dietetic Association (ADA)
216 West Jackson Boulevard
Suite 800
Chicago, IL 60606
312-899-0040

American Heart Association (AHA)
7320 Greenville Avenue
Dallas, TX 75231
214-373-6300

National Heart, Lung, and Blood Institute (NHLBI)
9000 Rockville Pike
Bethesda, MD 20892
301-496-4236

National Arthritis and Musculoskeletal and Skin Diseases Information Clearinghouse
Box AMS
9000 Rockville Pike
Bethesda, MD 20892
301-495-4484

National Osteoporosis Foundation (NOF)
2100 M Street, NW
Suite 602
Washington, DC 20037
202-223-2226

Sex Information and Education Council of the U.S. (SIECUS)
130 West 42nd Street
Suite 2500
New York, NY 10036
212-819-9770

Depression Awareness, Recognition, and Treatment Program
National Institute of Mental Health
D/ART Public Inquiries
5600 Fishers Lane
Room 15C-05
Rockville, MD 20857
301-443-4513

National Mental Health Association (NMHA)
Information Center
1021 Prince Street
Alexandria, VA 22314-2971
703-684-7722
800-969-6642

National Cancer Institute
Cancer Information Service
9000 Rockville Pike
Bethesda, MD 20892
800-4-CANCER
(800-422-6237)

American Cancer Society National Headquarters
1599 Clifton Road, NE
Atlanta, GA 30329
800-ACS-2345
(800-227-2345)

Further Resources

The Change: Women, Aging and the Menopause, Germaine Greer, New York: Knopf/Random House, 1992.

Choice Years, Judith Paige and Pamela Gordon. New York: Villard Books, 1991.

Managing Your Menopause, Wulf H. Utian, M.D., PhD., and Ruth S. Jacobowitz. New York: Fireside/Simon and Schuster, 1990.

The Menopause, Hormone Therapy, and Women's Health-Background Paper. Congress of the United States, Office of Technology Assessment, May 1992.

Menopause and Midlife Health, Morris Notelovitz and Diana Tonnesen, New York: St. Martin's Press, 1994.

Menopause News, ed. Judy Askew, 2074 Union St., San Francisco, CA 94123.

The Menopause Self-Help Book, Susan M. Lark, M.D. Berkeley: Celestial Arts, 1990.

The New Ourselves Growing Older, Paula Brown Doress and Diane Laskin Siegal. New York:Simon and Schuster, 1994 (in cooperation with the Boston Women's Health Book Collective).

The Silent Passage; Menopause, Gail Sheehy, New York:Random House, 1991.

Who, What, Where? Resources for Women's Health and Aging, National Institute on Aging, March 1992.

Section 4.2

Demystifying Menopause

DHSS Publication No. 94-1181, January 1994.

Generations past called it "change of life." Today we're more apt to call it what it is: menopause. Yet our understanding of this change in a woman's childbearing status may still be clouded by myth and mystification.

Natural menopause is the end of menstruation and childbearing capability that occurs in most women somewhere around age 50. Today women can expect to live about a third of their lives after menopause.

Technically, the term "menopause" refers to the actual cessation of menstrual periods. When a woman has not had a period for a year, then the date of her last menstrual period is retrospectively considered the date of her menopause. However, the term "menopause" has come to be used in a general sense in place of the more proper terms, "climacteric" or "peri-menopause," which encompass the years immediately preceding and following the last menstrual period.

To cut through some of the myth and mystery surrounding the hormonal changes that accompany menopause, it is necessary first to understand what happens in the cycle of a normally menstruating woman.

The menstrual cycle, averaging 28 days, is divided into two phases. The first is called the follicular, or pre-ovulatory, phase and lasts 10 to 17 days. The second is the luteal, or post-ovulatory, phase lasting 13 to 15 days (see illustration).

Hormone Activity During Menstrual Cycle

Figure 4.1 describes hormone activity during the menstrual cycle. The hypothalamus (the part of the brain that regulates many basic body functions) and the pituitary (a gland adjacent to the brain that secretes hormones regulating growth and the activity of other glands) are involved in the beginnings of the follicular phase.

The hypothalamus produces gonadotropin-releasing hormone (GRH), which stimulates the pituitary to release two gonadotropins–follicle-stimulating hormone (FSH) and luteinizing hormone (LH). FSH stimulates the development of follicles (sacs that hold the eggs) in the ovary. These follicles produce estrogen.

One follicle becomes dominant, increasing its estrogen production to aid in the maturation of the egg. In response to the estrogen, the endometrium (lining of the uterus or womb) thickens. The estrogen also goes to the pituitary resulting in a mid-cycle surge of LH. Ovulation—the release of the egg from the follicle—follows. The LH also transforms the ruptured follicle into the corpus luteum (tissue mass necessary to maintain pregnancy).

As the luteal phase begins, the corpus luteum produces both estrogen and progesterone. The progesterone makes the lining of the womb more receptive to the implanting egg. Progesterone also prevents the pituitary from releasing any more gonadotropins and halts further follicular growth. If conception does not occur, the corpus luteum disintegrates and the thickened lining of the womb is shed in menstruation.

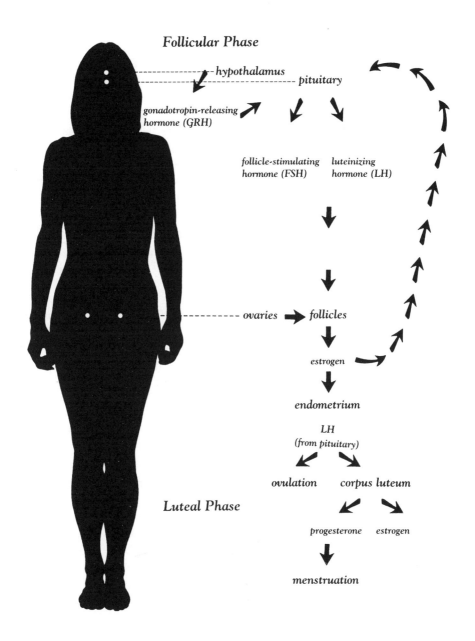

Figure 4.1. Hormone Activity during the Menstrual Cycle

Changing Cycle

Usually sometime in a woman's early to mid 40s—two to eight years before actual menopause—her menstrual cycle begins changing. Notably, levels of hormones such as estrogen, produced by the ovaries, decrease; ovulation (release of eggs from the ovaries) stops or becomes more infrequent; and the pattern of the menstrual cycle changes.

Initially this may mean heavier and/or more frequent periods. Later, periods may be scantier and less frequent. Lack of ovulation may cause some light bleeding or spotting between periods. However, not all women follow this pattern exactly. Some may experience simply a wide variability in the time and quantity of flow, and a few may have little or no change in menstrual cycle. For some women, the unpredictability of menstrual pattern changes is unsettling because social activities can no longer be planned around a specific cycle, and there is no period due date to help determine pregnancy status. And indeed, because most women continue to ovulate at least in some cycles, pregnancy is possible until a woman has actually passed menopause. In fact, in some cultures where women bear many children, it is not uncommon for a woman to give birth to her last child and never menstruate again.

In the vast majority of cases, menstrual irregularities in the years before menopause are simply manifestations of the normal transition in the woman's hormonal status. Sometimes, if these irregularities cause too many problems or if a woman's doctor suspects that the uterine lining is not being shed completely during menstruation as happens during a normal period, the doctor may suggest treatment with a synthetic progesterone, called a progestin, to make the cycle more regular. In cases of extremely heavy bleeding, the doctor may recommend surgery.

The age at which a woman has her last period is not known to be related to race, body size, or her age when she began to menstruate. The average age for menopause in American women is 50 to 52. But it is not abnormal for it to occur several years earlier or later. Some studies show that women who have had many children reach menopause earlier. And smokers may experience menopause an average of one to two years earlier than nonsmokers.

Even after menopause, women's bodies continue to produce estrogen, but far less of the hormone is made in the ovaries. Most postmenopausal estrogen is produced in a process in which the adrenal gland makes precursors of estrogen, which are then converted by stored fat to estrogen. However, far less estrogen is produced in this manner than is produced in the ovaries before menopause.

Hot Flashes

The most common symptom of menopause, the hot flush or flash, may begin before a woman has stopped menstruating and may continue for a couple of years after menopause. Although it is known that the hot flash (or "vasomotor flush," as doctors sometimes call it) is related to decreased estrogen levels, exactly how this occurs is not completely understood.

Many women describe the hot flash as an intense feeling of heat. Some say it actually feels like the temperature in the room has risen. Most commonly the sensation starts in the face, neck or chest and may extend to other parts of the body. It is usually accompanied by perspiration and may last a few seconds to several minutes. Increased heart rate and finger temperature have been documented during hot flashes.

About half of the women who have hot flashes visibly blush or have a patchy reddish flush of the face, neck and chest. For some women, the feeling of heat is followed by a feeling of being chilled. The hot flash may be particularly disturbing when it occurs during sleep. This problem, often involving profuse sweating, can awaken the women and is credited for much of the insomnia sometimes associated with menopause.

Up to 75 percent to 85 percent of women have hot flashes, but less than half of all women experiencing a natural menopause have symptoms severe enough to warrant medication. Obese women tend to have a lower incidence of hot flashes, possibly because they have higher levels of estrogen, converted from stored fat.

Many women find they can cope with hot flashes by dressing in layers that can be removed, wearing natural fabrics, drinking cold rather than hot beverages, keeping rooms cooler, and sleeping with fewer blankets.

Estrogen Replacement

For women who cannot get sufficient relief without drugs, hormone replacement therapy may be prescribed. The length of time that a woman is advised to continue taking hormones may vary from several months to several years, depending on her symptoms.

Often abbreviated ERT, estrogen replacement therapy may relieve at least two other postmenopausal problems related to lower estrogen levels: urogenital atrophy and osteoporosis. The first of these involves both the vagina and bladder. The vagina becomes foreshortened, thins, and lubricates less efficiently. Itching, burning and dryness may result. Intercourse may become painful and vaginal infections more frequent. A similar tissue thinning occurs in the bladder, sometimes resulting in urinary discomfort, which may include the sudden and/or frequent need to urinate.

Osteoporosis involves loss of bone mass. It occurs in the elderly of both sexes, but is particularly common in fair-skinned, short, thin women. Smoking is an additional risk factor. It is estimated that 25 of every 100 white women over 60 suffer spinal fractures as a result of osteoporosis.

Although osteoporosis is by no means a universal outcome of menopause, some estimates say that 60 percent of untreated white women will develop some symptoms. In addition to ERT, weight-bearing exercise and sufficient calcium intake—particularly if begun years before menopause—may help prevent the bone loss associated with this condition.

Other symptoms experienced by some menopausal women that are probably related to lower estrogen levels include joint pains and sensations of tingling, prickling or creeping of the skin.

Estrogen therapy can be taken in several different dosage forms: vaginal creams, oral tablets, transdermal patches (by which the drug is slowly absorbed through the skin), and intramuscular injection. The first three are the most common dosage forms. The vaginal cream is usually given to relieve local problems of the vagina and bladder.

Although many women report a lessening of symptoms such as headaches and depression when they take estrogen, studies have not consistently shown these to be related to hormone changes. Some believe that these symptoms may be more a byproduct of other factors, such as life changes that a woman may be going through around the age of 50, pre-conceived and possibly erroneous ideas of what menopause may be like, and a woman's response to society's undervaluation of aging women.

In any case, because of the rare but serious adverse effects associated with estrogen use, ERT would not be considered medically appropriate for other symptoms of lowered estrogen in the absence of hot flashes, urogenital atrophy, or the potential for osteoporosis.

Adding Progestin

The most serious adverse effect of non-contraceptive estrogen use is a higher risk of endometrial cancer (cancer of the inner lining of the uterus). For a number of years after this relationship was established in the mid-70s, ERT fell into some disfavor.

In the last few years, the use of ERT has again been on the rise, with doctors increasingly prescribing a progestin in the last 10 to 13 days of each estrogen cycle to prevent endometrial hyperplasia (abnormal increase in endometrial cells), a presumed precursor of cancer. It should be noted that FDA has not yet added this use to progestin labeling and is presently evaluating data about both progestins' possible protective effects against endometrial cancer and the possible but unknown cardiovascular risk, which may include an adverse effect on cholesterol.

Postmenopausal women who are on estrogen/progestin therapy may experience some menstrual-like bleeding (although it is usually far lighter than a normal menstrual period). For this reason, some women do not like to take progestins.

The weight of evidence from scientific studies is that there is not a higher incidence of breast cancer in women who take estrogen. However, women who have had breast cancer should not take ERT (except in cases where it is part of cancer treatment), because some tumors are dependent on estrogen for their growth. Others for whom estrogen is contraindicated are those who have a known or suspected estrogen-dependent tumor, may be pregnant, have undiagnosed abnormal genital bleeding, active thrombophlebitis (blood clots) or clotting disorders, or have previously had these when given estrogen.

Since there are some women with a variety of conditions for whom ERT may not be the best choice, the benefits and risks of ERT should be weighed carefully by each woman and her physician.

Less serious side effects of ERT include enlarged and tender breasts, nausea, skin discoloration, water retention, weight gain, headache, and heartburn.

A possibly beneficial side effect of estrogen is that it may raise the levels of the desirable kind of cholesterol known as high density lipoproteins (HDLs). Scientists think that postmenopausal women who take estrogens may have added protection against heart disease. However, when progestins are added, this effect may be canceled out.

The form of progestin most often prescribed for use with ERT, medroxyprogesterone (brand names Provera, Amen, Curretab and others), seems to only slightly lower HDL levels. ERT, both with and without added progestins, lowers total cholesterol. In contrast to oral contraceptives, which use a higher dose of hormones, ERT appears not to influence blood pressure in any significant way.

Some women who cannot take estrogens can receive a certain degree of relief from hot flashes by taking a progestin alone. But this hormone does not reverse urogenital atrophy, may increase inappropriate hair loss or gain, and may lead to abnormal bleeding.

If it is not advisable for a woman to take an estrogen or a progestin, a doctor may prescribe Bellergal-S, a combination of phenobarbital, ergotamine and belladonna alkaloids, which FDA has approved for relieving hot flashes. While not specifically approved for hot flashes, clonidine (Catapres and others), a heart drug, is sometimes prescribed for this purpose, and studies show that it gives some relief. Doctors may also prescribe other drugs for relief of symptoms such as insomnia, headache and depression.

As the proportion of women nearing menopause increases with the advancing age of "baby boomers," it is likely that more attention will be paid to the interests of menopausal women. This focus may provide impetus for a more complete scientific unraveling of the mysteries surrounding this stage of life, so that women may deal with it on a factual basis and be free to live the latter third of their lives in the fullest manner possible.

—by Judith Levine Willis

Part Two

Other Gynecological Concerns

Chapter 5

Endometriosis

Chapter Contents

Section 5.1

Endometriosis

NIH Publication No. 91-2413 (1991).

Endometriosis is a common, yet poorly understood disease. It can strike women of any socioeconomic class, age, or race. It is estimated that between 10 and 20 percent of American women of childbearing age have endometriosis. While some women with endometriosis may have severe pelvic pain, others who have the condition have no symptoms. Nothing about endometriosis is simple, and there are no absolute cures. The disease can affect a woman's whole existence—her ability to work, her ability to reproduce, and her relationships with her mate, her child, and everyone around her.

The National Institute of Child Health and Human Development (NICHD), part of the Federal Government's National Institutes of Health (NIH), conducts and supports research on the various processes that determine the health of children, adults, families, and populations. As part of NICHD's mandate in the reproductive sciences, NICHD has established a Reproductive Medicine Network linking several institutions across the country. While this cooperative effort focuses on other important issues such as infertility and various male and female reproductive disorders, developing an optimal treatment for endometriosis is one of its primary goals.

What Is Endometriosis?

The name endometriosis comes from the word "endometrium," the tissue that lines the inside of the uterus. If a woman is not pregnant this tissue builds up and is shed each month. It is discharged as menstrual flow at the end of each cycle. In endometriosis, tissue that looks and acts like endometrial tissue is found outside the uterus, usually inside the abdominal cavity.

Endometrial tissue residing outside the uterus responds to the menstrual cycle in a way that is similar to the way endometrium usually responds in the uterus. At the end of every cycle, when hormones cause the uterus to shed its endometrial lining, endometrial tissue growing outside the uterus will break apart and bleed. However, unlike menstrual fluid from the uterus, which is discharged from the body during menstruation, blood from the misplaced tissue has no place to go. Tissues surrounding the area of endometriosis may become inflamed or swollen. The inflammation may produce scar tissue around the area of endometriosis. These endometrial tissue sites may develop into what are called "lesions," "implants," "nodules," or "growths."

Endometriosis is most often found in the ovaries, on the fallopian tubes, and the ligaments supporting the uterus, in the internal area between the vagina and rectum, on the outer surface of the uterus, and on the lining of the pelvic cavity. Infrequently, endometrial growths are found on the intestines or in the rectum, on the bladder, vagina, cervix, and vulva (external genitals), or in abdominal surgery scars. Very rarely, endometrial growths have been found outside the abdomen, in the thigh, arm, or lung.

Physicians may use stages to describe the severity of endometriosis. Endometrial implants that are small and not widespread are considered minimal or mild endometriosis. Moderate endometriosis means that larger implants or more extensive scar tissue is present. Severe endometriosis is used to describe large implants and extensive scar tissue.

What Are the Symptoms of Endometriosis?

Most commonly, the symptoms of endometriosis start years after menstrual periods begin. Over the years, the symptoms tend to gradually increase as the endometriosis areas increase in size. After menopause, the abnormal implants shrink away and the symptoms subside.

The most common symptom is pain, especially excessive menstrual cramps (dysmenorrhea) which may be felt in the abdomen or lower back or pain during or after sexual activity (dyspareunia). Infertility occurs in about 30 to 40 percent of women with endometriosis. Rarely, the irritation caused by endometrial implants may progress into infection or abscesses causing pain independent of the menstrual cycle. Endometrial patches may also be tender to touch or pressure, and intestinal pain may also result from endometrial patches on the walls of the colon or intestine.

The amount of pain is not always related to the severity of the disease—some women with severe endometriosis have no pain; while others with just a few small growths have incapacitating pain.

Endometrial cancer is very rarely associated with endometriosis, occurring in less than 1 percent of women who have the disease. When it does occur, it is usually found in more advanced patches of endometriosis in older women and the long-term outlook in these unusual cases is reasonably good.

How Is Endometriosis Related to Fertility Problems?

Severe endometriosis with extensive scarring and organ damage may affect fertility. It is considered one of the three major causes of female infertility. However, unsuspected or mild endometriosis is a common finding among infertile women and how this type of endometriosis affects fertility is still not clear. While the pregnancy rates for patients with endometriosis remain lower than those of the general population, most patients with endometriosis do not experience fertility problems.

What Is the Cause of Endometriosis?

The cause of endometriosis is still unknown. One theory is that during menstruation some of the menstrual tissue backs up through the fallopian tubes into the abdomen, where it implants and grows. Another theory suggests that endometriosis may be a genetic process or that certain families may have predisposing factors to endometriosis. In the latter view, endometriosis is seen as the tissue development process gone awry.

Whatever the cause of endometriosis, its progression is influenced by various stimulating factors such as hormones or growth factors. In this regard, NICHD investigators are studying the role of the immune system in activating cells that may secrete factors which, in turn, stimulate endometriosis.

In addition to these new hypotheses, investigators are continuing to look into previous theories that endometriosis is a disease influenced by delayed childbearing. Since the hormones made by the placenta during pregnancy prevent ovulation, the progress of endometriosis is slowed or stopped during pregnancy and the total number of lifetime cycles is reduced for a woman who had multiple pregnancies.

How Is Endometriosis Diagnosed?

Diagnosis of endometriosis begins with a gynecologist evaluating the patient's medical history. A complete physical exam, including a pelvic examination, is also necessary. However, diagnosis of endometriosis is only complete when proven by a laparoscopy, a minor surgical procedure in which a laparoscope (a tube with a light in it) is inserted into a small incision in the abdomen. The laparoscope is moved around the abdomen, which has been distended with carbon dioxide gas to make the organs easier to see. The surgeon can then check the condition of the abdominal organs and see the endometrial implants.

The laparoscopy will show the locations, extent, and size of the growths and will help the patient and her doctor make better informed decisions about treatment.

What Is the Treatment for Endometriosis?

While the treatment for endometriosis has varied over the years, doctors now agree that if the symptoms are mild, no further treatment other than medication for pain may be needed. For those patients with mild or minimal endometriosis who wish to become pregnant, doctors are advising that, depending on the age of the patient and the amount of pain associated with the disease, the best course of action is to have a trial period of unprotected intercourse for 6 months to 1 year. If pregnancy does not occur within that time, then further treatment may be needed.

For patients not seeking a pregnancy where treatment specific for the management of endometriosis is required and a definitive diagnosis of endometriosis by laparoscopy has been made, a physician may suggest hormone suppression treatment. Since this therapy shuts off ovulation, women being treated for endometriosis will not get pregnant during such therapy, although some may elect to become pregnant shortly after therapy is stopped.

Hormone treatment is most effective when the implants are small. The doctor may prescribe a weak synthetic male hormone called Danazol, a synthetic progestin alone, or a combination of estrogen and progestin such as oral contraceptives.

Danazol has become a more common treatment choice than either progestin or the birth control pill. Disease symptoms are improved for 80 to 90 percent of the patients taking Danazol, and the size and the extent of implants are also reduced. While side effects with Danazol treatment are not uncommon (e.g., acne, hot flashes, or fluid retention), most of them are relatively mild and stop when treatment is stopped. Overall, pregnancy rates following this therapy depend on the severity of the disease. However, some recent studies have shown that with mild to minimal endometriosis, Danazol alone does not improve pregnancy rates.

It is important to remember that Danazol treatment is unsafe if there is any chance that a woman is pregnant. A fetus accidentally exposed to this drug may develop abnormally. For this same reason, although pregnancy is not likely while a woman is taking this drug, careful use of a barrier birth control method such as a diaphragm or condom is essential during this treatment.

Another type of hormone treatment is a synthetic pituitary hormone blocker called gonadotropin-releasing hormone agonist, or GnRH agonist. This treatment stops ovarian hormone production by blocking pituitary gland hormones that normally stimulate ovarian cycles.

These hormones are currently being tested using different methods of administration. One such treatment involves a drug that is administered as a nasal spray twice daily for 6 months and works by suppressing production of estrogen, which controls the growth of the endometrial tissue. Other treatments being developed in this category include daily or monthly hormone injections. One concern is the loss of bone mineral which occurs with this type of hormone therapy. This may limit the duration and frequency of this type of treatment.

While pregnancy rates for women with fertility problems resulting from endometriosis are fairly good with no therapy and with only a trial waiting period, there may be women who need more aggressive treatment. Those women who are older and who feel the need to become pregnant more quickly or those women who have severe physical changes due to the disease, may consider surgical treatment. Also, women who are not interested in pregnancy, but who have severe, debilitating pain, may also consider surgery.

Conservative surgery attempts to remove the diseased tissue without risking damage to healthy surrounding tissue. This surgery is called laparotomy and is performed in a hospital under anesthesia. Pregnancy rates are highest during the first year after surgery, as recurrences of endometriosis are fairly common. The specifics of the surgery should he discussed with a doctor.

Some patients may need more radical surgery to correct the damage caused by untreated endometriosis. Hysterectomy and removal of the ovaries may be the only treatment possible if the ovaries are badly damaged. In some cases, hysterectomy alone without the removal of the ovaries may be reasonable.

New surgical treatments are being developed that further utilize the laparoscope instead of full abdominal surgery. During routine laparoscopy, the surgeon can cauterize small areas of endometriosis. Other evolving techniques include using a laser during laparoscopy to vaporize abnormal tissue. This involves a shorter recovery time. Laparoscopy treatment is possible, however, only if the surgeon can see pelvic structures clearly through the laparoscope. These newer techniques should be performed by surgeons specializing in such delicate procedures. Although these techniques are promising, more study is needed to determine if they yield results comparable to conventional surgical management.

Where to Look for Answers

Because endometriosis affects each woman differently, it is essential that the patient maintains a good, clear, honest communication with her doctor. For the single truth about endometriosis is that there are no clear-cut, universal answers.

If pregnancy is an issue, then age may affect the treatment plan. If it is not an issue, then treatment decisions will depend primarily on the severity of symptoms.

Because these decisions can be difficult and confusing, there are organizations that provide information and offer support and help to those who are affected by this disease.

Endometriosis Association
8585 North 76th Place
Milwaukee, Wisconsin 53223
(414) 355-2200

The American College of Obstetricians and Gynecologists
409 12th Street, SW
Washington, DC 20024-2188
(202) 638-5577

American Fertility Society
2140-11th Avenue South
Suite 200
Birmingham, Alabama 35205-2800
(205) 933-8494

Section 5.2

Endometriosis: Coping with a Mysterious Disorder

DHSS Publication No. 92-1191, 1992.

Whether the hero is Sherlock Holmes, Miss Marple, or Charlie Chan, a fictional whodunit can be fun. A real-life mystery is another story. In increasing numbers, women are learning they have a real, mysterious, and often painful and disabling condition of the reproductive organs: endometriosis.

In endometriosis, fragments of the endometrium, the lining of the uterus, become implanted elsewhere in the body. (When the implants grow into the uterine muscle layer, the disorder is called adenomyosis.) Like the endometrium itself, the implanted fragments build up tissue each month, then break down and bleed. Though the endometrium is shed during menstruation, blood from an implant outside the uterus has no way to leave the body. Consequently, internal bleeding, inflammation, and scar tissue can result.

Endometriosis is associated with ectopic (outside the uterus) pregnancy and can cause pain, heavy or irregular menstrual bleeding, and infertility. In fact, endometriosis is estimated to cause as much as 30 percent of all reported infertility in women.

While treatment can decrease symptoms and increase fertility for some women, the condition usually recurs, and its cause and progression are baffling. Why some women get it and others do not is a major part of the mystery that researchers are trying to solve.

Any menstruating woman, even a teenager, can develop endometriosis. Of the nearly 3,000 cases registered with the international Endometriosis Association in Milwaukee, 41 percent of the women had their first symptoms before they were 20. Today, estimates of the number of American women who have endometriosis range up to 5 million—a remarkable increase over the 20 cases that were reported worldwide in 1921. And, according to Robert Badwey, M.D., an obstetrician-gynecologist in suburban Washington, D.C., "For whatever reason—greater incidence, better diagnostic techniques, or both—we're much more aware of endometriosis now than even a *few* years ago."

The first definitive report in Western culture on endometriosis was given in 1921 by John Sampson, M.D. He believed that, during menstruation in certain women, tissues from the uterine lining back up through the fallopian tubes into the abdominal cavity, where they become implanted.

Over the years, Sampson's theory has been generally accepted. In 1984, however, scientists reported in *Obstetrics and Gynecology* that menstrual backup through the tubes is not limited to women with endometriosis. Lead investigator Jouko Halme, M.D., of the University of North Carolina School of Medicine at Chapel Hill, wrote that, because 90 percent of the women with open tubes and no sign of endometriosis "showed evidence of retrograde menstruation, it [Sampson's theory] cannot explain why only some women have developed the disease." Research is being conducted to determine how other factors may be involved.

One theory is that some women may have an immune system disorder that can cause the production of antibodies against their own endometrium. This "autoimmune response" appears in a number of women with endometriosis.

Certain women probably are predisposed to inheriting endometriosis, says Lyle Breitkopf, M.D., a gynecologist who works with the New York City chapter of the Endometriosis Association.

"I've seen it in first-degree relatives—in sisters, including identical twins, and in grandmother-mother-daughter situations," he says.

Some physicians believe that part of the increase in reported cases of endometriosis can be attributed to the trend toward postponing having children until later in a woman's reproductive years. Other experts point out that an association between deferred childbearing and endometriosis has not been proven. In many women, the condition subsides during pregnancy and the breast-feeding period that follows. A few women have reported that symptoms actually worsen during pregnancy.

Endometriosis can afflict many areas of the body: the ovaries, the fallopian tubes, the ligaments supporting the uterus, the area between the uterus and rectum, the bladder, and other abdominal tissues. In rare instances, it is found in sites outside the abdomen. One of the theories put forward to explain its occurrence in distant sites is that endometrial tissue may travel through the lymph or blood vessel systems.

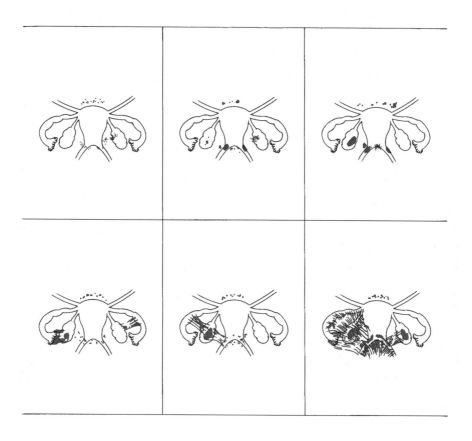

Figure 5.1. *Endometriosis is depicted here in stages from minimal to severe, but not necessarily as it would progress in any one patient. The disorder is minimal in the upper left drawing. The upper middle picture shows filmy adhesions and deep endometriosis. On the upper right, deep endometriosis has developed; adhesions partially obliterate the area between the uterus and rectum—the culdesac. On the lower left, the left ovary is fixed to a fallopian tube. The lower middle drawing shows deep endometriosis on the left ovary; adhesions fix the ovary to both a tube and ligament. In the lower right drawing, endometriosis is severe, with the culdesac completely obliterated and both ovaries and left tube fixed to other tissue. Conception would be very unlikely to occur in this stage of endometriosis.(Drawings were made from the Revised American Fertility Society Classification of Endometriosis: 1985.)*

Normally, an increased level of hormones each month triggers the release of an egg from the ovary. Finger-like tissues on one of the fallopian tubes grasp the egg, and little hair-like "cilia" within the tube transport it toward the uterus. If no fertilization occurs, the endometrium breaks down and is shed during menstruation.

Abnormal implants outside the uterus behave very much like the endometrium itself, in that they also respond to the hormonal changes controlling menstruation. They, too, build up, then break down and bleed. But blood outside the uterus has no way to leave the body, so it is absorbed by the surrounding inflamed tissue. Subsequently, as the cycle recurs month after month without interruption by pregnancy, the implants may increase in size. They may seed new implants and form scar tissue and adhesions (scarring that connects one organ to another). Sometimes, cysts called *endometriomas* form and may rupture, often causing excruciating pain.

Severe endometriosis can lead to infertility in several ways. When it occurs in the ovaries, it can produce cysts that prevent an egg from being released. If it occurs in the tubes, the implants can block the passage of the egg. And adhesions can fix the ovaries and tubes in place so that the egg is not grasped and moved into one of the tubes. In 60 percent of reported cases, both ovaries are affected.

The association between mild endometriosis and the inability to conceive is less clear. One theory involves substances called prostaglandins, which are normally present in endometrial and other tissue. It is believed that as implants outside the uterus break down, they release prostaglandins that concentrate in the abdominal fluid. Some scientists believe this could alter ovarian function or cause the fallopian tubes to contract irregularly and thereby not transport the egg correctly.

Symptoms of endometriosis vary from patient to patient. For some women, pain occurs before or during menstruation and gets progressively worse. Others report pain at any time during the month. There may be a sharp pain at ovulation or during intercourse or a dull pain after intercourse. If the bladder or intestines are involved, urination or defecation can be painful, and blood may appear in the urine or stool. There may be premenstrual staining. As the disease progresses, there may be heavy menstrual flow. True to the unpredictable nature of endometriosis, the severity of its symptoms may have little to do with the extent of its progression. Patients with relatively few implants may have severe pain. Patients with widespread implants may have no pain.

Sometimes endometriosis is hidden and is detected by chance during examination for another condition. One reason may be that a symptom, such as pain, may not be recognized as unusual. As Mary Lou Ballweg, executive director of the Endometriosis Association, puts it: "Perhaps they were told by Mom, who may have had the same problems, that menstrual pain is normal, so they just live with it and don't consult a doctor until the symptoms become unbearable." According to Ballweg, "97 percent of the women in a study from our data registry reported pain as a symptom." Moreover, she says, while some women with endometriosis have apparently normal menstrual periods for several years before beginning to have discomfort and pain, others report they've nearly always had difficult menstrual periods.

Women with symptoms should consult a gynecologist. Left untreated, endometriosis usually worsens.

When a woman visits her physician, she should be sure to explain all her symptoms. After taking a thorough patient history, the physician ordinarily will perform rectal and pelvic examinations to try to locate abnormalities, such as tender or immobile nodules or thickened masses. Such findings may corroborate the suspicion of endometriosis but, in most cases, the only way to confirm a diagnosis is for the physician to take a closer look with a relatively simple surgical procedure called laparoscopy.

In the procedure, usually performed on an outpatient basis, a light-transmitting, flexible, telescope-like device called a laparoscope is inserted into the abdomen through a tiny incision. The device allows close visual inspection of the suspected diseased tissue. The physician may extract a tissue specimen through the laparoscope for laboratory analysis. If endometriosis is verified, the physician will base therapy on several factors: symptoms, the extent of disease, the patient's age, and whether—and how soon—the patient wants to have children.

For extreme cases, major surgery may be necessary to remove all or part of the reproductive organs. A hysterectomy-salpingo-oophorectomy—in which the uterus, tubes and ovaries are surgically removed—results, of course, in permanent infertility.

Unfortunately, such surgery doesn't necessarily mean the woman's endometriosis is cured. According to Karen Lamb, R.N., Ph.D., who conducted a study of the Endometriosis Association's case registry, "Of the 189 women who had a hysterectomy-oophorectomy, 30 to 35 percent reported surgery offered neither relief nor cure, and 44 percent of those receiving estrogen replacement therapy for post-menopausal symptoms had a return of endometriosis symptoms."

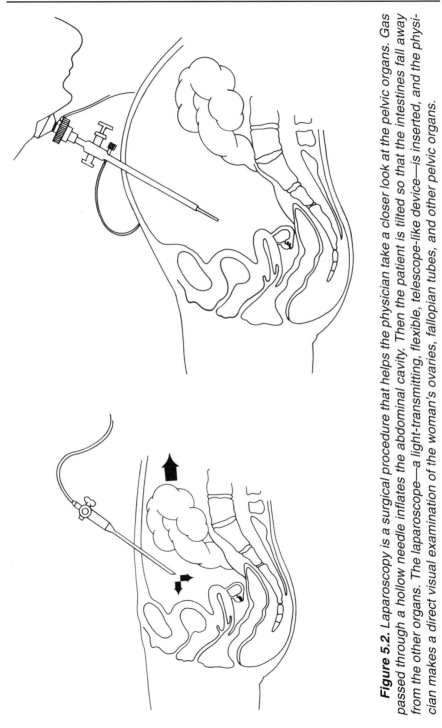

Figure 5.2. Laparoscopy is a surgical procedure that helps the physician take a closer look at the pelvic organs. Gas passed through a hollow needle inflates the abdominal cavity. Then the patient is tilted so that the intestines fall away from the other organs. The laparoscope—a light-transmitting, flexible, telescope-like device—is inserted, and the physician makes a direct visual examination of the woman's ovaries, fallopian tubes, and other pelvic organs.

Ballweg notes that one question raised by the study is whether more women would have had a successful outcome if implants on the bowel and bladder had been removed. "Only recently," she says, "a few surgeons have developed good techniques for removing endometrial implants from these areas."

Women faced with the possible removal of their reproductive organs should consider carefully what it may mean for them and discuss it at length with their physicians, their loved ones, and perhaps a counselor. Ballweg suggests talking to other women who have had the disease to see how they decided what to do. Even when a woman gets a second medical opinion, she says, "what it boils down to in most cases is the woman herself having to make a decision based on very personal issues, such as having a child and her own needs related to her work and her marital relationship or sexuality."

Treating Endometriosis

The Food and Drug Administration has approved several drugs for treating endometriosis.

A synthetic hormonal drug called danazol can be used to shrink the implants. A study of danazol at Harvard Medical School in Boston showed decreased symptoms in 89 percent of the patients and actual reduced disease (fewer or smaller implants) in 94 percent. Over five years, 33 percent of patients had recurring disease. Of 56 patients who wanted children, 26 became pregnant; 15 also had surgery, however, so the extent of danazol's influence isn't clear. Although most patients complained of masculinizing side effects—such as weight gain, decreased breast size, and deepened voice—only one patient in the study discontinued the therapy because of the side effects.

Any woman taking danazol should keep in close touch with her physician to watch for problems because some effects may be irreversible. Long-term effects of the drug are unknown. Also, it's important to avoid pregnancy while taking hormonal drugs because of their unknown potential for causing birth defects.

In 1990, FDA approved a nasal spray formulation called Synarel (nafarelin acetate) to alleviate symptoms and cause the endometrial implants to shrink or stop growing. Of 247 women treated with Synarel for six months, 85 percent showed a partial or complete reduction in the size of implants. Six months after treatment was discontinued, symptoms reappeared in half of those who had been helped.

The side effects of Synarel are largely the same as women experience during menopause. Menstruation stops or diminishes. Other side effects include hot flashes, vaginal dryness, headaches, and nasal irritation. Synarel shouldn't be used longer than six months because the shutdown of estrogen may cause bone loss. Women at risk of osteoporosis should discuss with their doctors the risks and benefits of using the drug.

Last year, FDA approved another endometriosis treatment: an injectable drug similar to Synarel called Lupron Depot (leoprolide acetate), which was previously approved to treat advanced prostate cancer. Endometriosis patients receive injections of Lupron Depot once a month for six months. The manufacturer reports that in clinical trials, Lupron's effectiveness was comparable to danazol. Side effects were similar to those associated with Synarel, and the same precautions that apply to Synarel should be observed by patients taking Lupron.

Also, oral contraceptives produce some changes in the body similar to those caused by pregnancy, so they may be given to curb the disease's progression. If needed, pain medication may be prescribed.

Surgery that preserves the reproductive organs may be performed to remove diseased tissue and correct misaligned organs. Sometimes, surgery and drug therapy are used together.

Recurrence rates after treatment need further study, Ballweg says.

Another treatment combines laparoscopy with laser surgery to remove the diseased tissue. According to Colin Pollard of FDA's Center for Devices and Radiological Health, which regulates both laparoscopes and lasers, the laser is connected to the laparoscope and positioned in such a way that its intense light beam is directed through the laparoscope onto the tissue to destroy it. While removing implants with major abdominal surgery requires about a week of hospitalization and a month or more of home recovery, the laser-laparoscopy surgery is usually done on an outpatient basis and requires only about a week's recovery time at home. Also, laser surgery may be better than conventional surgery in preserving fertility, because it destroys less tissue and does not cause scar tissue to form.

Chronic endometriosis can be frustrating and disabling. Its pain can threaten a patient's sexual life, social activities, and career. Its resultant disorders and infertility are heartbreaking. And, there are unanswered questions as to its cause, prevention and treatment. Still, more than 2,000 scientific papers have been written on the subject, and scientists, clinicians, and other professionals are working to unravel the mysteries of endometriosis.

Patients can help by reporting their experiences with the disease to the Endometriosis Association's data registry program. The association also offers patient support and educational literature. To report, to locate the nearest chapter, or to learn more about endometriosis, write to:

Endometriosis Association,
8585 N. 76th Place,
Milwaukee, WI 53223,
or call (1-800) 992-3636.

—by Dixie Farley

Section 5.3

On the Teen Scene—Endometriosis: Painful but Treatable

FDA Consumer 93-1205, January/February 1993.

"The pain was so sharp I thought I'd ruptured my appendix, but the doctor said, no, it wasn't that. It was between my periods, so I didn't connect it with menstruation. I was 16."

"Over the next 10 years, I had more and more of these 'pain attacks,' and my periods gradually became heavier and more painful."

"When I was pregnant with my first child, I was virtually pain-free. But shortly after he was born, each month around ovulation, I went to bed in tears from horrible pain. And I bled so much during menstruation I didn't dare leave the house. I went back to the doctor. It was endometriosis."—A woman from Des Moines, Iowa.

Endometriosis is a mysterious, often painful, and disabling condition in which fragments of the lining of the uterus (womb) become embedded, or implanted, elsewhere in the body.

Of the more than 3,000 patients registered with the research program of the international Endometriosis Association in Milwaukee,

41 percent report having symptoms as teenagers. About 5 million American women and girls, some as young as 11 have endometriosis according to the association.

"These girls have terrible pain," says Lyle Breitkopf, M.D., a gynecologist in New York City. "Typically, they come to the school nurse month after month—maybe six to eight of their 12 menstrual cycles—needing something for pain or being sent home vomiting, writhing on the floor.

For the woman from Des Moines, 25 years with endometriosis led to removal of her uterus, fallopian tubes, and ovaries a number of years ago. For many women today, new medicine and less drastic surgery reduce endometriosis symptoms and preserve reproductive organs. FDA has approved several drugs to treat endometriosis and regulates medical devices, such as lasers, used in surgical treatment.

A teen who thinks she may have endometriosis should be examined by a gynecologist. The sooner treatment begins, the better it is for the patients, says Breitkopf. "When we find them at an early stage, we can arrest the condition more easily and keep after it so it doesn't progress as far."

Doctors don't know why endometriosis only strikes certain women.

Some probably inherit it, says Breitkopf. "I've seen it in sisters, including identical twins, and in grandmother-mother-daughter situations."

According to Robert Badwey, M.D., a gynecologist in suburban Washington, D.C., "For whatever reason—greater incidence, better diagnostic techniques, or both—we're much more aware of endometriosis now than even a few years ago."

What's Happening in the Body?

Normally, an increased level of hormones each month triggers the release of an egg from the ovary. Finger-like tissues on one of the fallopian tubes grasp the egg, and tiny hair-like "cilia" inside the tube transport it toward the uterus. The egg is not fertilized, so the uterine lining breaks down and is shed during menstruation.

Though not in the uterus, the abnormal implants of endometriosis also respond to hormonal changes controlling menstruation. Like the lining, these fragments build tissue each month, then break down and bleed. Unlike blood from the lining, however, blood from implants outside the uterus has no way to leave the body. Instead, it is absorbed by surrounding tissue, which can be painful.

As the cycle recurs month after month, the implants may get bigger. They may seed new implants and form scar tissue and adhesions (scarring that connects one organ to another). Sometimes, a collection of blood called a sac or cyst forms. If a cyst ruptures, it often causes excruciating pain.

Symptoms vary from patient to patient. Severity of symptoms frequently has little to do with the extent of the implants. For instance, some women with just a few implants have severe pain, while some with many implants have little or no pain.

For some, pain starts before or during menstruation and gets worse as the period progresses. Others report pain at a variety of times during the month. There may be a sharp pain at ovulation when the egg, trying to move into the fallopian tube, causes a cyst on the ovary to burst. (Many women normally feel a twinge of pain at ovulation. Pain caused by a ruptured endometriosis cyst is severe.)

Patients whose implants affect the bladder or intestines often report painful urination or bowel movements and, sometimes, blood in the urine or stool.

Endometriosis sometimes causes premenstrual staining and, as the period progresses, heavy menstrual flow.

Often, endometriosis remains hidden a long time. A symptom such as pain at menstruation may not be seen as unusual, explains Mary Lou Ballweg, executive director of the Endometriosis Association.

"Perhaps a young woman is told by Mom, who had the same problems, that menstrual pain is normal," Ballweg says. "So she just lives with it and doesn't see a doctor until the symptoms become unbearable. Some young women with endometriosis have apparently normal menstrual periods for years before having discomfort and pain. Others report they've nearly always had difficult periods."

As many as 30 percent of women who report infertility problems have endometriosis.

Severe endometriosis can lead to infertility in different ways. In the ovaries, it can produce cysts that prevent the egg's release. In the fallopian tubes, implants can block the passage of the egg. Also, adhesions can fix ovaries and tubes in place so that projections on the tubes can't grasp the egg and move it into the tube. The effect of mild endometriosis on infertility is less clear.

Women with endometriosis may have a higher rate of "ectopic" pregnancy, a potentially life-threatening condition in which the fertilized egg begins to develop outside the womb.

The only way a doctor can be sure a woman has endometriosis is by surgical examination using laparoscopy, a fairly simple procedure usually done without an overnight hospital stay. The doctor makes a tiny incision and inserts a lighted, flexible, telescope-like device called a laparoscope that allows a close look at the tissue.

New Drugs

Among the drugs approved to treat endometriosis is a synthetic hormone called Danocrine (danazol), used to shrink the abnormal implants. A study at Harvard Medical School in Boston showed Danocrine improved symptoms in 89 percent of the patients and reduced the size or number of implants in 94 percent. In a third of the patients, the condition recurred within five years. Most patients complained of side effects such as weight gain, decreased breast size, and deepened voice, but only one patient stopped the treatment because of the effects.

In 1990, FDA approved a nasal spray called Synarel (nafarelin acetate) to relieve symptoms and shrink the implants or stop them from growing. Of 247 women treated with Synarel for six months, 85 percent had their implants shrink or disappear and their symptoms relieved. Six months after treatment stopped, symptoms reappeared in half of those who had been helped. The side effects are mainly those of menopause, such as hot flashes, vaginal dryness, and lighter, less frequent, or no menstruation. Other effects include headaches and nasal irritation.

Last year, FDA approved an injectable drug named Lupron Depot (leuprolide acetate) for treatment of endometriosis. It is similar to Synarel. Patients get injections once a month for six months. In clinical studies, Lupron's effectiveness was about the same as Danocrine's, the manufacturer reported. Side effects were similar to those with Synarel.

People taking endometriosis drugs need to watch for problems such as difficulty breathing or chest or leg pain, which may indicate a blood clot and should be reported to the doctor immediately. Frequent checkups are needed to monitor effects such as possible thinning of the bones. A patient should immediately report any new or worsened symptoms to the doctor. However, it's *normal* for endometriosis symptoms to temporarily worsen when a woman begins taking medicine.

Surgery

Sometimes medicine is not enough. Surgery may be needed to remove diseased tissue or to correct misaligned organs.

One method to remove diseased tissue combines laparoscopy with laser surgery. The laser is connected to the laparoscope and positioned so that its intense light beam is directed through the laparoscope onto the tissue to destroy it. The procedure usually is done without an overnight hospital stay and requires only about a week's recovery time at home.

"You're always reluctant to perform surgery or use medication on teenage patients," says Breitkopf. "But these young women are in terrible pain, and they can be helped. They really need to see a gynecologist so the endometriosis can be stemmed at the lowest possible stage of development."

Recurrence rates after treatment need further study, Ballweg says.

The monthly pain and heavy menstrual periods of chronic endometriosis can be frustrating, especially during the teenage years, when social and school activities are so important. Today, with diagnosis and treatment, a young woman's life can often return to normal.

Glossary

Endometriosis. A disorder in which fragments of the uterine lining (called the endometrium) implant elsewhere in the body, where they bleed—similar to menstruation, only the blood is absorbed by the body. The name is a combination of three Greek terms: *endo*=within, *metri*=uterus (womb), and *osis*=condition.

Gynecologist. A doctor who specializes in disorders of women's reporpductive organs.

Infertility. The inability to conceive a baby.

Laparoscope. A lighted, flexible, telescope-like device inserted into the body through a tiny incision to allow the doctor a close look at tissue.

Laser. Its letters stand for **L**ight **a**mplification by **s**timulated **e**mission of **r**adiation. Radiation here means electromagnatic energy, which

includes light. Doctors use lasers with laparoscopes to remove endometriosis implants.

Ovulation. The discharge of an egg from an ovary.

Uterus. The technical term for "womb", where a fertilized egg attaches
to the lining to grow. If the egg is not fertilized, the lining is shed as
menstruation.

— by Dixie Farley

Chapter 6

Uterine Fibroids

Uterine fibroids, one of the most common noncancerous gynecological conditions occurring in reproductive-age women, are estimated to affect more than 1 out of 5 women under 50 and account for 3 out of every 10 hysterectomies performed annually in the United States.

A fibroid, or myoma, is a noncancerous mass of muscle and connective tissue in the uterus (womb). No one knows what causes fibroids, but scientists believe their growth may be stimulated by the female sex hormone estrogen.

"A fibroid can be as small as a pinhead or as large as a watermelon," says Gene Williams, M.D., a medical officer in the obstetrics and gynecological devices branch of FDA's Center for Devices and Radiological Health. "It can cause no symptoms or a lot of symptoms. To the woman who has one, a fibroid may feel like a rock-hard bulge in the lower abdomen."

Every year, about 175,000 American women—most of them 35 to 55—undergo hysterectomy, or surgical removal of the uterus, as treatment for fibroids. According to American College of Obstetricians and Gynecologists guidelines, a fibroid that makes a woman's uterus bigger than it would be at 12 weeks of pregnancy, even if the woman is suffering no other symptoms, is an indication for a hysterectomy.

However, the practice of routinely recommending hysterectomy for fibroids has come under increasing scrutiny from both consumer organizations and doctors concerned about the high rate of hysterectomy in

DHSS Publication No. 94-1181, January 1994.

the United States. By age 60, more than a third of American women have had a hysterectomy, a rate higher than in any other Western country.

Blue Cross/Blue Shield of Illinois, in a study of all the hysterectomies performed in the state between 1987 and 1989, concluded that one-third were unnecessary.

Most of the unnecessary surgeries, the insurer found, were performed for fibroids and other benign (noncancerous) conditions.

Fibroid Types

Fibroids are classified by their position in the uterus. Intramural fibroids, the most common type, grow inside the uterine wall. Subserous or subserosal fibroids grow outward from the uterine wall into the abdominal cavity. Submucous fibroids grow inward from the uterine wall, taking up space within the uterus itself. This type of fibroid is the most likely to cause symptoms of heavy, prolonged menstrual bleeding. A fibroid can be as big as 20 centimeters (nearly 8 inches) in diameter and can weigh more than 20 pounds.

Small fibroids usually cause few if any symptoms. But, as a fibroid grows larger, it may press on the bladder and the ureters, the pair of tubes that connect the bladder to the kidneys. Pressure on the bladder can cause urinary frequency; pressure on the ureters can lead to kidney and urinary tract infections. Fibroids can sometimes be a cause of miscarriages and infertility.

A woman with a moderate-to-large fibroid may also notice a protruding stomach and a sensation of heaviness in the abdomen. For many women, the most distressing symptom is prolonged, heavy bleeding at the time of their menstrual periods, as well as spotty vaginal bleeding outside of the normal menstrual cycle. Women who lose too much blood may become anemic.

Sometimes a fibroid develops a thin stalk "like a balloon on a string," says David Barad, M.D., head of reproductive endocrinology at New York's Montefiore Medical Center. This is called a pedunculated fibroid. In some cases, the stalk can become twisted, cutting off its own blood supply, and causing severe pain.

Fibroids tend to grow in spurts, with periods of rapid growth punctuated by periods of no or very slow growth. As a woman approaches menopause, a fibroid may begin to grow rapidly. After menopause, however, fibroids stop growing and may start to shrink.

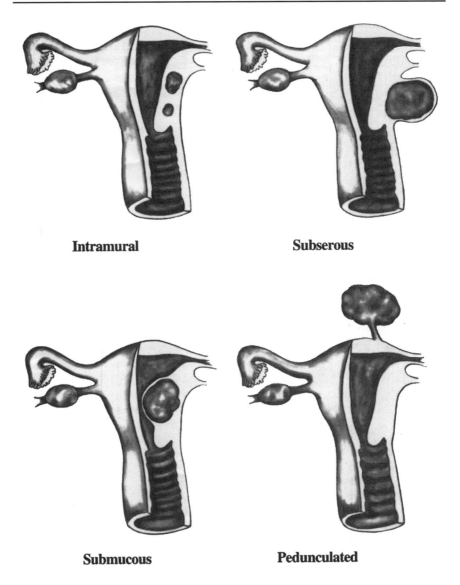

Intramural

Subserous

Submucous

Pedunculated

Figure 6.1. Fibroid Types. Fibroids are classified by their position in the uterus. Intramural fibroids (top left) are the most common type and grow inside the uterine wall. Subserous fibroids (top right) grow outward from the uterine wall into the abdominal cavity. Submucous fibroids (bottom left) grow inward from the uterine wall and are the most likely type to cause heavy, prolonged menstrual bleeding. Sometimes fibroids become pedunculated (bottom right), developing a thin stalk and looking like a balloon on a string. The stalk may twist, causing severe pain.

Options Increase

The practice of routinely recommending hysterectomy for fibroids has come under increasing scrutiny from both consumer organizations and doctors. New medications and less-invasive surgeries have made more treatment options available to women whose fibroids cause them problems. A number of doctors interviewed for this article say the most important consideration in treating a fibroid should be how the patient feels about her condition and what level of intervention she is comfortable with.

"The physician should look objectively at the patient's symptoms, inform her of the treatment choices, and give her the autonomy to decide what she wants to do," says David Barad, M.D., director of reproductive endocrinology and infertility services at Montefiore Medical Center, Bronx, New York, and an associate professor at the Albert Einstein College of Medicine.

"There are probably hundreds of thousands of women who have fibroids on their uteruses that don't need to have anything done to them. At the other end of the spectrum, if a woman who has completed her family has a large fibroid that is causing distressing symptoms — like painful cramps, heavy menstrual bleeding, and anemia — she would be a candidate for hysterectomy."

In the March 1993 issue of the *American Journal of Obstetrics and Gynecology*, Andrew J. Friedman, M.D., and Susan T. Haas, M.D., of Harvard Medical School, write that the recommendation for surgery when fibroids make a woman's uterus larger than a 12-week pregnancy is based on three main concerns:

- Ovarian cancer might go undetected because the presence of a fibroid makes it difficult for the doctor to feel the ovaries during a pelvic examination.

- A rapidly growing fibroid may signal uterine cancer.

- A growing fibroid may produce more debilitating symptoms and add to the risks of surgery later on.

Friedman and Haas, advocating a less aggressive approach to fibroid treatment, respond to these concerns this way:

- The development of ultrasound (the use of high-frequency sound waves to produce an image of a part of the body) makes it

90

possible to look at a woman's ovaries even when a fibroid prevents a manual examination. In any case, ovarian cancer is rare before age 50, and most hysterectomies for fibroids are done on women ages 35 to 44.

- Ultrasound and magnetic resonance imaging can be used to screen for uterine cancer, also rare in women under 50.

- Studies of hysterectomies done because of fibroids have not shown that removing a larger uterus poses a greater risk of surgical complications. "Watchful waiting" and treatment of problematic symptoms with medication or minimally invasive surgery may be just as effective as hysterectomy.

Exploring Drug Therapy

Many doctors prescribe drugs chemically similar to gonadotropin releasing hormone (GnRH) to treat fibroids. GnRH, produced by the pituitary gland, stimulates the production of estrogen. The drugs, known as GnRH analogs, block release of the hormone, thereby preventing the production of estrogen. These drugs, which include leuprolide (Lupron), nafarelin (Synarel), and goserelin (Zoladex), are approved by FDA to treat endometriosis in women and prostate cancer in men. Although FDA has not approved these drugs for treatment of fibroids, as with other approved medications, doctors may prescribe them if in their professional judgment a patient will benefit from them.

"Placing a woman on these drugs creates a false menopause," says Lisa Rarick, M.D., a medical officer in the division of metabolism and endocrine drug products of FDA's Center for Drug Evaluation and Research. "Her periods stop. The lack of estrogen usually causes the fibroid to shrink, just as they do after natural menopause. Sometimes other symptoms such as pressure or pain, can be relieved by the shrinkage."

Side effects of GnRH analogs include many of the symptoms experienced by women during menopause: "hot flashes," vaginal dryness, and bone loss. Because of these side effects, the drugs are not approved for use for longer than six months. And once the medication is stopped, the fibroid usually starts to grow again.

Some gynecologists are now experimenting with combining GnRH analogs with hormone replacement therapy to "add back" lost estrogen. "This is not generally accepted clinical use as yet," says Barad. "We don't know that simply adding back estrogen will address all the safety considerations of long-term use of GnRH analogs."

91

Barad and others have found a useful role for GnRH analogs as preoperative therapy to shrink fibroids and stop heavy bleeding. "Both anesthesia and surgery are easier and safer if you can first make the fibroid smaller and stop the heavy bleeding so the patient isn't anemic," says Barad.

The drug danazol (Danocrine) which is chemically similar to the male sex hormone testosterone, may also be prescribed to stem heavy menstrual bleeding caused by a fibroid. Like the GnRH analogs, danazol is approved for treatment of endometriosis but not for treatment of fibroids. Its main side effect is to increase male characteristics, such as facial hair and deepening of the voice; however, not all patients experience this side effect.

New Surgical Techniques

The development of endoscopes, lasers, and electrosurgical devices has led to new, less-invasive surgical techniques to remove fibroids. An endoscope is a thin fiberoptic tube that surgeons insert into the body. It can transmit an image to a television-like screen. Specialized endoscopes for viewing the abdominal cavity are called laparoscopes. Endoscopes designed to view the inside of the uterus are known as hysteroscopes. A laser is a device that uses a thin, intense light beam to "cut" or vaporize tissue, while electrosurgery or electrocautery devices use electricity to destroy tissue by applying heat.

These devices can be combined in several ways to perform a variety of procedures. Some devices combine the visualization and surgical functions in one instrument, such as the hysteroscopic resectoscope, which consists of a hysteroscope with an electrosurgery device built into it. This device is often used to remove submucous fibroids, the type most likely to cause symptoms of heavy menstrual bleeding).

The most appropriate procedure for each patient will depend on factors such as the size and position of the fibroid, the severity of symptoms, and future childbearing plans. Hysterectomy, by removing the uterus, makes it impossible to become pregnant or carry a baby.

Endometrial ablation, in which an electrosurgical device is used to remove the lining of the womb, may be recommended if a woman's major fibroid-related symptom is heavy, debilitating menstrual bleeding. This procedure also makes pregnancy impossible.

Myomectomy, or surgical removal of a fibroid leaving the uterus in place, may be an alternative to hysterectomy, particularly for women who still want to have children. In determining whether to recommend a myomectomy, a doctor will take into consideration the woman's overall health as well as the number and location of the fibroids, says Grant Bagley, M.D., of FDA's Office of Health Affairs.

"A myomectomy can be a very simple procedure or it can be very complicated," says Bagley. "A thorough discussion is needed with each patient as to whether their particular case will be difficult."

According to Barad of Montefiore, myomectomies can result in higher than average blood loss and scarring of the uterus that can adversely affect a woman's chances of becoming pregnant. "The operation you are performing to preserve reproductive potential may actually have the opposite effect." However, Bagley says newer techniques can be used to limit blood loss and preserve fertility.

If the fibroid is approachable from inside the uterus, a myomectomy may be performed using a hysteroscope. This procedure may be done in a physician's office if the fibroids are small. In some cases, patients can resume normal work and leisure activities within about a week.

A woman who has discomfort and heavy menstrual bleeding caused by a large fibroid, and who does not want to become pregnant, may opt to have a hysterectomy. A traditional abdominal hysterectomy is major surgery, requiring a four to five-day hospital stay and a recuperation period of about six weeks.

Women with relatively smaller fibroids may be able to have a vaginal hysterectomy instead. In this procedure, the uterus is removed through the vagina, thereby avoiding a large abdominal incision. Some doctors will prescribe GnRH analogs for several months before surgery to try to shrink the woman's uterus so that a vaginal hysterectomy can be performed instead of an abdominal one. In some cases, a vaginal hysterectomy is done with the assistance of a laparoscope. Most patients will have a shorter hospital stay and recovery period for a vaginal hysterectomy than for an abdominal procedure.

Physicians differ in their approach to the treatment of fibroids, Rarick points out. "Some will only do hysterectomies. Others will do everything they can to preserve the uterus."

And Williams advises: "Patients need to ask questions and be aware of all their options."

One Woman's Decision

In 1983, Diane Trent (not her real name), 42, began experiencing pain on the left side of her abdomen during her monthly period. Then

93

she began to have extremely heavy periods lasting as long as two weeks. She went to see her gynecologist, who performed a pelvic examination and told her she had a fibroid in her uterus. The doctor recommended a hysterectomy.

Trent requested an ultrasound examination, which showed that the fibroid was about 7 centimeters (23/4 inches) in diameter. She decided she only wanted to undergo a hysterectomy as a last resort and asked her doctor if there was a less drastic option.

In response, the gynecologist performed an endometrial biopsy, which showed no cancer, and a dilation and curettage (D&C), a procedure that involves dilating the cervix (neck of the womb) and scraping the uterine lining. The D&C stemmed Trent's heavy bleeding for a while. But after a few months the problem recurred. At times, she says, the bleeding "was so disabling that I couldn't go to work." Because the fibroid was pressing on her bladder, she had to urinate frequently.

Many women in Trent's situation would have opted for a hysterectomy. Instead, Trent consulted a reproductive endocrinologist, who agreed to monitor the fibroid's growth.

After three years, it had grown to 10 centimeters (4 inches) in diameter—about the size of a grapefruit. Her new doctor now recommended a hysterectomy.

"My feeling was that this was not life threatening and I didn't know what the long-term outcome of surgery would be," Trent says. "I decided I would rather put up with some discomfort that I knew would go away eventually." So she found another specialist who was willing to continue monitoring the fibroid.

The mass did not enlarge during the next five to six years. Trent is now 52. Since she reached menopause about two years ago, the fibroid has shrunk slightly. She continues to have an ultrasound examination every year. Her doctor says the fibroid should keep shrinking slowly, but it will never disappear completely.

Lisa Rarick, M.D., a medical officer in FDA's Center for Drug Evaluation and Research, says Trent's experience illustrates that the "best" treatment for a fibroid may be what the patient is most comfortable with.

"The issue is whether you can live with the symptoms. It's very individual. It depends how uncomfortable you are and how you feel about having surgery."

—by Eleanor Mayfield

Chapter 7

Ovarian Cysts

Benign Ovarian Cysts

Noncancerous ovarian cysts are a very common condition among women of reproductive age. But before diagnosing a condition as a benign ovarian cyst, doctors rule out cancer.

Normally, the follicle (or cyst) created by the ovaries each month bursts harmlessly when ovulation occurs. Sometimes, however, this normal physiologic process goes awry. The follicle, instead of bursting and releasing its egg, may continue to swell with fluid, or the corpus luteum (tissue that secretes hormones to prepare for pregnancy) may fail to dissolve even though the egg has not been fertilized. In either of these situations, the result is a "functional," or physiologic, cyst—a fluid-filled sac that may be as small as a grape or as large as a grapefruit.

Functional cysts are the most common ovarian cysts. In a premenopausal woman, such a cyst is always benign (noncancerous) and will frequently disappear spontaneously within a couple of months. Sometimes a functional cyst ruptures, spilling ovarian fluid into the abdominal cavity and causing pain. As the body absorbs the fluid, however, the pain subsides, and surgery is rarely necessary.

Ovarian cysts may be diagnosed by pelvic examination or by ultrasound imaging.

An excerpt from DHSS Publication No. 94-1181, January 1994.

A woman who has a functional cyst may have abdominal cramps, nausea, and menstrual irregularity. However, many women have no symptoms at all.

A gynecologist who diagnoses a cyst of less than 6 centimeters (2 1/4 inches) in diameter in a premenopausal woman who is ovulating will usually want to observe the patient for a couple of menstrual cycles to see if the cyst goes away by itself, says Lisa Rarick, M.D., a medical officer in FDA's Center for Drug Evaluation and Research.

If the cyst doesn't disappear spontaneously, the doctor may recommend that the woman take birth control pills to suppress ovulation. Most birth control pills are combinations of two female sex hormones, estrogen and progestin. In some cases, progestin-only pills (also called "mini-pills") may be prescribed instead of combination pills. Both combination birth control pills and mini-pills work by preventing the release from the brain of other hormones that stimulate ovulation. Deprived of hormonal stimulation, a functional ovarian cyst will often shrink and eventually disappear.

An ovarian cyst that doesn't disappear after a couple of months may be a benign semisolid cyst. This kind of cyst is usually diagnosed by ultrasound imaging. The most common semisolid cyst is a dermoid cyst, so called because it is made up of skin-like tissue; it can usually be removed by laparoscopic surgery. Occasionally, an ovary containing a dermoid cyst becomes twisted on itself, causing severe pain. Surgical removal of the affected ovary, or oophorectomy, may be necessary if this happens.

Any cyst that is 6 centimeters in diameter—about the size of a peach—or larger in a premenopausal woman should be investigated immediately as a possible malignancy, says Rarick, as should a cyst of any kind in a woman who has completed menopause.

While some doctors will recommend surgical examination of a large ovarian cyst, many gynecologists will examine the mass through a laparoscope, says Rarick. "It's possible to use a needle to puncture the cyst or aspirate its contents. The cyst can even be removed through the laparoscopic incision."

Polycystic ovarian disease, also known as Stein-Leventhal syndrome, is a benign condition characterized by multiple small cysts on the ovaries. This disease has a distinct set of symptoms that may appear as early as adolescence and may include menstrual irregularity, abnormal growth of body hair, lack of breast development, obesity, and infertility.

Standard treatments for polycystic ovarian disease are the drugs clomiphene (Clomid, Milophene, Serophene) and menotropins (Pergonal), which stimulate ovulation. At one time, the standard treatment was surgical wedge resection, which involved removing part of the affected ovary. This procedure is now considered outmoded because it creates scars on the ovary that can cause infertility.

—by Eleanor Mayfield

Chapter 8

Hysterectomy

A hysterectomy is an operation to remove the uterus *(womb)*. Most hysterectomies are not emergency operations, so you have time to think about your options. This section is designed to help you understand the options and their meaning for you.

Functions of the Uterus and Ovaries

The uterus cradles and nourishes a fetus from conception to birth, and aids in the delivery of the baby. It also produces the monthly menstrual flow, or period.

The ovaries have two major functions. One is the production of eggs or ova, which permit childbearing. The second is the production of hormones or chemicals which regulate menstruation and other aspects of health and well-being, including sexual well-being.

If the egg that is released during a woman's normal monthly cycle is not fertilized, the lining of the uterus is shed by bleeding *(menstruation)*.

After a hysterectomy, a woman can no longer have children and menstruation stops. The ovaries generally continue to produce hormones, although in some cases they may have reduced activity.

Some hysterectomies also include removal of the ovaries, so the supply of essential female hormones is greatly reduced. This can have various effects, as discussed later.

New York State Department of Health, Publication No. 1421, March 1993.

Whether or Not to Have a Hysterectomy

Hysterectomy is one treatment for a number of diseases and conditions. If you have cancer of the uterus or ovaries or hemorrhage *(uncontrollable bleeding)* of the uterus, this operation may save your life. In most other cases, a hysterectomy is an elective procedure. The operation is done to improve the quality of life—to relieve pain, heavy bleeding or other chronic conditions and discomfort.

But there may be other ways of treating or dealing with these problems. So,—together with your doctor—you should weigh all the alternatives and effects of the different choices to help you decide what is right for you.

Reasons for a Hysterectomy or Alternatives

Reasons why hysterectomies may be recommended fall into three categories:

- to save lives;
- to correct serious problems that interfere with normal functions;
- to improve the quality of life.

The following describe the more common reasons for recommending hysterectomies.

Cancer of the Uterus or Ovary

Cancerous organs and, in some cases, adjoining organs and structures, are removed in order to stop the spread of this life-threatening disease.

Fibroids

These are common noncancerous *(benign)* tumors of the uterus and they are the most frequent reason for recommending a hysterectomy. They grow from the muscular wall of the uterus and are made up of muscle and fibrous tissue. Many women over 35 have fibroids, but usually have no symptoms.

In some women, however, fibroids *(myomas)* may cause heavy bleeding, pelvic discomfort and pain and occasionally pressure on other organs. These symptoms may require treatment, but not always a hysterectomy. For example, there are some promising new experimental drugs that may temporarily shrink the tumors. However, these drugs may have serious side effects and are generally very costly. There is also a type of abdominal surgery *(myomectomy)* that removes the myoma without removing the uterus. These treatments may be sufficient or they may offer temporary relief and enable a woman to postpone having a hysterectomy, especially if she still wishes to bear children.

Some women choose to do nothing since fibroids will often shrink in size as a woman goes through menopause.

Endometriosis

Another common reason for recommending a hysterectomy is endometriosis. This is a noncancerous condition in which cells similar to the uterine lining grow like islands outside of the uterus. This growth occurs most commonly in the ovaries, fallopian tubes, bladder, bowel and other pelvic structures, including the uterine wall. These cells may cause pain and discomfort by bleeding at the time of menstruation. Endometriosis may also cause scarring, adhesions and infertility.

Symptoms can vary greatly and some women choose to do nothing, or find that drug therapy, pain relief medication or more localized surgery are effective. When these are not effective, hysterectomy may be the treatment of choice.

Prolapse

As a woman ages, the vaginal supports begin to lose their muscle tone and sag downward *(prolapse)*. With prolapse, the bladder and/or rectum may be pulled downward with the uterus. This happens to most women to some degree. For the vast majority, the sagging is minor and produces no symptoms.

If the prolapse worsens, some women experience a heavy or dragging feeling in the pelvic area, problems controlling bladder and/or bowel function, and occasionally, protrusion of one of the organs through the vaginal opening.

Some women get relief from a number of these symptoms by doing special *(Kegel)* exercises to strengthen the pelvic muscles, by taking hormone therapy or by using a plastic or metal ring *(pessary)* which may help to hold the uterus in place. None of these treats the underlying problem.

A hysterectomy with repair of supporting structures is usually recommended in more serious cases. A woman has to decide for herself if the discomfort is great enough to have a hysterectomy.

Cancer of the Cervix

Precancerous changes in the cervix are often found on routine Pap smears. These lesions or abnormalities must be treated, but rarely with a hysterectomy. When detected early and treated effectively, most of these conditions *do not* progress to invasive, life-threatening cancer. They can be treated conservatively. Most can be treated on an outpatient basis.

It is only in the case of invasive cancer of the cervix that hysterectomy may be the treatment of choice.

Pre-cancer of the Uterus

A precancerous change can occur when the lining *(endometrium)* of the uterus overgrows. Hyperplasia of the endometrium means an "overgrowth" of the lining of the uterus. It causes irregular and/or excessive bleeding. It can usually be treated with hormone therapy. In more severe cases or cases that do not respond to hormone treatment, hyperplasia of the endometrium may lead to cancer of the uterus. In these cases, hysterectomy would be the treatment of choice.

Pelvic Adhesions

Irritation of the lining of the abdomen may cause adhesions *(scarring)* which bind affected organs to each other. The adhesions can result from endometriosis, infection or injury. The symptoms may include severe pain, bowel and bladder problems and infertility.

Pain relief medication or less drastic surgery, such as laser therapy, can be effective in some cases. In very serious cases, hysterectomy may be recommended. However, a hysterectomy itself can cause adhesions.

Unusually Heavy Bleeding

It is normal for the amount and length of menstrual flow to vary from woman to woman. There may also be differences in menstrual flow from one cycle to the next. If bleeding that is unusually heavy or frequent for you occurs, this may be due to a variety of causes. The most common causes are fibroids and hormonal changes.

Because there can be many reasons for unusually heavy bleeding, getting an accurate diagnosis is vital before deciding on a course of treatment. Depending on the diagnosis, drug therapy or minor surgery may be indicated. Rarely, there can be hemorrhage of the uterus in which case a hysterectomy can be life saving.

Pelvic Pain

This is a common symptom. As with heavy bleeding, there can be a number of causes for pelvic (lower belly) pain. These include endometriosis, fibroids, ovarian cysts, infection or scar tissue. Pain in the pelvic area may not be related to the uterus. Therefore, a careful diagnosis is essential before considering whether to have a hysterectomy.

Benefits and Risks of Hysterectomy

General Considerations

A hysterectomy may be life-saving in the case of cancer. It can relieve the symptoms of bleeding or discomfort related to fibroids, severe endometriosis or uterine prolapse. On the other hand, you may prefer to seek alternatives to surgery for these symptoms or other problems related to the uterus and pelvic organs.

Symptoms like pelvic pain or unusual bleeding may not necessarily be related to the uterus. An accurate diagnosis will help you to determine the potential benefits and risks of a hysterectomy.

The risks of hysterectomy include the risks of any major operation, although its surgical risks are among the lowest of any major operation.

Hysterectomy patients may have a fever during recovery, and some may have a mild bladder infection or wound infection. If an infection occurs, it can usually be treated with antibiotics. Less often, women may require a blood transfusion before surgery because of anemia or during surgery for blood loss. Complications related to anesthesia may occur.

As with any major abdominal or pelvic operation, serious complications such as blood clots, severe infection, adhesions, postoperative *(after surgery)* hemorrhage, bowel obstruction or injury to the urinary tract can happen. Rarely, even death can occur.

In addition to the direct surgical risks, there may be longer-term physical and psychological effects, potentially including depression and loss of sexual pleasure. If the ovaries are removed along with the uterus prior to menopause *(change of life)*, there is an increased risk of osteoporosis and heart disease as well. These will he discussed later along with possible treatments.

In making a decision, you should also consider that a hysterectomy is not reversible. After a hysterectomy, you will no longer be able to bear children and you will no longer menstruate. You need to evaluate the impact these changes would have on you.

Talk about your concerns with your doctor or a counselor and your partner. You may want to bring your partner to your doctor's office to discuss concerns before having the operation.

Removal of Tubes and Ovaries

Should your ovaries be removed along with your uterus if you have a hysterectomy?

If you have a diagnosis of uterine cancer, the ovaries should be removed because the hormones they secrete may encourage the growth of the cancer. They also may have to be removed in severe endometriosis because they produce the hormones that are responsible for endometriosis.

The fallopian tubes are generally removed when the ovaries are removed because they are adjoining structures and their sole purpose is to serve as a passageway between the ovaries and the uterus.

In cases other than uterine cancer or endometriosis, there is controversy among doctors about the advantages and disadvantages of removing ovaries and tubes as part of a hysterectomy.

Some doctors believe that healthy ovaries should be removed as part of a hysterectomy in women who are over a certain age, when normal ovarian hormonal activity may be diminishing. It is done as a preventive measure to reduce the risks of developing ovarian cancer. This is because ovarian cancer is very difficult to detect at an early stage and is often resistant to the best medical treatments.

Other doctors disagree because this cancer is not common and because removal of the ovaries does not always guarantee women will not develop ovarian cancer. (Rarely, the cells that cause ovarian cancer can be present in the body even after the ovaries are removed.) In addition, ovaries produce several hormones which are beneficial to women. They protect against serious diseases such as heart disease and osteoporosis and contribute to sexual pleasure.

As a woman ages, the ovaries gradually reduce their production of hormones. When menstruation ends, at the menopause, the ovaries markedly diminish production of estrogen, and this results in decreased protection against heart disease and osteoporosis. For a period of time after menopause, the ovaries continue to produce androgen, a hormone which is primarily critical for maintaining women's sexual desire. Normally, androgen may produce additional facial hair as well. Removing the ovaries causes menopause to occur more abruptly. The symptoms of menopause include hot flashes, night sweats, insomnia, fatigue, depression and vaginal dryness.

After ovaries are removed—or when menopause occurs—hormone replacement therapy often helps. Hormone replacement therapy cannot exactly duplicate the hormonal activity of the ovaries, but will reduce the risks of heart disease and osteoporosis, and reduce menopausal symptoms like hot flashes and vaginal dryness. It may also contribute to sexual pleasure. However, there are some women who cannot be placed on hormone replacement therapy. For example, some women with liver disease or a history of hormone-dependent tumors, such as breast cancer may not be able to take these hormones.

Sexuality

Every person reacts differently, and reactions are a combination of emotional and physical responses. We still have much to learn about the effects of hysterectomy on sexual function.

Some women say they enjoy sex more after a hysterectomy, particularly if they had a lot of bleeding and pain beforehand. Some women feel more relaxed not worrying about getting pregnant.

Some women who have hysterectomies experience diminished sexual enjoyment. There may be a number of reasons for this which are only partially understood. For some women, uterine contractions and pressure against the cervix add to sexual pleasure. Others may feel less pleasure or reduced desire due to loss of certain hormones, especially after removal of ovaries. In addition, loss of hormones can cause vaginal dryness and make sex uncomfortable. Hormone replacement therapy may relieve some of these symptoms. A vaginal gel or lubricant can reduce vaginal dryness.

For some women, reduction in sexual pleasure is temporary while they and their partners adjust. Because sexual feelings are so individual, it may be difficult to predict exactly how a hysterectomy will affect your feelings.

Emotional Effects

Some women report having a strong emotional reaction, or feeling down, after a hysterectomy. Most feel better after a few weeks, but some women do feel depressed for a long time. Other women experience a feeling of relief after a hysterectomy.

No longer being able to bear children can cause emotional problems for some women. Some women feel changed or feel they have suffered a loss. Talking things over with your physician, your partner, a friend or a counselor often helps. It may help to talk with a friend or another woman who has had a hysterectomy before and after your operation.

Alternatives to Hysterectomy

Alternatives to hysterectomy have their own benefits and risks. A myomectomy for fibroids, for example, is more localized therapy and does not involve removal of the uterus. However, like hysterectomy, it does involve general anesthesia and is a major operation. A myomectomy is a technically more difficult operation than a hysterectomy, and there may be increased risk of bleeding and infection. With this procedure, tumors may remain or recur which may lead to further surgery in the future, sometimes a hysterectomy.

Laparoscopy is a common procedure which enables the physician to visualize and treat a number of gynecologic conditions such as endometriosis through one or more minute incisions in the abdomen. It usually requires one day surgery and general anesthesia. Laser therapy or microsurgical techniques can be utilized with laparoscopy.

Each drug therapy has its own side effects and you should review these with your physician. Some therapies are more experimental and their benefits and risks may not be as well understood. You need to carefully review with your doctor what is known about any therapy you choose.

More localized therapy, like a myomectomy in the case of fibroids or laser or drug treatment in the case of endometriosis, may be valuable as an initial procedure for you, with the option of a hysterectomy later. Or you may choose to simply bear with your symptoms for a while and see what happens over time since the bleeding and discomfort related to endometriosis or fibroids may diminish as a woman enters menopause.

In considering a hysterectomy, you may wish to get a second opinion. A second opinion means that a second doctor will review your medical history, examine you and advise you as to whether he or she agrees with your primary doctor's treatment recommendation. It is an opportunity for you to discuss your condition with another expert. Many health insurance plans require and pay for a second opinion before any major surgery. If you don't know another doctor to ask for a second opinion, your insurance company or the county medical society *(listed in the white pages of the phone book)* can give you the names of appropriate doctors in your area. It is preferable to request a physician who is board certified in obstetrics and gynecology.

Finally, because every woman is unique and because a hysterectomy was recommended to you because of your individual needs, it is important that you discuss your personal risks and benefits with your doctor before deciding whether to have a hysterectomy. As with other surgery, different doctors make different judgements about when to recommend this operation.

Different Types of Hysterectomies

All hysterectomies are major operations involving removal of at least the uterus. Some types of hysterectomies involve removing other organs as well. It is important to talk with your doctor about the kind of hysterectomy recommended for you.

Total Hysterectomy

This operation involves removing both the body of the uterus and the cervix, which is the lower part of the uterus. The cervix is usually removed to prevent subsequent cervical cancer. A hysterectomy can sometimes be done through the vagina *(vaginal hysterectomy)*; at other times, a surgical incision in the lower belly *(abdominal hysterectomy)* is preferable. For example, if you have large fibroid tumors, it is difficult to safely remove the uterus through the vagina.

Vaginal hysterectomy, when it can safely be performed, generally involves fewer complications, a shorter recovery period and no visible scar.

In a total hysterectomy and bilateral (both sides) salpingo-oophorectomy, the ovaries and fallopian tubes are removed, along with the uterus and cervix. "Complete hysterectomy," which is sometimes used to refer to this procedure, is not a medical term.

Subtotal Hysterectomy

In this operation, only the upper part of the uterus is removed, but the cervix is not. Tubes and ovaries may or may not be removed. This procedure is always done through the abdomen.

Radical Hysterectomy

This procedure is reserved for serious disease such as cancer. The entire uterus and usually both tubes and ovaries as well as the pelvic lymph nodes are removed through the abdomen. Since cancer is unpredictable, other organs or parts of other systems are sometimes removed as well.

Hospitalization and Recovery

Presurgical routines vary from hospital to hospital. Generally:

- Blood and urine samples are taken.
- Sometimes enemas are given.
- The abdominal and pelvic areas may be shaved.

After the operation, the hospital stay is usually less than a week, depending on the type of hysterectomy and whether there are any complications.

Since hysterectomy is a major operation, discomfort and pain from the surgical incision are most pronounced during the first few days after surgery, but medication is available to minimize these symptoms.

By the second or third day, most patients are up walking. Normal activity can usually be resumed in four to eight weeks. Each patient is an individual, so the pace of recovery will vary.

Sexual activity can usually be resumed in six to eight weeks.

During recovery, you may need to rest frequently at first. Plan ahead and ask friends, neighbors or relatives to help you when you get home. It will probably take a while to feel peppy.

Many women find that special exercises can help them recover faster and feel better.

You can discuss both presurgical procedures and your recovery, including useful exercises, with your doctor.

Questions to Ask Your Doctor

- Why do I need to have a hysterectomy?

- What organ or organs will be removed and why?

- Will my ovaries be left in place? If not, why?

- Will my cervix be removed? If so, why?

- Are there alternatives for me besides a hysterectomy?

- What are the advantages, risks, benefits of each?

- What will be the physical effects of a hysterectomy?

- Are these permanent?

- What will happen to my figure, my weight, my breasts?

- How will it affect my sex life?

- Will I experience menopause *(change of life)*? Can the symptoms of menopause be treated? What are the risks and benefits of such treatment?

- Will the operation be a vaginal or abdominal hysterectomy? And why?

- What can I expect in the hospital? pre-operative procedures? length of stay? anesthesia? infection? transfusion? urinary catheter?

- What kind of care will I need after my hysterectomy?

- How should I prepare for coming home from the hospital?

- How soon can I go back to work? Try heavy housework?

- When can I resume sexual activity?

Chapter 9

Vaginitis

Chapter Contents

Section 9.1

Vaginitis, Important Information for Your Good Health

NIH Publication No. 93-3512, July 1993.

Vaginitis is a medical term that is used to refer to *any* infection or inflammation of the vagina. The symptoms of vaginitis are common and most women will have at least one form of vaginitis in their lifetime. Even though vaginitis is so common, many women know little about it.

The term "yeast infection" is what most women think of when they hear the word vaginitis. However, a yeast infection is only *one kind* of vaginal infection. Vaginitis can be caused by several different organisms, sometimes at the same time, as well as by hormonal changes, allergies, or irritations.

Because vaginitis can have many causes, it is important to see your doctor or other health care professional so that the proper cause can be identified and the correct treatment can be prescribed. Once started, the medication should be used exactly according to your doctor's instructions in order to cure the vaginitis. The symptoms may go away before you finish the medication. Even so, you should complete the therapy to help ensure a cure.

Vaginitis can sometimes be a sign of other health problems. Knowing more about the signs and symptoms of this common condition will help you and your health care provider make a proper diagnosis.

What is vaginitis?

"Vaginitis" is a word that is used to describe disorders that cause infection or inflammation ("itis" means inflammation) of the vagina. Vulvovaginitis refers to inflammation of both the vagina and vulva (the external female genitals). These conditions can result from an infection caused by organisms such as bacteria, yeast, or viruses, as well as by irritations from chemicals in creams, sprays, or even clothing that are in contact with this area. In some cases, vaginitis results from organisms that are passed between sexual partners.

How do I know if I have vaginitis?

The common symptoms of vaginitis are itching, burning, and vaginal discharge that is different from your normal secretions. The itching and burning can be inside the vagina or on the skin or vulva just outside the vagina. Discomfort during urination or sexual intercourse may also occur. If everyone with vaginitis had these symptoms, then the diagnosis would be fairly simple. However, it is important to realize that as many as 4 out of every 10 women with vaginitis may not have these typical symptoms. Frequently, a routine gynecologic exam will confirm vaginitis even if symptoms are not present. This is one reason why it is important to have a gynecologic exam at least every 2 years.

Is vaginal discharge normal?

A woman's vagina normally produces a discharge that is usually described as clear or slightly cloudy, nonirritating, and odor-free. During the normal menstrual cycle the amount and consistency of discharge vary. At one time of the month there may be a small amount of a very thin or watery discharge and at another time, a more extensive, thicker discharge may appear. All of these descriptions could be considered normal.

A vaginal discharge that has an odor or that is irritating is usually an abnormal discharge. The irritation might be itching or burning or both. The burning could feel like a bladder infection. The itching may be present at any time of the day but it is often most bothersome at night. Both of these symptoms are usually made worse by sexual intercourse. It is important to see a doctor or clinician if there has been a *change* in the amount, appearance, or smell of the discharge.

What are the most common types of vaginitis?

The six most common types of vaginitis are:

- *Candida* or "yeast" vaginitis
- Bacterial vaginosis
- *Trichomoniasis* vaginitis

- *Chlamydia* vaginitis
- Viral vaginitis
- Noninfectious vaginitis

Although each of these causes of vaginal infection can have different symptoms, it is not always easy for a patient to figure out which type of vaginitis she has; in fact, diagnosis can even be tricky for an experienced clinician. Part of the problem is that sometimes more than one type of vaginitis can be present at the same time. Often vaginitis is present without any symptoms at all.

To help you better understand these six major causes of vaginitis, let's look briefly at each one of them and how they are treated.

What are Candida or "yeast" infections?

Yeast infections of the vagina are what most women think of when they hear the term "vaginitis." They are caused by one of the many species of fungus called *Candida. Candida* normally live in small numbers in the vagina as well as in the mouth and digestive tract of both men and women.

Yeast infections produce a thick, white vaginal discharge with the consistency of cottage cheese. Although the discharge can be somewhat watery, it is odorless. Yeast infections usually cause the vagina and the vulva to be very itchy and red.

Since yeast is normal in a woman's vagina, what makes it cause an infection? Usually this happens when a change in the delicate balance in a woman's system occurs. For example, a woman may take an antibiotic to treat a urinary tract infection and the antibiotic kills her "friendly" bacteria that normally keep the yeast in balance; as a result the yeast overgrows and causes the infection. Other factors which can upset the delicate balance include pregnancy which changes hormone levels and diabetes which allows too much sugar in the urine and vagina.

Risk Factors for Vaginal Candida Infections

- Recent course of Antibiotics
- Uncontrolled Diabetes
- Pregnancy
- High Estrogen Contraceptives
- Immunosuppression

- Thyroid or Endocrine Disorders
- Corticosteroid Therapy

What is bacterial vaginosis?

Although "yeast" is the name most women know, bacterial vaginosis is actually the most common vaginal infection in women of reproductive age. Bacterial vaginosis will often cause a vaginal discharge. The discharge is usually thin and milky and is described as having a "fishy" odor. This odor may become more noticeable after intercourse. Redness or itching of the vagina are not common symptoms of bacterial vaginosis. It is important to note that many women with bacterial vaginosis have no symptoms at all and the vaginitis is only discovered during a routine gynecologic exam. Bacterial vaginosis is caused by a combination of several bacteria. These bacteria seem to overgrow much the same way as *Candida* will when the vaginal balance is upset. The exact reason for this overgrowth is not known. Since bacterial vaginosis is caused by bacteria, not by yeast, it is easy to see that different methods are needed to treat the different infections. A medicine that is appropriate for yeast is not effective against the bacteria that causes bacterial vaginosis.

What are **trichomoniasis, chlamydia,** *and viral vaginitis?*

Trichomonias, commonly called "trich" (pronounced "trick"), is caused by a tiny single-celled organism known as a "protozoa." When this organism infects the vagina it can cause a frothy, greenish-yellow discharge. Often this discharge will have a foul smell. Women with trichomonal vaginitis may complain of itching and soreness of the vagina and vulva, as well as burning during urination. In addition, there can be discomfort in the lower abdomen and vaginal pain with intercourse. These symptoms may be worse after the menstrual period. Many women, however, do not develop any symptoms. It is important to understand that this type of vaginitis can be transmitted through sexual intercourse. For treatment to be effective, the sexual partner must be treated at the same time as the patient.

Another primarily sexually transmitted form of vaginitis is caused by the germ known as *Chlamydia*. Unfortunately, most women do not have symptoms. This makes diagnosis difficult. A vaginal discharge is sometimes present with this infection but not always. More often a woman might experience light bleeding especially after intercourse.

She may have pain in the lower abdomen and pelvis. Chlamydial vaginitis is most common in young women (18 to 35 years) who have multiple sexual partners. If you fit this description, you should request screening for *Chlamydia* during your annual checkup. The best "treatment" for *Chlamydia* is prevention. Use of a condom will decrease your risk of contracting not only *Chlamydia*, but other sexually transmitted diseases as well.

Viruses are a common cause of vaginitis. One form caused by the *herpes simplex virus* (HSV) is often just called "herpes" infection. These infections are also spread by sexual intimacy. The primary symptom of herpes vaginitis is pain associated with lesions or "sores." These sores are usually visible on the vulva or the vagina but occasionally are inside the vagina and can only be seen during a gynecologic exam. Outbreaks of HSV are often associated with stress or emotional upheaval.

Another source of viral vaginal infection is the human papillomavirus (HPV). HPV can also be transmitted by sexual intercourse. This virus can cause painful warts to grow in the vagina, rectum, vulva, or groin. These warts are usually white to gray in color, but they may be pink or purple. However, visible warts are not always present and the virus may only be detected when a Pap smear is abnormal.

Many of the germs that cause vaginitis can be spread between men and women during sexual intercourse. Use of a barrier contraceptive such as a condom can help reduce your risk of contracting these and more serious germs such as the human immunodeficiency virus (HIV) which can lead to AIDS.

What is noninfectious vaginitis?

Occasionally, a woman can have itching, burning, and even a vaginal discharge without having an infection. The most common cause is an allergic reaction or irritation from vaginal sprays, douches, or spermicidal products. The skin around the vagina can also be sensitive to perfumed soaps, detergents, and fabric softeners.

Another noninfectious form of vaginitis results from a decrease in hormones because of menopause or because of surgery that removes the ovaries. In this form, the vagina becomes dry or "atrophic." The woman may notice pain, especially with sexual intercourse, as well as vaginal itching and burning.

How do you treat vaginitis?

The key to proper treatment of vaginitis is proper diagnosis. This is not always easy since the same symptoms can exist in different forms of vaginitis. You can greatly assist your health care practitioner by paying close attention to exactly which symptoms you have and when they occur, along with a description of the color, consistency, amount, and smell of any abnormal discharge. Do not douche before your office or clinic visit; it will make accurate testing difficult or impossible.

Because different types of vaginitis have different causes, the treatment needs to be *specific* to the type of vaginitis present. When a woman has had a yeast infection diagnosed by her doctor, she is usually treated with a prescription for a vaginal cream or suppositories. If the infection clears up for some period of time but then the exact same symptoms occur again, a woman can obtain, with her doctor or pharmacist's advice, a vaginal cream or suppository without a prescription that can completely treat the infection. The important thing to understand is that this medication may only cure the most common types of *Candida* associated with vaginal yeast infections and will not cure other yeast infections or any other type of vaginitis. If you are not absolutely sure, see your doctor. You may save the expense of buying the wrong medication and avoid delay in treating your type of vaginitis.

When obtaining these over-the-counter medicines, be sure to read all of the instructions completely before using the product. Be sure to use all of the medicine and don't stop just because your symptoms have gone away. Be sure to see your health care practitioner if:

- All of the symptoms do not go away completely.
- The symptoms return immediately or shortly after you finish treatment.
- You have any other serious medical problems such as diabetes.
- You might be pregnant.

Other forms of infectious vaginitis are caused by organisms that need to be treated with oral medication and/or a vaginal cream prescribed by your doctor. Products available without a prescription will probably not be effective. As with all medicine, it is important to follow your doctor's instructions as well as the instructions that come with the medication. Do not stop taking the medicine when your symptoms go away. Do not be embarrassed to ask your doctor or health care practitioner questions. Good questions to ask include: Is it okay to douche while on this vaginal cream? Should you abstain from sexual intercourse during treatment? Should your sexual partner(s) be treated at the same time? Will the medication for this vaginitis agree with your other medication(s)? Should you continue the vaginal cream or suppositories during your period? Do you need to be reexamined and if so, when?

"Noninfectious" vaginitis is treated by changing the probable cause. If you have recently changed your soap or laundry detergent or have added a fabric softener, you might consider stopping the new product to see if the symptoms remain. The same instruction would apply to a new vaginal spray, douche, sanitary napkin, or tampon. If the vaginitis is due to hormonal changes, estrogen may be prescribed to help reduce symptoms.

How can I prevent vaginitis?

There are certain things that you can do to decrease the chance of getting vaginitis. If you suffer from yeast infections, it is usually helpful to avoid garments that hold in heat and moisture. The wearing of nylon panties, pantyhose without a cotton panel, and tight jeans can lead to yeast infections. Good hygiene is also important. Many doctors have found that if a woman eats yogurt that contains active cultures (read the label) she will get fewer infections.

Because they can cause vaginal irritation, most doctors do not recommend vaginal sprays or heavily perfumed soaps for cleansing this area. Likewise, repeated douching may cause irritation or, more importantly, may hide a vaginal infection.

Safe sexual practices can help prevent the passing of diseases between partners. The use of condoms is particularly important.

If you are approaching menopause, have had your ovaries removed, or have low levels of estrogen for any reason, discuss with your doctor the use of hormone pills or creams to keep the vagina lubricated and healthy.

Summary

- "Vaginitis" is a medical term that describes an infection or irritation of the vagina and/or vulva by yeast, bacteria, viruses, other organisms, or chemical irritants.

- When present, symptoms of different types of vaginitis overlap which can make diagnosis difficult. In addition, more than one cause of vaginitis can be present at the same time in the same woman.

- Proper diagnosis by your doctor or health care practitioner is the key to proper treatment. Yeast, bacteria, viruses, and other organisms each require a specific type of therapy. Use of the wrong medication will not help and will only delay proper treatment.

- All vaginitis is not caused by yeast. The use of a nonprescription medication or other treatment may make the proper diagnosis more difficult if yeast is not the cause of the infection.

- Some forms of vaginitis are sexually transmitted and can co-exist with other more serious sexually transmitted diseases. The proper use of condoms can be helpful in preventing some forms of vaginitis.

- Follow complete instructions in treating your vaginal infection. If symptoms do not clear completely or if they reoccur, see your doctor or health care practitioner for further instructions.

Section 9.2

Controlling "Yeast Infections"

DHSS Publication No. 94-1181, January 1994.

Intense itching is usually the hallmark of a vaginal yeast infection. Once a woman has experienced it, she's not likely to forget it.

Nearly 75 percent of all women will have at least one such infection in their lifetime. Many are plagued by recurring yeast infections, which are most frequent between the ages of 16 and 35.

Yeast is a term for single-celled fungi. The technical name for the variety of fungus often present in the human body is candida, and the technical name for infections caused by these fungi is candidiasis. Such infections occur not only in the vagina, but also in other parts of the body in both sexes.

In December 1990, the Food and Drug Administration approved the over-the-counter (nonprescription) sale of the first of several products for treating vaginal yeast infections in women previously diagnosed by their doctors as having them.

A woman who has had one vaginal yeast infection can usually recognize its symptoms if it recurs. And a woman who has had several infections has no doubt about what's wrong when the next yeast infection starts.

There are several symptoms, but, according to Michael Spence, M.D., director of the Public Health and Preventive Medicine Program at Hahnemann University in Philadelphia, "If a woman does not itch, it's unlikely that she has a yeast infection."

Another symptom is a thick, mostly odorless discharge. But this can be misleading because, according to Spence, "Discharge in and of itself is not diagnostic. If you have a white discharge with an intense irritating itch, you may have an infection. Unfortunately, many women will, in response to increased estrogen at mid-cycle and the increased production of cervical mucus, develop a white, curdy discharge. That is not a yeast infection."

While not all women experience the following symptoms of a vaginal yeast infection, it's possible to have:

- vaginal soreness or irritation
- a rash on the vulva around the vagina
- pain or discomfort during intercourse
- abdominal pain
- soreness of the vulva or vagina
- burning during urination
- and even vaginal bleeding in some cases in addition to itching and discharge.

Causes of Yeast Infection

Candidiasis is caused by one of four varieties of candida: *Candida albicans, Candida glabrata, Candida tropicalis, and Candida krusei.* By far the most common—causing nearly 80 percent of vaginal yeast infections—is *Candida albicans.*

Most people have these organisms in the genital or intestinal tract to some degree at various times. It's the overgrowth of the fungus that causes problems.

According to Spence, there are a number of causes of the uncontrolled growth, usually related to some type of immune suppression. Sometimes there's been a significant change in diet. Other times it's due to use of antibiotics to treat another infection, such as strep throat or acne.

Broad-spectrum antibiotics such as penicillin or tetracycline can kill or suppress helpful bacteria in the genital tract, allowing yeast to grow unchecked, according to Philip Mead, M.D., Professor of Obstetrics and Gynecology at the University of Vermont College of Medicine.

It's even possible that an underlying disorder, like diabetes, is the root cause of the infection. "Whenever you see a fungal infection in a woman, these are the things that come immediately to mind," says Spence.

When physicians see recurrent yeast infections without another cause, they have to wonder about HIV disease. Because HIV (the virus that leads to AIDS) involves a lowering of the immune system, it could significantly impair a woman's ability to combat yeast, says Spence.

"Yeast infections can be passed back and forth between partners in unprotected intercourse, but because yeast is frequently present anyway, a sexual partner is more likely to pick up the infection if his or her immune system is also depressed," says Mead.

Immunity can become depressed by a number of factors besides HIV infection. Illness or infection of any kind weakens the immune system. Physical or mental stress can also wreak havoc, leaving the immune system less able to combat yeast infections. Lack of sleep, poor nutrition, and taking any medication, including birth control pills, can upset the body' s balance, allowing yeast to thrive. Pregnant women also have a tendency to have more yeast infections, as the immune system becomes temporarily altered by hormonal surges.

Diagnosis

Diagnosing vaginal yeast infections can be tricky, especially at first. Several other disorders, including inflammation of the cervix or sexually transmitted diseases such as trichomoniasis (a parasitic infection) or herpes, can have similar symptoms.

According to Mead, clinical diagnosis of yeast infections starts with a slide of vaginal secretions examined under the microscope. "Those slides [can be] very specific. If you see the yeast organisms, you can assume that's the diagnosis."

(Slides are actually examined for a particular stage of the fungus form called mycelia. While yeast is a commonly present form of fungus, mycelia is the variation of the fungus type that can grow out of control and cause infection problems.)

It's possible to have a yeast infection that doesn't show up in the limited examination of a single slide smear. Mead says that if a woman has a negative slide smear, but still has significant symptoms, her physician is likely to order a culture.

For example, there is one variety of candida—*Candida glabrata*— that causes symptoms but does not characteristically show up under the microscope. For that, a culture may be necessary. "A culture is more sensitive," says Mead. "It should pick up virtually anything."

While studies have shown that women are able to correctly identify recurring vaginal yeast infections most of the time, there is still some concern about misdiagnosing and mistreating other problems that may mimic symptoms. Through package and product labeling of products sold without prescription, FDA and pharmaceutical companies are working to make sure that women with an infection that differs even slightly from the symptoms of a previous yeast infection return to their doctors.

Over-the-Counter Availability—With Warnings

Until 1990, drugs to treat vaginal yeast infections were available only by prescription. In December 1990, after receiving the advice of a number of experts, FDA gave Schering-Plough HealthCare the go ahead to market and sell over-the-counter its antifungal medication Gyne-Lotrimin, a brand name for clotrimazole. It has been joined by several other products that are either clotrimazole or another antifungal, miconazole nitrate. (The first miconazole nitrate drug to be allowed to be sold OTC for vaginal yeast infections was Advanced Care Products' Monistat 7.)

Both clotrimazole and miconazole nitrate are from the same antifungal drug family and work very similarly by breaking down the cell wall of the yeast organism, causing it to dissolve completely.

The products are supplied in one of two ways: as vaginal inserts or suppositories or as a cream with a special applicator. Both formulations are for use at bedtime every night for seven nights.

While most women note improvement within just a few days, it's important to finish the seven-day treatment to make sure all of the trouble-making fungus has been disabled. Women who don't see rapid improvement of their symptoms are likely to have a problem other than a vaginal yeast infection.

"The benefit [of OTC sale of these products] is that they are readily available for women to purchase without having to go to a physician," says Joseph Winfield, M.D., a medical officer in FDA's anti-infective drugs division. Ready availability of OTC treatments means that women no longer have to suffer while waiting for an appointment, or rearrange work and family life to find time to go to the doctor's office for a recurrent infection.

"Vaginal candidiasis is a rather common occurrence," says Winfield. "It doesn't present any life-threatening condition to the individual [with an infection] and it's okay to treat over the counter—but only for women [who] have had an infection diagnosed by a physician previously. As those same symptoms recur, they should be able to treat themselves."

In October 1992, FDA required additions to printed information accompanying OTC products for vaginal yeast infections. One significant addition to the patient package insert was a notice that recurrent vaginal yeast infections, especially those that do not clear up easily with proper treatment, may also be the result of serious medical conditions, including HIV infection. The labeling also says: *If you experience vaginal yeast infections frequently (they recur within a two-month period) or if you have vaginal yeast infections that do not clear up easily with proper treatment, you should see your doctor promptly to determine the cause and to receive proper medical care.*

"While it is true that women who are HIV-infected are much more likely to have chronic vaginal yeast infections," says Mead, "most women with recurrent vaginal yeast infections aren't HIV-positive [HIV-infected]."

In addition to the HIV notice, the following warnings also appear on information accompanying the products:

- Do not use if you have abdominal pain, fever or foul-smelling vaginal discharge. You may have a condition that is more serious than a yeast infection. Contact your doctor immediately.

- Do not use if this is your first experience with vaginal itch and discomfort. See your doctor.

- If there is no improvement within three days, you may have a condition other than a yeast infection. Stop using this product and see your doctor.

- If symptoms recur within a two-month period, contact your doctor.

- Do not use during pregnancy except under the advice and supervision of a doctor.

- This medication is for vaginal yeast infections only. It is not for use in the mouth or the eyes. If accidentally swallowed, seek professional assistance or contact a Poison Control Center immediately.

- Keep this and all other drugs out of the reach of children. This product is not to be used in children less than 12 years of age.

Prevention

In general, candida likes warm, moist places. It's not possible to prevent every yeast infection, but a few simple steps can help reduce the number of infections women get.

Wear loose, natural-fiber clothing and underwear with a cotton crotch. As much as possible, avoid pantyhose, tights or leggings, nylon underwear, and tight jeans. Limit the use of deodorant tampons and feminine hygiene products if you feel an infection beginning, as they can interfere with the helpful bacteria in the vagina. Keep genitals dry after bathing or swimming (don't stay in a wet swimsuit for hours).

Seasonal changes can affect the likelihood of getting an infection, too. During high-heat, high-humidity periods, it's easier to get a yeast infection. Heavy winter clothing, which prevents easy release of perspiration and moisture, can also spell trouble.

Other Yeast Infections

Even though vaginal yeast infections are the most common type of candida infections, there are other ways in which yeast can cause problems.

Thrush is the name given to an oral yeast infection. It is most often seen in infants or in people with severely suppressed immune systems—as in AIDS. Its symptoms are painful sores in the mouth and throat that appear as creamy white patches and reveal red sores when scraped. Left untreated, thrush may spread to the throat and esophagus. (Other infections can cause similar symptoms, so anyone with these symptoms should have their condition accurately diagnosed by a health professional.)

Other candida infections can occur nearly anywhere on the body where there is a skin fold: under the arms, under the breasts, between the toes. The skin around the fingernails can be affected.

Candida infections have been reported in women who wear artificial fingernails. Fungal infections can start in the space between the artificial and natural nail if they become separated. The nails may become discolored by infection and may require drug treatment.

The drugs used to treat these other candida infections are similar, but not always identical to those used for vaginal yeast infections. Most of the treatments are from the "azole" drug family (clotrimazole, fluconazole). Some drugs are oral medications, although those are most often used only for stubborn or persistent infections. A fairly new drug (approved by FDA in January 1990), fluconazole is effective in a single dose by tablet or intravenous injection, but is most often used only in serious fungal infections, such as those in persons with HIV disease.

It's important to note that over-the-counter products for vaginal yeast infections are not appropriate for other types of fungal infections. Those products are only for the uses stated on the package. For any other yeast infection, see your doctor.

—by Amy Roffman

Chapter 10

The Pap Smear Test

The Controversial Pap Test

About 70 years ago, George Papanicolaou, M.D., observed that cervical cancer could be detected by studying cells taken from a woman's genital tract. His finding was put to use 25 years later with the development of the Pap test, named after him.

In the decades since then, the Pap test has become a routine part of gynecologic examinations and one of the most widely used procedures for detecting cancer. The American Cancer Society credits the Pap smear—so called because cells are "smeared" on a glass slide—and regular gynecologic check-ups with cutting deaths from cervical cancer by 70 percent over the last 40 years. Although 6,000 women will die from it this year, four decades ago cervical cancer claimed the lives of 20,000 American women annually. For years, Pap test results have reassured millions of women that they are either free of cervical cancer or it has been detected at an early stage, with a high probability of cure.

Recently, though, the Pap test has been surrounded by controversy. Reports suggest that 10 to 40 percent of cervical cancers or the cell abnormalities that precede them may be missed because of sloppy laboratory work or poor tissue sampling. The reports have prompted medical organizations and the federal government to investigate quality control in Pap testing and propose stricter standards to ensure

DHSS unnumbered publication entitled "What Is a Pap Smear?" and *FDA Consumer*, September 1989.

127

more reliable test results for cervical cancer and other diseases and conditions.

Meanwhile, researchers are trying to devise more accurate ways to detect the early signs of cervical cancer and to zero in on who is at risk for it. At the same time, health and medical groups once at odds over guidelines for cervical cancer screening have joined forces to develop unified recommendations for how often women should have a Pap test.

The Best Screening Tool for Cancer

"For all the problems that have come to the forefront, the Pap smear is still by far the best screening tool we have for any cancer" says William Creasman, M.D., professor and head of the Department of Obstetrics and Gynecology at the University of South Carolina and head of the cancer screening task force of the American College of Obstetricians and Gynecologists.

The American Cancer Society estimates that in 1989, 47,000 American women will be diagnosed with uterine cancer. Of these, 13,000 will be found to have cancer of the cervix—the neck of the uterus, which opens into the vagina. The remaining 34,000 women will be diagnosed with cancer of the body of the uterus or of the endometrium, its lining.

Cervical cancer develops slowly over years, and when caught early is very curable. In the very earliest stages of cervical cancer, cells on the surface of the cervix change in structure—a condition known as dysplasia. In some early cases, the lesion alone can be excised, but often effective treatment calls for hysterectomy—surgical removal of the entire uterus.

In the next step, abnormal cells develop into a localized cancer ("carcinoma *in situ*"). Carcinoma *in situ* is virtually 100 percent curable by surgery—either conization, in which a cone of tissue surrounding the cancer is removed, or a total hysterectomy. The choice of procedure often depends on whether the woman wants to have children. For patients diagnosed early but with more invasive cancer, the survival rate is from 80 to 90 percent, and treatment involves radiation, hysterectomy or both. The five-year survival rate for all cervical cancer patients is 66 percent, according to the American Cancer Society, which implies that some cases are not being found and treated early.

Properly done, the Pap test is highly effective in detecting abnormal cervical cells before they become cancerous. (It is only about 50 percent effective in detecting endometrial cancer. Because endometrial cancer afflicts mostly middle-aged or older women, the American Cancer Society recommends that women at risk of this disease have tissue samples taken at menopause. Their risk factors include infertility, obesity, failure to ovulate, and prolonged estrogen therapy.)

A Labor-Intensive Test

The accuracy of the Pap test depends on meticulous care in each of its steps, from cell collection, preparation, and staining on the slide to the interpretation of each specimen.

The test is a "uniquely labor intensive complex process" compared with other medical and laboratory tests, and its outcome "depends entirely on human judgment," states Leonard G. Koss, M.D., pathologist at the Albert Einstein College of Medicine, the Bronx, N.Y., in a recent issue of the *Journal of the American Medical Association.* Improperly done, the value of the test is "seriously compromised," notes the American Medical Association in a recent report on quality control in Pap testing.

The Pap smear is a seemingly easy procedure. A hollow tube-like instrument called a speculum is inserted into the vagina to expand the cervix. Then a cotton-tipped swab, wooden spatula, or cervical brush is used to collect cells from the opening of the cervix and its inner and outer surfaces. The cells are quickly pressed on a glass slide and "fixed" to prevent them from drying and changing appearance.

The doctor or nurse must take important information about the patient, such as age and obstetric and gynecologic history, which is forwarded along with the slide to the testing laboratory. There the sample is examined under a microscope by specially trained technologists who search for abnormalities among the 50,000 to 300,000 cells on each slide. Any suspicious slides are sent on to a pathologist, who classifies the smear as one of five types ranging from completely normal to definite cancer and determines whether further testing is needed.

Koss estimates that from 10 to 20 percent of Pap smears are inadequate from the first step. "It is generally assumed that obtaining a cervical smear is an easily executed, clinically simple procedure," says Koss. "This is not true."

Some practitioners don't do it properly—either not collecting enough cells, collecting them from the wrong place, or fixing them improperly on the slide—and so a flawed sample is sent for screening. And some laboratories, perhaps fearful of losing the physicians business, do not reject poor samples, according to Creasman.

Screening of the samples may be inadequate, too. In November 1987, the *Wall Street Journal* reported that so-called "Pap mills" around the country screen smears much too quickly and in haphazard ways that may fail to reveal abnormalities. The *Journal's* report set off congressional and professional reviews of the quality control of medical testing and prompted legislation to tighten regulations of laboratories that do Pap screening.

Koss estimates that each smear requires at least five minutes of study. The American Society of Cytotechnology suggests that no technologist screen more than 12,000 smears annually—or 50 a day. Yet, the Wall Street Journal reported laboratories in which individual workers screened as many as 35,000 slides in a single year.

New Quality Control Regulations

The American College of Obstetricians and Gynecologists believes that up to 40 percent of Pap smears may fail to disclose cancer or the cellular abnormalities that can lead to it. As many as half of those errors may result from inadequate sampling; the rest are apparently caused by shortcomings in the laboratories.

Currently, the federal Centers for Disease Control requires that cytology laboratories engaged in interstate commerce (and thus subject to federal regulation) must re-screen 10 percent of negative Pap smears as a means of quality control. New York state licenses laboratories only after a mandatory examination of the cytotechnologists. A California law forbids that state's cytotechnologists from screening more than 75 slides a day.

And Congress last year amended the 20-year-old Clinical Laboratory Improvement Act to require quality standards for the estimated 12,000 labs receiving Medicare and Medicaid funding or engaging in interstate commerce. Congress also ordered the Health Care Financing Administration (HCFA) to regulate doctors' office laboratories that examine Pap smears.

In effect, HCFA officials say, the new rules will cover nearly all commercial laboratories and should go a long way toward improving cervical cancer detection. Among the requirements: proficiency testing for examiners and laboratories and a ceiling on the number of slides to be screened by each technician.The new regulations will take effect Jan. 1, 1990.

Out of the controversy comes hope for greater survival. Increased attention to quality control, a new consensus on Pap test guidelines, and research on who is at risk and how testing can be improved could eventually lower deaths from cervical cancer still further. "We certainly could knock the incidence of invasive disease down to a greater degree," says Creasman. "But we'll never get rid of it entirely because some women won't get Pap smears or won't get them done when they should."

Who Should Be Tested—And How Often?

For years, women and their doctors have been confused about how often Pap testing should be done because health organizations made different recommendations. Last year, seven medical, professional and scientific organizations announced new uniform guidelines for Pap testing.

The organizations, including the American Cancer Society and the American College of Obstetricians and Gynecologists (ACOG), determined that all women who are or have been sexually active or are over 18 should have an annual Pap test and pelvic examination. After three consecutive normal results, they said, the test could be done less often—if the woman and her doctor agree. However, the groups advised that all women at high risk for cervical cancer should have annual Pap tests.

Who Is at High Risk?

Studies show that women who become sexually active early in their teen years, who have multiple sex partners, who have their first child before the age of 20, and who have many pregnancies are at higher than average risk. Also at higher risk are women whose sex partners have other partners.

The risk of cervical cancer is much lower in women in monogamous relationships, and studies indicate that the disease occurs much less often in celibate women. But recent studies show that half of all married women and from 70 to 80 percent of married men have had multiple sex partners. About half of all teenagers have had more than one sexual partner by the time they reach 16, according to ACOG. In effect, then, the consortium of medical groups recommends that nearly all women who are sexually active have annual Pap tests regardless of age, according to Creasman.

"If a woman is in any of these high-risk groups she should have annual Pap tests and cervical exams," says George Morley, M.D., the president of ACOG. "To do any less is to play Russian roulette with her life. The annual Pap test will be her early warning system to protect her health and perhaps her life."

Viruses and DES May Add to Risk

Women whose mothers took the hormone diethylstilbestrol (DES) during pregnancy are at a higher risk of cervical cancer. Prescribed in the late 1940s and 1950s to prevent miscarriage, DES was found to cause cervical and vaginal cancer in some women born to mothers who used it. The drug is no longer prescribed for that purpose.

Most experts now believe that the family of human papilloma viruses (HPV)—which cause genital warts—also cause cervical cancer, and they suggest that women who have had this sexually transmitted disease should have yearly Pap tests.

Some specialists estimate that most women who develop cervical cancer are infected with HPV. The incidence of HPV caused genital warts has been increasing dramatically the last few years, suggesting an eventual increase in cervical cancer. Although a link between cervical cancer and herpes virus type 2 has also been suggested, it is far less certain than that between HPV and the disease.

In a study reported earlier this year in the *Journal of the American Medical Association,* University of Utah scientists noted another possible risk factor for cervical cancer: passive or active smoking. The researchers found that women who don't smoke but who are exposed to cigarette smoke for three hours or more a day were nearly three times more likely to get the disease. Women who smoke are more than three times as likely to get the disease. The Utah study has not yet been duplicated.

In the past, some doctors have suggested that women over 60 or 65 need not get Pap tests, but the new guidelines have no such cutoff. After three years of negative tests, older women, like younger ones, should discuss with their doctors how often they should have a Pap test.

Creasman also recommends that women who have had hysterectomies for treatment of a malignant cervical lesion should have an annual Pap test to make sure that the tumor has not recurred. If the hysterectomy was for a benign lesion the risk is much lower and testing can be done every two to three years, he says.

Most important, say experts, is that every woman should discuss her risks with her physician and the two of them then should decide how often she should be tested.

Pap Test Saves Lives

Some instances of precancerous cell changes are missed in Pap tests because changes in the cells are too slight for technologists to detect. Several companies are now working on tests that detect the human papilloma virus in cervical tissue before precancerous lesions develop. The first such test, called Virapap, was approved by the Food and Drug Administration in January 1989 for use in high-risk women as an adjunct to the Pap smear.

Efforts are also under way to find better ways of reading the Pap smear. One technique involves using a computerized microscope to measure dye absorbed by cells—a potential clue to cancer or the cellular changes that precede it.

Still, Creasman believes there is nothing on the immediate horizon that will replace the Pap test. "We've been waiting for years to get a computer to do it . . . and we're still waiting."

Says ACOG President Morley: "Our main defense against death from the disease is prevention. We can prevent death through early detection. We detect the disease through regular pelvic examinations and Pap tests. The earlier we detect it, the greater the chances for cure."

It may not be perfect, but the Pap test saves lives.

Where Goes That Smear?

Until better tests for cervical cancer come along and new federal guidelines controlling quality of laboratory testing are in place, William Creasman, M.D., head of the cancer screening task force for the American College of Obstetricians and Gynecologists, says women should question their physicians closely about Pap testing. He recommends the following:

- Ask where your tissue sample will be sent. Is the laboratory certified by a professional organization like the College of American

Pathologists? If the lab does testing for Medicare- or Medicaid-funded patients, chances are it is accredited.

- Is the lab near your doctor? A doctor and laboratory that are close geographically are probably more likely to communicate. Also, if a lab is far away, it suggests that samples are being sent that far to save money—not a good practice when your life is at stake.

The most important thing to remember, say experts, is that cervical cancer is one of the most curable of all cancers because the cellular changes that lead to it are slow to develop and can be detected by a Pap test.

For additional information on cervical cancer and the pap smear test see Volume 10 of the Health Reference Series, entitled Cancer Sourcebook for Women.

—by Ellen Hale

Questions and Answers about the Pap Smear Test

What is a Pap smear?

- A test which may be done as a part of a pelvic exam.

- A test to prevent cancer of the cervix—the opening of the uterus. It can find abnormal cells of the cervix before they become cancer.

- The health care provider takes cells from the cervix through the vagina during a pelvic exam.

- The Pap smear is not a test for pregnancy or for sexually transmitted diseases like gonorrhea or chlamydia or AIDS.

When is the best time for a Pap smear?

- Once a year if 18 or older.
- Once a year if you ever had sex (penis in the vagina).
- More often if your Pap smear is abnormal.

How do I get ready for a Pap smear?

- Do not have sex (sexual intercourse, penis in the vagina) for 2 days before the test.

- Do not wash the vagina or douche for 2 days before the test.

- Do not put anything in the vagina for 2 days before the test. No tampons, sponges, douches, cervical caps, diaphragms, creams, foams, condoms or penis.

How will I know if I have an abnormal Pap Smear?

- The health care provider sends the Pap smear to a lab.
- The clinic will let you know if the lab reports that the cells are not normal.

If I have an abnormal pap smear, will I get cancer?

- You will need follow up.
- If not treated, it takes about 3 to 10 years for severe, abnormal changes to become cancer.
- Mild changes often do not need treatment.
- If not treated, some women will get better.
- Regular Pap smears and treatment when needed can prevent most cancer of the cervix.

What can I do to help avoid cancer of the cervix?

- Get regular Pap smears.
- Do not smoke.
- Eat healthy foods including dark green leafy vegetables and red/orange/yellow fruits and vegetables.
- Do not have sex at a young age (before age 18).
- Abstain or do not have sex.
- Limit your number of sex partners.
- Talk with sexual partner about his past and current sexual partners.
- Use a condom for all penis in the vagina sex.
- Do not have sex with men with genital warts or other sexually transmitted diseases.

- Do not have sex without a condom with men whose past partners have had cervical cancer.

What if I have questions about my Pap smear?

- Talk with your health care provider at the family planning clinic.
- Don't be afraid to ask any question you have.

Chapter 11

Vulvar Self-Exam

Your Guide to the Benefits of Vulvar Self-Examination

The "vulva" refers to the external female genital organs—very special area of a woman's body so vital to healthy female identity and sexual function.

Yet...how often do most women correctly examine the vulva? Would you know the right way to check the vulva...what to look for? Could you find the early signs of important changes which mean the start of serious infection or even cancer of the vulva?

If you're not in the habit of doing vulvar self-exams...or if you're not sure of the importance or the right way to do self-exams...Find out how a simple self-exam of the vulva can alert you to a problem before serious infection develops...before cancer develops.

Unfortunately, physicians are seeing an increasing number of women with cancer (and precancerous conditions) of the vulva in all age groups, but especially in younger women. Infectious diseases of the vulva (especially viral infections such as genital warts and herpes) are also increasing.

Genital warts (sometimes called "condyloma accuminata") will cause an estimated 1 million women to seek medical attention this year. Most women who discover genital warts DO NOT have cancer. However, the same virus that causes genital warts (human papilloma virus) has been linked to cancer of the female genitals.

Atlanta Reproductive Health Centre, ©1993 Used by permission.

Why Vulvar Self-Exams?

The Importance of Early Detection

Women may have early infections or precancerous growths, but may not be aware of changes in the vulva until the disease becomes more advanced. As you would expect, more serious cases require more extensive treatment...which could even mean a major loss of vulvar tissue to survive.

Yet, if caught early, your physician can better treat as well as prevent the spread of infection or growths on the vulva. The key is early detection.

A simple self-exam of the vulva is the most important habit you can start now to help you notice important changes in the vulva... changes which need to be reported and discussed with your physician.

Who Should Perform VSE?

All women who are sexually active...and even women who are not sexually active but are over 18 years old.

How Often Should VSE Be Performed?

Once a month, just as recommended for breast self-exams; or any time you have symptoms related to the vulva. Women with any history of vulvar disease are encouraged to perform vulvar self-exams more often. (Vulvar self-exams are best performed between menstrual periods.)

Important Note: most changes or new growths on the vulva will not be cancerous and will need only minor checking and treatment. But, you should report all changes to your physician to determine the best care at the first sign of a problem.

How to Perform a VSE...Where To Look

Find a comfortable, well-lighted place to sit such as a bed or a carpet. Hold a mirror in one hand. Then, use the other hand to separate and expose the parts of the vulva surrounding the opening of the vagina. Once you have a good viewing position, examine the main parts of the vulva as follows:

1. Check the "mons pubis" (the area above the vagina around the pubic bone where the pubic hair is located). Look carefully for any bumps, warts, ulcers, or changes in skin color (pigmentation, especially newly developed white, red, or dark areas). Then, use the finger tips to check any visible change and to sense any bump just below the surface you might feel but not see.

2. Check the "clitoris" and surrounding area (directly above the vagina) by looking and by touch.

3. Examine the "labia minora" (the smaller folds of skin just to the right and left of the vaginal opening). Look and touch by holding the skin between thumb and fingers.

4. Look closely at the "labia majora" (the larger folds of skin just next to the labia minora). Examine both right and left just as you did the labia minora.

5. Move down to the "perineum" (the area between the vagina and the anus). Check thoroughly.

6. Finally, examine the area surrounding the anal opening as before by looking and by touch.

Remember the basic rule: vulvar diseases are most easily, safely, and successfully treated when discovered early. Now you know and now you have yet another good way to help protect your own health—the monthly vulvar self-examination—a good habit to start today.

What to Look For in the Examination

If you find any new growths or changes, report them to your physician as soon as possible. Some examples include:

- A new mole, wart, or growth of any kind.
- New areas of "pigmentation" (skin color) especially newly developed white, red, or dark skin areas.
- Ulcers or sores, except for any minor injury with a known cause.
- Areas of continuing pain, inflammation, or itching.

From Women Who Know

"I only wish someone had told me about vulvar self-examination years ago." *Female patient who required major surgery for advanced cancer of the vulva.*

"I believe vulvar self-examination saved my life." *Female patient who discovered early vulvar cancer and was successfully treated with minor surgery.*

From a Concerned Physician

"Early detection and treatment of vulvar diseases can save lives as well as female identity and sexual function. Vulvar Self-Examination (VSE) is the key to early detection if only women will discover it and practice it."

For Additional Information

R. Allen Lawhead, Jr., M.D.
Director of Gynecologic Oncology
Cancer Center of Georgia, GBMC
285 Boulevard, Suite 430
Atlanta, GA 30312
Phone: (404) 265-3614

The information in this patient education brochure is based on "A Health Care Professional's Guide to Vulvar Self-Examination," by R. Allen Lawhead, Jr., M.D. This brochure was developed and produced by Bluestone Vista, Inc.. in cooperation with Dr. Lawhead. This brochure is designed to encourage the practice of Vulvar Self-Examination, and is not intended as a substitute for proper consultation and care from a qualified physician or other health care professional.

Chapter 12

Sexually Transmitted Diseases (STDs) in Women

Chapter Contents

Section 12.1

Protect Yourself from STDs

Reprinted with permission for the American Social Health Association, a nonprofit organization dedicated to stopping STDs and their harmful consequences.

How do STDs cause special problems for women?

- Some STD infections show no signs. Often a woman does not know she has an STD because the infection is hidden inside her body.

- Some STDs cause lasting damage to the female reproductive organs. This might keep a woman from having babies when she wants to.

Can STDs hurt babies?

Yes. A pregnant woman who has an STD can pass the disease to her baby. Thousands of infants die or suffer birth defects each year because of STD infections they get from their mother during pregnancy or birth.

What about AIDS?

AIDS is caused by a virus. People who have the AIDS virus (also known as HIV, human immunodeficiency virus) may seem to be healthy for months or years after getting the virus. But they can spread the virus to others without knowing it. Later they might become very sick and develop AIDS.

A woman could get pregnant without knowing she carries the AIDS virus. If she does, she could pass the virus to her baby. It may also be possible to pass this virus through breast milk.

People who have had any STD are more likely to get the AIDS virus than people who have not had an STD.

What should I do if I'm planning to get pregnant?

- See your doctor or health clinic for a check-up and get tested for STDs. Most STDs can be cured.

- Get tested. Even if the STD cannot be cured, your doctor can treat your symptoms and can take steps to protect your baby. There is no cure for AIDS, but a test can help you and the doctor to manage your care and the care of your baby.

Can STDs keep me from having children?

Yes. STDs such as gonorrhea and chlamydia often cause damage that makes it hard or impossible for a woman to get pregnant.

These STDs can lead to pelvic inflammatory disease (PID), which often causes severe pain in the abdomen. PID can scar the tubes that carry the egg to the uterus. If these tubes are blocked by scars, the egg cannot grow properly. Women with scarred tubes often have a tubal or ectopic pregnancy. During an ectopic pregnancy, the egg will grow outside the uterus. This condition can cause death and requires immediate surgery.

How can I avoid getting an STD?

Your risk for getting an STD increases with the number of sexual partners you have. You can avoid all STDs if you don't have sexual contact with anyone and don't share drug needles. But *you can greatly decrease your risk if you have only one partner (this person must not have sex with anyone but you and must not have an STD) and if you use condoms (rubbers).*

If you are not sure that your partner is free from STDs, use condoms during any sexual contact. Make sure the condom is used from start to finish during vaginal sex, oral sex, or anal sex. Other products will provide protection for many sexual practices, and the National STD Hotline (1-800-227-8922) can answer questions about this.

Use spermicides with a condom. Spermicides alone can't be trusted to prevent disease, but they can give protection in case a condom breaks. Spermicides are available in a foam or a cream and must cover the entire vagina. Follow the directions on the package, and do not use spermicides for oral sex. Spermicides may not protect against STDs when used for anal sex.

Get checked. If you have sex with more than one person, see a doctor or health clinic often. Doctors can test for hidden STDs like chlamydia. Since some STDs are linked to the risk of cervical cancer, get a Pap smear often, too.

How do drug needles spread STDs?

Even a small amount of blood can carry many viruses. Many cases of AIDS are spread when a person is injected with needles or syringes that have been used by a person with the AIDS virus. Hepatitis and some other diseases also are spread this way. If you must use or lend needles, make sure they are cleaned in bleach. In clinics and doctors' offices in the United States, needles are never used twice.

Gonorrhea

How Women Suffer. Symptoms are often unseen. But without treatment, gonorrhea can keep you from having babies and can cause arthritis.

How Babies Suffer. Eye infection that could lead to blindness. Since babies get gonorrhea during birth, treatment during pregnancy will protect your baby.

Special Considerations. Gonorrhea and chlamydia can cause pelvic inflammatory disease (PID) in women. PID can scar the tubes that carry the egg to the uterus, and this can make it hard to have children. PID can also lead to ectopic pregnancy, and this can threaten your life.

Chlamydia

How Women Suffer. Chlamydia symptoms are often unseen. But without treatment, chlamydia can keep you from having babies.

How Babies Suffer. Eye infection or pneumonia. Since babies get chlamydia when born, treatment during pregnancy will protect your baby.

Special Considerations. Chlamydia and gonorrhea symptoms are similar, but the drugs that cure gonorrhea will not cure chlamydia.

Genital Herpes

How Women Suffer. Genital herpes symptoms are often unseen, but a person with genital herpes may develop very painful blisters or bumps near or inside the vagina or rectum. There is no cure for herpes, and the symptoms can return again and again.

How Babies Suffer. May cause very painful blisters on the skin. May damage the eyes, the brain, and other internal organs. Can lead to retardation. While herpes is rare in babies, about one in six babies who get it will not survive. Since babies most often get herpes at delivery, there are ways to protect your baby from herpes if you know you have it.

Special Considerations. If you think you or your partner could have herpes, be sure to tell your doctor or health clinic. A doctor can tell if you need a cesarean section delivery to protect the baby. More than half of babies born with herpes come from mothers who don't know about their own herpes infection.

Drug treatment will control herpes outbreaks, but this treatment may not be safe during pregnancy. Even after birth, keep your baby from touching your herpes sores. Do not let people who have herpes sores on the lip kiss your baby.

Syphilis

How Women Suffer. Usually a painless sore appears near or inside the vagina, the mouth or rectum. Often the sore, rash, or growth is not seen. These sores may appear to heal by themselves, but the disease is still in the body.

How Babies Suffer. Eye damage, dental and bone deformities, blindness, brain damage, death. Symptoms might appear at birth or months or years later. Early treatment will protect your baby.

Special Considerations. Infection might lead to miscarriage. Without treatment, the disease stays in the body for years and can cause severe damage or death. It can be cured at any time with antibiotics, but some damage may be permanent.

145

AIDS

How Women Suffer. HIV, the AIDS virus, usually leads to AIDS. AIDS makes it difficult for the body to fight disease, and often leads to death.

How Babies Suffer. Many babies whose mothers have the AIDS virus will get it from their mothers and develop AIDS during early childhood. Treatment during pregnancy can help protect your baby. Babies can get the AIDS virus before birth, during birth, or possibly through breast milk.

Special Considerations. A woman may have the virus but not have symptoms. There is no cure yet, but treatment can keep you healthier. Testing will help you prevent the spread of the AIDS virus to your baby or others. People with the AIDS virus should consult their doctor about the risks of pregnancy. The virus usually causes no symptoms, but blood tests can find it.

STD Warning Signs

You can get an STD whether you're pregnant or not. If you have any of these symptoms, see your doctor:

- excess discharge or unusual smell from the vagina
- irritation, discomfort, itching, swelling, soreness, or pain in or around the vagina or rectum
- genital sores, blisters, rashes, bumps, or growths (even if they don't hurt)
- painful urination
- swollen glands in the groin
- abdominal pain, especially during sex
- bleeding from the vagina when you're not having a period.

Signs often appear where you are infected. If you have oral sex, you could show symptoms in the mouth.

If you have an STD, you may also have these symptoms:

- swelling, soreness, or redness in the throat
- fever, chills, and aches
- sores or white patches inside the mouth.

If you think you have an STD:

- See a doctor or health clinic right away. It is important for your doctor to know if you have an STD or if you are pregnant. If you have an STD, make sure your sexual partner is tested and treated.

- Follow the doctor's instructions carefully. If the doctor prescribes medicine, take all of it. The infection can still cause problems even if the symptoms go away.

- Don't have sex until you and your partner are completely cured. Until you're well, you can give the disease to your partner.

Sex and Disease

One out of every 20 Americans will get a Sexually Transmitted Disease (STD) this year.

One out of five already has one.

These diseases will cause serious health problems for women.

But you can protect yourself... and your baby.

You can get a sexually transmitted disease (STD) if you have sexual contact with someone who has an STD. This includes vaginal, anal, and oral sex. These diseases are spread by both men and women.

STDs are caused by germs that live on the skin or in body fluids like semen, vaginal secretions, or blood. These germs can enter a person's body through the vagina, the mouth, the anus, an open sore, or a cut. Some germs like those that cause herpes or genital warts, can even infect a person through the skin of the genitals or anywhere on the body.

Many kinds of STDs can seriously damage your health if you don't get treatment. Some STDs, like AIDS, can kill you or your baby.

More Information about STDs

Check the following sources for additional information:

- your doctor

- your local health department or free STD clinic

147

- the National STD Hotline at 1-800-227-8922, toll-free. The hotline is open from 8 A.M. to 11 P.M., (Eastern time) Monday through Friday.

- Call the National AIDS Hotline (1-800-342-AIDS) any day, 24 hours a day.

This brochure is published by the American Social Health Association (ASHA). ASHA is a private, nonprofit organization dedicated to stopping all STDs and their harmful consequences to individuals, families, and communities. ASHA produces educational materials on sexual health; operates national hotlines for STDs, AIDS, and herpes; advocates for strong public health programs to prevent the spread of STDs; and funds research to find better treatments.

For more information on our programs or other materials, please write to us at the address below.

American Social Health Association
P.O. Box 13827
Research Triangle Park, NC 27709
Phone: (919) 361-8422

Section 12.2

General Information on Pelvic Inflammatory Disease

NIH/NIAID, August 1992.

The most serious and common complication of sexually transmitted diseases (STDs) among women is pelvic inflammatory disease (PID), an infection of the upper genital tract. PID can affect the uterus, ovaries, fallopian tubes, or other related structures. Untreated, PID can lead to infertility, tubal pregnancy, chronic pelvic pain, and other serious consequences.

Each year in the United States, more than 1 million women experience an episode of acute PID, with the rate of infection highest among teenagers. More than 100,000 women become infertile (cannot become pregnant) each year as a result of PID, and a large proportion of the 70,000 ectopic (tubal) pregnancies occurring every year are due to the consequences of PID. In 1990 alone, an estimated four billion dollars were spent on PID and its complications.

Cause

PID occurs when disease-causing organisms migrate upwards from the vagina and cervix into the upper genital tract. Many different organisms can cause PID, but most cases are associated with gonorrhea and chlamydial infections, two very common STDs. Scientists have found that bacteria normally present in the vagina and cervix may also play a role.

Investigators are learning more about how these organisms cause PID. The gonococcus probably travels to the fallopian tubes, where it causes sloughing of some cells and invades others. It is believed to multiply within and beneath these cells. The infection then may spread to other organs, resulting in more inflammation and scarring.

149

Chlamydia and other bacteria may behave in a similar manner. It is not known how other bacteria that normally inhabit the vagina (e.g., organisms such as *Gardnerella vaginalis* and *Bacteroides*) gain entrance into the upper genital tract. It appears that the cervical mucus plug and secretions, believed to prevent the spread of microorganisms to the upper genital tract, are less effective during ovulation and menstruation. In addition, the organisms may gain access more easily during menstruation, if menstrual blood flows backward from the uterus into the fallopian tubes, carrying the organisms with it. This may explain why symptoms of PID caused by gonorrhea or chlamydia more often begin immediately after menstruation rather than at any other time during the menstrual cycle.

Symptoms

The major symptoms of PID are lower abdominal pain and abnormal vaginal discharge. Other symptoms such as fever, pain in the right upper abdomen, painful intercourse, and irregular menstrual bleeding can occur as well. PID, particularly when caused by chlamydia, may produce only minor symptoms or no symptoms at all, even though it can seriously damage the reproductive organs.

Risk Factors for PID

- Women with sexually transmitted diseases—especially gonorrhea and chlamydia—are at greater risk of developing PID; a prior episode of PID increases the risk of another episode because the body's defenses are often damaged during the initial bout of upper tract infection.

- Sexually active teenagers are more likely to develop PID than are older women.

- The more sexual partners a woman has, the greater her risk of developing PID.

- IUD insertion, induced abortion, and other procedures during which instruments are passed through the cervix into the uterus increase the risk of PID.

Recent data indicate that women who douche once or twice a month are more likely to have PID than those who douche less than once a month. Douching may flush bacteria into the upper genital tract. Douching may also ease symptoms of an infection, delaying effective treatment.

Diagnosis

PID can be difficult to diagnose. If symptoms such as lower abdominal pain are present, the doctor will perform a physical exam to determine the nature and location of the pain. Additional evaluation should be conducted to determine if the patient has a fever, abnormal vaginal or cervical discharge, and evidence of cervical infection with gonorrhea or chlamydia. If the findings of this exam suggest that PID is likely, current guidelines advise doctors to begin treatment.

If more information is necessary, the doctor may order other tests, such as a sonogram, endometrial biopsy, or laparoscopy to distinguish between PID and other serious problems that may mimic PID. Laparoscopy is a surgical procedure in which a tiny, flexible tube with a lighted end is inserted through a small incision just below the navel. This procedure allows the doctor to view the internal abdominal and pelvic organs as well as take specimens for cultures or pathologic studies, if necessary.

Treatment

Because culture specimens from the upper genital tract are difficult to obtain and because multiple organisms are usually responsible for an episode of PID, at least two antibiotics are given so that they will be effective against a wide range of infectious agents. The infection may still be present after the symptoms are gone, so it is important to finish taking all of the medicine, even if symptoms go away. Patients should be re-evaluated by their physician 2 to 3 days after treatment is begun to be sure the antibiotics are working to cure the infection.

About one-fourth of women with suspected PID must be hospitalized. This may be recommended if the patient is severely ill, if she cannot take oral medication and needs intravenous antibiotics, if she is pregnant or is an adolescent, or if the diagnosis is uncertain and may include an abdominal emergency such as appendicitis.

Many women with PID have sex partners who have no symptoms. Because of the risk of reinfection, however, sex partners should be treated. Even if they do not have symptoms, they may be infected with organisms that can cause PID.

Consequences of PID

Women with recurrent episodes of PID are more likely than women with a single episode to suffer long-term consequences, such as infertility, tubal pregnancy, or chronic pelvic pain. Infertility occurs in approximately 20 percent of women who have had PID.

However, most women with tubal infertility never have had symptoms of PID. Organisms such as chlamydia can silently invade the fallopian tubes and result in scarring, which blocks the normal passage of eggs into the uterus.

A woman who has had PID has a six- to tenfold increased risk of tubal pregnancy, in which the egg can become fertilized but cannot pass into the uterus to grow. Instead, the egg usually attaches in the fallopian tube that connects the ovary to the uterus. The fertilized egg cannot grow normally in the fallopian tube. This type of pregnancy is life-threatening to the mother, and almost always fatal to her fetus. It is the leading cause of maternal death in African-American women.

In addition, untreated PID results in chronic pelvic pain and scarring in about 20 percent of patients. These conditions are difficult to treat but are sometimes improved with surgery.

Another complication of PID is the risk of repeat episodes. As many as one-third of women who have had PID will have the disease at least one more time. With each episode of reinfection, the risk of infertility is increased.

Prevention

You can play an active role in protecting yourself from PID by taking the following steps:

- If you think you have a sexually transmitted disease, get tested. Early treatment may prevent the development of PID.

- To prevent sexually transmitted diseases that can cause PID, use a barrier contraceptive such as a diaphragm and ask your partner to use a latex condom (rubber).

Research

Although much has been learned about the biology of the microbes that cause PID and the ways in which they damage the body, there is still much to learn. Scientists supported by the National Institute of Allergy and Infectious Diseases (NIAID) are studying the effects of antibiotics, hormones, and substances that boost the immune system on the interactions between STD organisms and fallopian tube tissue. These studies may lead to insights about how to prevent infertility or other complications of PID. Vaccines to prevent gonorrhea and chlamydial infection are also under development.

Meanwhile, the search continues for faster and more accurate ways to detect PID, particularly in women with "silent" or asymptomatic PID.

Section 12.3

Women and HIV Infection

NIH/NIAID, February 1995.

AIDS is the fourth leading cause of death for women aged 25 to 44 in the United States. In fact, the disease is the primary cause of death in women of this age group in 15 major U.S. cities.

The number of women infected by HIV is steadily increasing. As of December 31, 1994, more than 58,000 AIDS cases have been reported among adult and adolescent women. The majority are black or Hispanic. Epidemiologists believe that the actual number of women with AIDS is greater because many women whose immune systems are severely compromised by HIV infection remain undiagnosed and unreported. CDC revised the definition of AIDS in January 1993 to add three new conditions, one of which is specific to women—invasive cervical cancer. The other conditions—bacterial pneumonia, pulmonary tuberculosis and having counts of CD4+ T cells, the immune system cells infected by HIV, of 200 or less—also are important for women.

NIAID Epidemiologic Studies of Women with HIV/AIDS

For the National Institute of Allergy and Infectious Diseases (NIAID), HIV infection in women is a major research focus. NIAID supports studies of the natural history, symptoms and transmission of HIV infection in women to learn more about the disease and to design better clinical trials of potential therapies and vaccines. Such studies are carried out in the United States and in 14 other countries: Brazil, Dominican Republic, Jamaica, Mexico, Haiti, India, Kenya, Malawi, Rwanda, Senegal, Thailand, Uganda, Zambia and Zaire.

More Information Needed

In December 1990, the U.S. Public Health Service (PHS) sponsored a national conference on women and HIV infection. A steering committee, which included women living with HIV as well as health and social service providers, made recommendations to the PHS that have helped guide NIAID's research. The conference attendees noted the increasing number of women with HIV infection and underscored the need for targeted studies of women. Recognizing this need, NIAID began several HIV/AIDS studies focusing on women, as well as encouraging women to enroll in the institute's clinical trials of promising HIV/AIDS therapies.

The Women's Interagency HIV Study (WIHS) and the HIV Epidemiology Research Study (HERS)

WIHS is a large long-term study that explores the natural history of HIV infection in U.S. women. Specifically, WIHS researchers comprehensively investigate the impact of HIV among women aged 13 and older. The primary research areas of WIHS are:

- the spectrum and predictors of AIDS-defining and other HIV-related conditions

- predictors of several diseases of the female reproductive system including cervical neoplasia, genital infections and cervical disease related to human papilloma virus (HPV)

- markers and predictors of HIV disease progression related to the immune system, the virus, hormones and clinical symptoms;

- trends in substance abuse, sexual behavior, health care use, and social and economic factors.

In addition, NIAID provides support for the CDC-funded HIV Epidemiology Research Study (HERS). Researchers at the four HERS sites, Baltimore, Md., Detroit, Mich., New York City, N.Y. and Providence, R.I., began recruiting women in 1992 and now approximately 800 HIV-infected and 400 HIV-uninfected high-risk women are enrolled. HERS and WIHS are conducted in tandem.

In 1993, NIAID selected four WIHS sites: New York City, N.Y., Washington, D.C., San Francisco, Calif. and Los Angeles, Calif. NIAID added two more sites in 1994: one in Chicago, Ill., and a second one in New York City, N.Y. The investigators began recruiting women in October 1994, with a projected enrollment of 2,000 HIV-infected and 500 HIV-uninfected high-risk women by the end of 1995.

WIHS and HERS have a common Statistical and Clinical Coordinating Center in Boston, Mass. The National Institute of Child Health and Human Development (NICHD) supports the WIHS site in Los Angeles. Additional WIHS support comes from the National Institute of Dental Research (NIDR) and the Agency for Health Care Policy and Research, part of PHS.

Observational Database

A large amount of information has been collected on HIV-infected individuals since September 1990 through the NIAID-supported Observational Database (ODB), a component of the community-based clinical trials network, the Terry Beirn Community Programs for Clinical Research on AIDS (CPCRA).

The CPCRA researchers are attempting to characterize the full spectrum of HIV infection and to provide an epidemiologic profile of the infection in both men and women. Information is collected on transmission, symptoms, current treatments and factors associated with disease progression.

Because participating women receive care from community physicians, the ODB also offers a snapshot of routine clinical practice. Women enrolled in the ODB who meet eligibility requirements have the opportunity to participate in CPCRA treatment protocols.

HIV Transmission to Women

To date, the majority of women with AIDS in the United States—
some 48 percent—became infected by sharing needles with HIV-infected
injection drug users. Recently, however, the number of women acquiring HIV through heterosexual contact with infected men has risen
dramatically and now totals more than 36 percent of all cases of
women with AIDS. During unprotected heterosexual intercourse with
an infected partner, women appear to be more easily infected than men.

The NIAID-supported Heterosexual AIDS Transmission Study
(HATS) was, in part, a collaborative project with CDC. HATS began
in December 1988 and ended in 1994. One HATS study, conducted at
the State University of New York in Brooklyn, examined the risk factors influencing heterosexual transmission of HIV to women. In pur-
suit of an explanation for the higher risk of HIV transmission among
female cocaine users, these HATS researchers found that knowledge,
perceptions and reported behavioral changes did not differ between
cocaine-using women and non-users in an inner-city group. However,
the cocaine users had more sexual partners and more cases of sexually transmitted diseases (STDs).

In the same HATS study, scientists found higher rates of HPV infection in a group of younger inner-city women than in older women
with comparable sexual practices. More than 40 million Americans
are infected with HPV, which causes genital warts, one of the most
common STDs in the United States. Age-related differences in younger
women's cervical tissue can facilitate HPV infection and may heighten
susceptibility to infection with HIV.

The risk of becoming infected, or infecting others, with HIV is substantially increased if one has an STD. A later study at SUNY Brooklyn is tracking the acquisition of STDs in women with HIV infection
and following the natural course of their HIV disease. This study,
called the Women's AIDS Cohort Study (WACS), has enrolled 450 HIV-
infected and high-risk uninfected women. NIAID merged WACS with
WIHS in June 1994.

WACS investigators found that women with HIV, once diagnosed,
reduce their number of sex partners, increase condom use and show
a trend towards stopping use of illegal drugs.

Controlling STDs is crucial to preventing the spread of HIV infection. NIAID is comparing different approaches of detection and treatment of STDs to identify those methods with the greatest potential
for reducing HIV transmission.

Additionally, NIAID supports basic research that will lead to the development of topical antimicrobial agents, compounds that might be used safely and effectively in the vagina to kill viruses. The institute also supports studies assessing the ability of nonoxynol-9, an agent found in many spermicides, to destroy the bacteria that cause gonorrhea and chlamydia.

Symptoms and Diagnosis

Because many women do not perceive themselves at risk for HIV infection, symptoms that could serve as warning signals of infection may go unheeded. Recurrent yeast infections (vaginal candidiasis) often occur in the early stages of HIV infection in women. Pelvic inflammatory disease, abnormal changes or dysplasia in cervical tissue that precede cancer, genital ulcers, genital warts and severe mucosal herpes infections also may occur among women with HIV infection. These symptoms should signal doctors to offer women HIV testing accompanied by counseling.

Limited access to health care contributes to the late diagnosis of HIV infection in women and their consequential higher death rates. Women whose infections are detected early survive as long as infected men, according to preliminary findings from one NIAID-supported study.

However, HIV-infected women are one-third more likely to die without an AIDS-defining condition than are HIV-infected men, according to a CPCRA study reported in the *Journal of the American Medical Association*, December 28, 1994. The investigators could not identify why the women had a greater risk of relatively early death, but suggest that important factors may involve poorer access to or use of health care resources among HIV infected women as compared to men, domestic violence and lack of social supports for women.

Early diagnosis of HIV infection allows women to take full advantage of antiretroviral therapies and forestall the development of AIDS-related infections and malignancies. Health care workers need to be alert to early signs of HIV infection in women and, conversely, women need to consider HIV testing in light of their risk status.

NIAID Clinical Studies

NIAID supports three clinical trials networks through the Division of AIDS to identify effective therapies for men, women and children with HIV infection and the subsequent opportunistic infections that develop from it.

The AIDS Clinical Trials Group (ACTG) is a network of 57 sites based at major academic institutions with the ability to carry out sophisticated large-scale research studies. CPCRA complements the ACTG by building on the expertise of primary care providers, involving them in the design and conduct of scientifically sound, community-based clinical trials.

The Division of AIDS Treatment Research Initiative (DATRI) conducts unusual or intensive studies of high priority to the NIAID that are not easily performed within the other clinical trials networks. Through the NIAID Division of Intramural Research, the institute also conducts basic and clinical research toward the development of treatments and vaccines for men, women and children with HIV infection.

The CPCRA, ACTG and WIHS each receive advice from members of communities affected by HIV through Community Constituency Groups (CCGs). In the case of the ACTG, CCG members are selected from community advisory boards that provide direction to, and oversight of, clinical trials at the local level. CCG members serve as full and active members on all committees of the ACTG and CPCRA to ensure community input into NIAID's scientific agenda.

No NIAID-sponsored studies exclude women. However, some sites experience difficulty recruiting and retaining women in clinical studies. The Women's Health Committee of the ACTG ensures that the network's scientific agenda reflects women's issues. As part of their mandate, the committee reviews the eligibility requirements for ACTG studies to determine whether certain criteria, such as weight or blood iron, contribute to the difficulties in enrolling women in studies.

The Patient Care Committee of the ACTG has evaluated other possible barriers that may prevent women from participating in clinical trials. They found many women with HIV lack access to health care and have few options to support themselves and their children. The Women, Children and People of Color Interest Group of CPCRA also has explored this issue. Researchers in both networks work closely with church groups, social workers and others at the grassroots level to find solutions to these problems.

Additionally, funds are available to clinical trials sites for ancillary services to do gynecologic assessments and to help provide child care, transportation and linkage to social services when needed. Some measures of success of such efforts have been seen in ACTG and CPCRA. Since 1986, women's overall enrollment has climbed greatly.

In 1994, women accounted for 22 percent of the adults in CPCRA, and 18 percent of those in ACTG.

Antiretroviral Therapies

Treatment for people with HIV infection consists of the use of one or more of several antiretroviral drugs. Treatment guidelines are similar for women who are not pregnant and for men with HIV infection. Studies have shown that the drug zidovudine (AZT) is as beneficial to women as men and should be considered by physicians once a person's number of white blood cells, called CD4+ T cells, drops below 500 cells per cubic millimeter of blood. Limited data are available on the use of the drug didanosine (ddI) and other antiretroviral therapies in women.

Ongoing studies will determine the effects of antiretroviral drugs on pregnant women and their children. Obstetricians from the ACTG Women's Health Committee work closely with the ACTG's Pediatric Committee to develop trials for pregnant women. Thus far, AZT seems to be well-tolerated when used by pregnant women and has not caused malformations, fetal distress or premature birth in their babies.

Other Studies

Two ACTG studies address cervical dysplasia in women. One trial is comparing topical vaginal 5-fluorouracil maintenance therapy to standard therapy to prevent the recurrence of cervical dysplasia in women with HIV infection.

Treatments to fight several gynecologic conditions including genital ulcer disease, fungal infections and pelvic inflammatory disease are under consideration for future ACTG clinical trials. NIAID-funded sites receive resources and training for clinical staff to conduct routine gynecologic exams. Plans to include nested studies, as components of a larger study, are under way to allow investigators to collect additional information on participants' gynecologic conditions.

CPCRA recently completed recruitment of a trial specifically for women. This protocol is designed to determine if fluconazole can prevent yeast infections of the mouth, throat and vagina of women with HIV infection. Candida infections of the mucous membranes may represent the earliest recognized and most common opportunistic infections afflicting women with HIV infection. These infections, common and easily treatable in most women, can be severe in women with HIV.

DATRI researchers recently ended a study of laboratory methods for measuring the amount of HIV in vaginal and cervical secretions as compared to amount of virus in blood, immunologic markers and clinical status of women with HIV. Another DATRI study is being planned to examine the effects of antiretroviral therapy on HIV burden in infected women.

Perinatal Transmission

NIAID-supported studies have shown that in the United States, HIV is transmitted from mothers to infants about 24 percent of the time. Researchers base their findings on blood samples taken from babies through 6 months of age. Other studies have documented rates of transmission ranging from 13 to 40 percent. Rates in developing nations are higher.

How perinatal transmission occurs is still unclear. Studies indicate that babies can be infected during pregnancy, during birth and postpartum. In a large European study, breast feeding was associated with a 14 percent increase in the risk of transmission. In developing countries, the World Health Organization recommends that women with HIV infection continue to breast feed because the benefits outweigh the risks of HIV transmission to their children. Breast feeding is discouraged in the United States for women with HIV infection.

Other questions regarding women who have HIV and are pregnant include the effects of anti-HIV drugs on both the mother and the fetus, the influence of HIV on pregnancy and the effects of pregnancy on the course of HIV infection. Current NIAID studies such as the Women and Infants Transmission Study (WITS) will answer many of these questions.

NIAID with NICHD established WITS in September 1989. The study addresses specific questions relating to the natural history of HIV in pregnant and nonpregnant women, including gynecologic complications, changes in the immune system and progression of disease. WITS emphasizes the long-term follow-up of HIV-infected women after they have given birth. The study has successfully recruited a population of women of many ethnicities with HIV from the mainland United States and Puerto Rico.

A large number of social, demographic and behavioral risk factors among these women make it difficult to assess HIV-specific effects on pregnancy. However, one WITS analysis indicates that, regardless of the babies' HIV status, those whose mothers used cocaine during pregnancy had shorter gestations, lower birth weights, and smaller head circumference, and were shorter in length.

Investigators at the University of Medicine and Dentistry of New Jersey, funded by NIAID and the Walter Reed Army Institute of Research in Washington, D.C., are comparing the natural histories of the pregnancies of women with HIV with those of women who do not have HIV. The scientists also are examining any effects of illegal drug use on the pregnancies. This study is coordinated with a CDC-sponsored perinatal study at the same site.

Strategies to Prevent Perinatal Transmission

As more women of childbearing age become infected with HIV, experts expect a concurrent rise in the number of infected children.

The results from ACTG 076 have shown that AZT reduced the risk of transmission of HIV from infected pregnant women to their newborns by two-thirds. HIV-infected women in their 14th to 34th week of pregnancy who did not need AZT as part of their medical care received either AZT or placebo during pregnancy and labor. At birth, infants in the study continued their mother's treatment until six weeks of age. AZT produced no serious side effects, but long-term follow-up of the infants and mothers is ongoing to learn more about the risks and benefits of treatment.

Pregnant women are also participating in an NIAID clinical trial of two experimental AIDS vaccines. Investigators will assess whether the vaccines will reduce the amount of virus present in the pregnant women and improve their health, while simultaneously stimulating antibodies that will prevent the women from passing HIV infection to their babies.

Another strategy to prevent transmission is to administer antibodies to pregnant women in the form of immune globulin injections to bolster the immune system. A three-year study, sponsored by NIAID, NICHD and the National Heart Lung and Blood Institute (NHLBI), is evaluating HIVIG, an immunoglobulin preparation containing large quantities of antibodies to HIV. Participants also receive AZT. A control group in the study will receive IVIG, an intravenous immunoglobulin preparation that contains many other types of antibodies, and AZT. In an earlier study on chimpanzees, HIVIG prevented infection after the animals were exposed to the virus.

For More Information about Trials

NIAID provides major support for the AIDS Clinical Trials Information Service, at 1-800-TRIALS-A, to advise callers of the status of HIV clinical trials being conducted throughout the United States. The AIDS Treatment Information Service at 1-800-HIV-0440 provides information about federally approved treatment guidelines. Both services operate from 9 a.m. to 7 p.m. Eastern Time, Monday through Friday. English- and Spanish-speaking specialists are available.

NIAID, a component of the National Institutes of Health, supports research on AIDS, tuberculosis and other infectious diseases as well as allergies and immunology.

Part Three

Family Planning Decisions

Chapter 13

Birth Control

Chapter Contents

Section 13.1

Choosing a Contraceptive

DHSS Publication No. 94-1181, January 1994.

Choosing a method of birth control is a highly personal decision, based on individual preferences, medical history, lifestyle, and other factors. Each method carries with it a number of risks and benefits of which the user should be aware.

Each method of birth control has a failure rate—an inability to prevent pregnancy over a one-year period. Sometimes the failure rate is due to the method and sometimes it is due to human error, such as incorrect use or not using it at all. Each method has possible side effects, some minor and some serious. Some methods require lifestyle modifications, such as remembering to use the method with each and every sexual intercourse. Some cannot be used by individuals with certain medical problems.

Disease Prevention

For many people, the prevention of sexually transmitted diseases (STDs), including HIV (human immunodeficiency virus), which leads to AIDS, is a factor in choosing a contraceptive. Only one form of birth control currently available—the latex condom, worn by the man—is considered highly effective in helping protect against HIV and other STDs. FDA has approved the marketing of male condoms made from polyurethane as also effective in preventing STDs, including HIV. However, at press time, they were not yet being sold in this country. Reality Female Condom, made from polyurethane, may give limited protection against STDs but has not been proven as effective as male latex condoms. People who use another form of birth control but who also want a highly effective way to reduce their STD risks, should also use a latex condom for every sex act, from start to finish.

In April 1993, FDA announced that birth control pills, Norplant, Depo-Provera, IUDs, and natural membrane condoms must carry labeling stating that these products are intended to prevent pregnancy but do not protect against HIV infection and other sexually transmitted diseases. In addition, natural membrane condom labeling must state that consumers should use a latex condom to help reduce the transmission of STDs. The labeling of latex condoms states that, if used properly, they will help reduce transmission of HIV and other diseases.

Spermicides Used Alone

Spermicides, which come in many forms—foams, jellies, gels, and suppositories—work by forming a physical and chemical barrier to sperm. They should be inserted into the vagina within an hour before intercourse. If intercourse is repeated, more spermicide should be inserted. The active ingredient in most spermicides is the chemical nonoxynol-9. The failure rate for spermicides in preventing pregnancy when used alone is from 20 to 30 percent.

Spermicides are available without a prescription. People who experience burning or irritation with these products should not use them.

Barrier Methods

There are five barrier methods of contraception:

- male condoms
- female condoms
- diaphragm
- sponge
- and cervical cap

In each instance, the method works by keeping the sperm and egg apart. Usually, these methods have only minor side effects. The main possible side effect is an allergic reaction either to the material of the barrier or the spermicides that should be used with them. Using the methods correctly for each and every sexual intercourse gives the best protection.

Male Condom

A male condom is a sheath that covers the penis during sex. Condoms on the market at press time were made of either latex rubber or natural skin (also called "lambskin" but actually made from sheep intestines). Of these two types, only latex condoms have been shown to be highly effective in helping to prevent STDs. Latex provides a good barrier to even small viruses such as human immunodeficiency virus and hepatitis B. Each condom can only be used once. Condoms have a birth control failure rate of about 15 percent. Most of the failures can be traced to improper use.

Some condoms have spermicide added. This may give some additional contraceptive protection. Vaginal spermicides may also be added before sexual intercourse.

Some condoms have lubricants added. These do not improve birth control or STD protection. Non-oil-based lubricants can also be used with condoms. However, oil-based lubricants such as petroleum jelly (Vaseline) should not be used because they weaken the latex. Condoms are available without a prescription.

Female Condom

The Reality Female Condom was approved by FDA in April 1993. It consists of a lubricated polyurethane sheath with a flexible polyurethane ring on each end.

FEMALE CONDOM

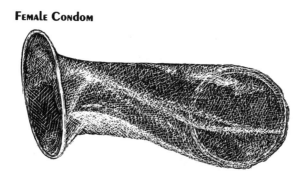

Figure 13.1.

One ring is inserted into the vagina much like a diaphragm, while the other remains outside, partially covering the labia. The female condom may offer some protection against STDs, but for highly effective protection, male latex condoms must be used. (The female condom should not be used at the same time as the male condom because they will not both stay in place.)

FDA Commissioner David A. Kessler, M.D., in announcing the approval, said, "I have to stress that the male latex condom remains the best shield against AIDS and other sexually transmitted diseases. Couples should go on using the male latex condom."

In a six-month trial, the pregnancy rate for the Reality Female Condom was about 13 percent. The estimated yearly failure rate ranges from 21 to 26 percent. This means that about 1 in 4 women who use Reality may become pregnant during a year.

Sponge

The contraceptive sponge, approved by FDA in 1983, is made of white polyurethane foam. The sponge, shaped like a small doughnut, contains the spermicide nonoxynol-9. Like the diaphragm, it is inserted into the vagina to cover the cervix during and after intercourse. It does not require fitting by a health professional and is available without prescription. It is to be used only once and then discarded. The failure rate is between 18 and 28 percent. An extremely rare side effect is toxic shock syndrome (TSS), a potentially fatal infection caused by a strain of the bacterium *Staphylococcus aureus* and more commonly associated with tampon use.

Diaphragm

The diaphragm is a flexible rubber disk with a rigid rim. Diaphragms range in size from 2 to 4 inches in diameter and are designed to cover the cervix during and after intercourse so that sperm cannot reach the uterus. Spermicidal jelly or cream must be placed inside the diaphragm for it to be effective.

The diaphragm must be fitted by a health professional and the correct size prescribed to ensure a snug seal with the vaginal wall. If intercourse is repeated, additional spermicide should be added with the diaphragm still in place. The diaphragm should be left in place for at least six hours after intercourse. The diaphragm used with spermicide has a failure rate of from 6 to 18 percent.

In addition to the possible allergic reactions or irritation common to all barrier methods, there have been some reports of bladder infections with this method. As with the contraceptive sponge, TSS is an extremely rare side effect.

[See Figure 13.2 on page 170.]

DiApHRAGM

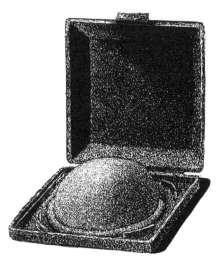

Figure 13.2.

Cervical Cap

The cervical cap, approved for contraceptive use in the United States in 1988, is a dome-shaped rubber cap in various sizes that fits snugly over the cervix. Like the diaphragm, it is used with a spermicide and must be fitted by a health professional. It is more difficult to insert than the diaphragm, but may be left in place for up to 48 hours. In addition to the allergic reactions that can occur with any barrier method, 5.2 to 27 percent of users in various studies have reported an unpleasant odor and/or discharge. There also appears to be an increased incidence of irregular Pap tests in the first six months of using the cap, and TSS is an extremely rare side effect. The cap has a failure rate of about 18 percent.

Hormonal Contraception

Hormonal contraception involves ways of delivering forms of two female reproductive hormones—estrogen and progestogen—that help regulate ovulation (release of an egg), the condition of the uterine lining, and other parts of the menstrual cycle. Unlike barrier methods, hormones are not inert, do interact with the body, and have the potential for serious side effects, though this is rare. When properly used, hormonal methods are also extremely effective. Hormonal methods are available only by prescription.

Birth Control Pills

There are two types of birth control pills: combination pills, which contain both estrogen and a progestin (a natural or synthetic progesterone), and "mini-pills", which contain only progestin. The combination pill prevents ovulation, while the mini-pill reduces cervical mucus and causes it to thicken. This prevents the sperm from reaching the egg. Also, progestins keep the endometrium (uterine lining) from thickening. This prevents the fertilized egg from implanting in the uterus. The failure rate for the mini-pill is 1 to 3 percent; for the combination pill it is 1 to 2 percent.

Combination oral contraceptives offer significant protection against ovarian cancer, endometrial cancer, iron-deficiency anemia, pelvic inflammatory disease (PID), and fibrocystic breast disease. Women who take combination pills have a lower risk of functional ovarian cysts.

The decision about whether to take an oral contraceptive should be made only after consultation with a health professional. Smokers and women with certain medical conditions should not take the pill. These conditions include:

- A history of blood clots in the leg, eyes, or deep veins of the legs
- Heart attacks, strokes or angina
- Cancer of the breast, vagina, cervix or uterus
- Any undiagnosed, abnormal vaginal bleeding
- Liver tumors
- Jaundice due to pregnancy or use of birth control pills.

Women with the following conditions should discuss with a health professional whether the benefits of the pill outweigh its risks for them:

- high blood pressure
- heart, kidney or gallbladder disease
- a family history of heart attack or stroke
- severe headaches or depression
- elevated cholesterol or triglycerides
- epilepsy
- diabetes.

171

Serious side effects of the pill include blood clots that can lead to stroke, heart attack, pulmonary embolism, or death. A clot may, on rare occasions, occur in the blood vessel in the eye, causing impaired vision or even blindness. The pills may also cause high blood pressure that returns to normal after oral contraceptives are stopped. Minor side effects, which usually subside after a few months' use, include: nausea, headaches, breast swelling, fluid retention, weight gain, irregular bleeding and depression. Sometimes taking a pill with a lower dose hormone can reduce these effects.

The effectiveness of birth control pills may be reduced by a few other medications, including some antibiotics, barbiturates, and antifungal medications. On the other hand, birth control pills may prolong the effects of theophylline and caffeine. They also may prolong the effects of benzodiazepines such as Librium (chlordiazepoxide), Valium (diazepam), and Xanax (alprazolam). Because of the variety of these drug interactions, women should always tell their health professionals when they are taking birth control pills.

Norplant

Norplant—the first contraceptive implant—was approved by FDA in 1990. In a minor surgical procedure, six matchstick-sized rubber capsules containing progestin are placed just underneath the skin of the upper arm. The implant is effective within 24 hours and provides progestin for up to five years or until it is removed. Both the insertion and the removal must be performed by a qualified professional.

Because contraception is automatic and does not depend on the user, the failure rate for Norplant is less than 1 percent for women

NORPLANT

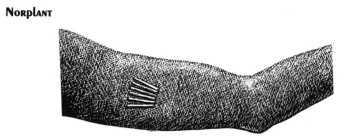

Figure 13.3.

who weigh less than 150 pounds. Women who weigh more have a higher pregnancy rate after the first two years.

Women who cannot take birth control pills for medical reasons should not consider Norplant a contraceptive option. The potential side effects of the implant include: irregular menstrual bleeding, headaches, nervousness, depression, nausea, dizziness, skin rash, acne, change of appetite, breast tenderness, weight gain, enlargement of the ovaries or fallopian tubes, and excessive growth of body and facial hair. These side effects may subside after the first year.

Depo-Provera

Depo-Provera is an injectable form of a progestin. It was approved by FDA in 1992 for contraceptive use. Previously, it was approved for treating endometrial and renal cancers. Depo-Provera has a failure rate of only 1 percent. Each injection provides contraceptive protection for 14 weeks. It is injected every three months into a muscle in the buttocks or arm by a trained professional. The side effects are the same as those for Norplant and progestin only pills. In addition, there may be irregular bleeding and spotting during the first months followed by periods of amenorrhea (no menstrual period). About 50 percent of the women who use Depo-Provera for one year or longer report amenorrhea. Other side effects, such as weight gain and others described for Norplant, may occur.

Intrauterine Devices

IUDs are small, plastic, flexible devices that are inserted into the uterus through the cervix by a trained clinician. Only two IUDs are presently marketed in the United States: ParaGard T380A, a T-shaped device partially covered by copper and effective for eight years; and Progestasert, which is also T-shaped but contains a progestin released over a one-year period. After that time, the IUD should be replaced. Both IUDs have a 4 to 5 percent failure rate.

It is not known exactly how IUDs work. At one time it was thought that the IUD affected the uterus so that it would be inhospitable to implantation. New evidence, however, suggests that uterine and tubal fluids are altered, particularly in the case of copper-bearing IUDs, inhibiting the transport of sperm through the cervical mucus and uterus.

**INTRAUTERINE
DEVICES**

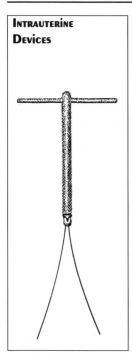

Figure 13.4.

The risk of PID with IUD use is highest in those with multiple sex partners or with a history of previous PID. Therefore, the IUD is recommended primarily for women in mutually monogamous relationships.

In addition to PID, other complications include perforation of the uterus (usually at the time of insertion), septic abortion, or ectopic (tubal) pregnancy. Women may also experience some short-term side effects—cramping and dizziness at the time of insertion; bleeding, cramps and backache that may continue for a few days after the insertion; spotting between periods; and longer and heavier menstruation during the first few periods after insertion.

The only non-contraceptive health benefit related to use of the IUD is decreased menstrual bleeding and less painful periods in women using a particular type of IUD in which the hormone progestin is infused into the uterus.

Periodic Abstinence

Periodic abstinence entails not having sexual intercourse during the woman's fertile period. Sometimes this method is called natural family planning or "rhythm." Using periodic abstinence is dependent on the ability to identify the approximately 10 days in each menstrual cycle that a women is fertile. Methods to help determine this include:

The basal body temperature method. The basal body temperature method is based on the knowledge that just before ovulation a woman's basal body temperature drops several tenths of a degree and after ovulation it returns to normal. The method requires that the woman take her temperature each morning before she gets out of bed. There are now electronic thermometers with memories and electrical resistance meters that can more accurately pinpoint a woman's fertile period.

174

The cervical mucus method. The cervical mucus method, also called the Billings method, depends on a woman recognizing the changes in cervical mucus that indicate ovulation is occurring or has occurred.

Periodic abstinence has a failure rate of 14 to 47 percent. It has none of the side effects of artificial methods of contraception.

Surgical Sterilization

Surgical sterilization must be considered permanent. Tubal ligation seals a woman's fallopian tubes so that an egg cannot travel to the uterus. Vasectomy involves closing off a man's vas deferens so that sperm will not be carried to the penis.

Vasectomy is considered safer than female sterilization. It is a minor surgical procedure, most often performed in a doctor's office under local anesthesia. The procedure usually takes less than 30 minutes. Minor post-surgical complications may occur.

Tubal ligation is an operating-room procedure performed under general anesthesia. The fallopian tubes can be reached by a number of surgical techniques, and, depending on the technique, the operation is sometimes an outpatient procedure or requires only an overnight stay. In a mini-laparotomy, a 2-inch incision is made in the abdomen. The surgeon, using special instruments, lifts the fallopian tubes and, using clips, a plastic ring, or an electric current, seals the tubes. Another method, laparoscopy, involves making a small incision above the navel, and distending the abdominal cavity so that the intestine separates from the uterus and fallopian tubes. Then a laparoscope—a miniaturized, flexible telescope—is used to visualize the fallopian tubes while closing them off.

Both of these methods are replacing the traditional laparotomy.

Major complications, which are rare in female sterilization, include: infection, hemorrhage, and problems associated with the use of general anesthesia. It is estimated that major complications occur in 1.7 percent of the cases, while the overall complication rate has been reported to be between 0.1 and 15.3 percent.

The failure rate of laparoscopy and mini-laparotomy procedures, as well as vasectomy, is less than 1 percent. Although there has been some success in reopening the fallopian tubes or the vas deferens, the success rate is low, and sterilization should be considered irreversible.

—by Merle Goldberg

175

Type	Male Condom	Female Condom	Spermicides Used Alone	Sponge	Diaphragm with Spermicide	Cervical Cap with Spermicide
Estimated Effectiveness	About 85%	An estimated 74–79%	70–80%	72–82%	82–94%	At least 82%
Risks	Rarely, irritation and allergic reactions	Rarely, irritation and allergic reactions	Rarely, irritation and allergic reactions	Rarely, irritation and allergic reactions; difficulty in removal; very rarely, toxic shock syndrome	Rarely, irritation and allergic reactions; bladder infection; very rarely, toxic shock syndrome	Abnormal Pap test; vaginal or cervical infections; very rarely, toxic shock syndrome
STD Protection	Latex condoms help protect against sexually transmitted diseases, including herpes and AIDS	May give some protection against sexually transmitted diseases, including herpes and AIDS; not as effective as male latex condom	Unknown	None	None	None
Convenience	Applied immediately before intercourse; used only once and discarded	Applied immediately before intercourse; used only once and discarded	Applied no more than one hour before intercourse	Can be inserted hours before intercourse and left in place up to 24 hours; used only once and discarded	Inserted before intercourse; can be left in place 24 hours, but additional spermicide must be inserted if intercourse is repeated	Can remain in place for 48 hours, not necessary to reapply spermicide upon repeated intercourse; may be difficult to insert
Availability	Nonprescription	Nonprescription	Nonprescription	Nonprescription	Rx	Rx

Figure 13.5. Birth Control Guide. Efficacy rate given in this chart are estimates based on a number of different studies. they should be understood as yearly estimates, with those dependent on conscientious use subject to a greater chance of human error and reduced effectiveness. For comparison,

Pills	Implant (Norplant)	Injection (Depo-Provera)	IUD	Periodic Abstinence (NFP)	Surgical Sterilization
97%–99%	99%	99%	95–96%	Very variable, perhaps 53–86%	Over 99%
Blood clots, heart attacks and strokes, gallbladder disease, liver tumors, water retention, hypertension, mood changes, dizziness and nausea; not for smokers	Menstrual cycle irregularity; headaches, nervousness, depression, nausea, dizziness, change of appetite, breast tenderness, weight gain, enlargement of ovaries and/or fallopian tubes, excessive growth of body and facial hair; may subside after first year	Amenorrhea, weight gain, and other side effects similar to those with Norplant	Cramps, bleeding, pelvic inflammatory disease, infertility; rarely, perforation of the uterus	None	Pain, infection, and, for female tubal ligation, possible surgical complications
None	None	None	None	None	None
Pill must be taken on daily schedule, regardless of the frequency of intercourse	Effective 24 hours after implantation for approximately 5 years; can be removed by physician at any time	One injection every three months	After insertion, stays in place until physician removes it	Requires frequent monitoring of body functions and periods of abstinence	Vasectomy is a one-time procedure usually performed in a doctor's office; tubal ligation is a one-time procedure performed in an operating room
Rx	Rx; minor outpatient surgical procedure	Rx	Rx	Instructions from physician or clinic	Surgery

60 to 85 percent of sexually active women using no contraception would be expected to become pregnant in a year. This chart should not be used alone, but only as a summary of information in the preceding article.

Section 13.2

Cervical Cap

Excerpts from *FDA Consumer*, September 1988.

The cervical cap is a small rubber device that is inserted into the vagina to block sperm from entering the cervix (the opening to the uterus). Like the diaphragm, the cap is a prescription device that comes in several sizes and must be fitted by a trained health worker. Also like the diaphragm, the cap is used with a spermicide. The cervical cap is however different from the diaphragm in some notable ways. The flexible thimble-shaped latex cap, about 1 1/2 inches in diameter, fits tightly over the cervix and is held in place by suction. The larger diaphragm, about 3 inches wide, is placed between the pubic bone and the vaginal wall and kept in place by tension. A spermicidal cream or gel is used with both devices, but the cap requires less of such substances and is, therefore, thought by some to be less messy than the diaphragm. The major advantage the cap offers over the diaphragm, however, is a greater degree of sexual spontaneity. While the diaphragm must be removed after 24 hours, the cap can stay in place up to 48 hours. Also, the cap does not require additional applications of spermicide with each act of intercourse, as does the diaphragm.

Some women report that the cap is more difficult to use than the diaphragm. The cap containing spermicide is inserted into the vagina by grasping the cap, dome down, between two fingers of one hand and compressing the rim. The cap is pushed as far as it will go along the back wall of the vaginal canal, and then the rim must be pressed around the cervix until it seals. The cap is removed by tilting the rim away from the cervix, thus breaking the suction; or it can be grasped between two fingers and pulled downward. Thus, insertion and removal require manual dexterity and knowledge of anatomy, and may be difficult for some women even after detailed instruction.

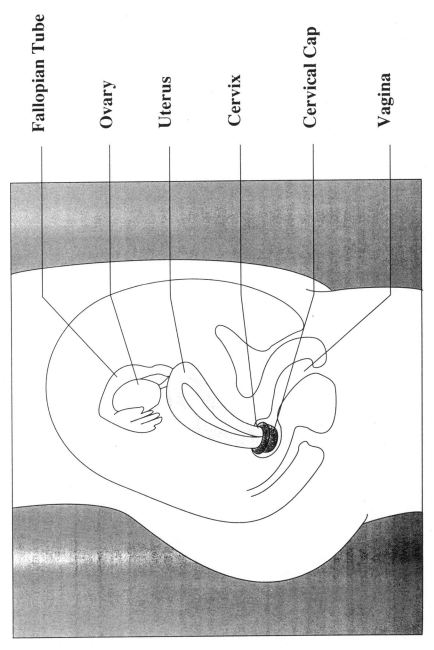

Figure 13.6.

Fallopian Tube

Ovary

Uterus

Cervix

Cervical Cap

Vagina

179

Cap Testing

Women activists in the late 1970s began a campaign for FDA approval of the cap, which many saw as having important advantages over the pill, the IUD, and other methods of contraception, including the diaphragm. At that time, Secretary of Health, Education, and Welfare Patricia Harris requested that FDA and the National Institutes of Health (NIH) help expedite testing the cap and making it available to women. FDA worked with women's groups to help them develop study protocols and issued nearly 100 "investigational device exemptions," under which approximately 50,000 women were fitted with a cervical cap or a diaphragm by a trained professional or lay health worker. The women's groups obtained informed consent from the study participants and submitted to FDA the data they collected on safety and efficacy of the cap.

The largest single study was funded by NIH's National Institute of Child Health and Human Development and headed by Gerald S. Bernstein, an obstetrician-gynecologist at the University of Southern California. Involving more than 1,000 women at eight California clinics, the study went from July 1981 to March 1986. The women were randomly assigned to use either the Prentif cervical cap (581 women) or the Ortho diaphragm (572 women). All were given instructions for use and were followed with periodic gynecologic exams and Pap tests. (A Pap test is an examination of cells taken from the cervix. Abnormal cells may indicate cancer or a precancerous condition, but not always; they can also result simply from an infection or other easily treated condition.)

Bernstein's study showed the diaphragm and cervical cap were equally effective in preventing pregnancy. One-year overall pregnancy rates were 17.4 percent for cap users and 16.7 percent for diaphragm users.

Effectiveness rates, however, can be expressed more definitively in terms of "user failures" or "method failures." For instance, a pregnancy that results because the woman left her cervical cap or diaphragm in the dresser drawer is determined to be a user failure. A pregnancy that results despite consistent and correct use of the method, on the other hand, can be ascribed to method failure. In Bernstein's study, user failure at the end of 12 months was 11.7 percent for the cap and 12.6 percent for the diaphragm. Method failure was 6.4 percent for the cap and 4.6 percent for the diaphragm. (The percentages for method and user failure add up to more than the total overall pregnancy rate for each device because of the statistical methods used in analyzing the data.)

The September-October 1987 issue of *Studies in Family Planning* reports the lowest method failure rate found for oral contraceptives that contain both estrogen and progestin is 0.1 percent, with an overall failure (pregnancy) rate of 3 percent; the lowest method failure rate for the IUD is 1 percent, with an overall pregnancy rate of 6 percent.

Drawbacks of the Cap

Experience with the cervical cap revealed some drawbacks, both with user convenience and possible health consequences. Of greatest concern was the change in Pap test results from normal to abnormal. In Bernstein's study, 4 percent of women using the cap converted to abnormal results after wearing the cap for three months, compared with 1.7 percent of women using a diaphragm. After the first three months, however, the conversion rates were similar for both devices. Because of this finding, FDA approved the cap with the condition that post-approval studies be conducted to obtain more data on the Pap test results of cap wearers and to try to determine what risk factors may predispose them to cervical cell changes. Also, the directions for the device specify that it is to be prescribed only for women with normal Pap tests and that all users have a repeat test after three months. If the repeat test is positive, the device should no longer be used.

There is no established association between use of the cap and development of toxic shock syndrome (TSS), a rare but sometimes fatal condition that afflicts mainly women. The label warns, however, that, as with any product that blocks the vagina—such as a tampon or a diaphragm—the risk of TSS may be increased. Therefore, women with a history of TSS and those with vaginal or cervical infections are advised not to use the cap. A woman should not wear the cap during a menstrual period or for six weeks after giving birth or having a miscarriage or abortion. The label also warns that use of the cap should be discontinued if the woman or her partner experiences burning or irritation of the genitals.

Some women in the studies had difficulty inserting or removing the cap, and in some it became dislodged occasionally. Also, because the cap comes in only four sizes, some women could not be properly fitted. Some noticed an unpleasant odor with the cap, usually when the device was worn for more than a few days. Removing the cap and cleaning it should alleviate the problem.

The cervical cap adds to the choices of birth control practices available to women and men. It should be remembered that the safest and most effective method for one woman, or couple, may not be the best for another. It is also important to remember that cervical caps and diaphragms may not protect against sexually transmitted diseases, including AIDS. The best barrier against these diseases is the condom—used properly and consistently. Lifestyle and medical history must be carefully considered in determining the contraceptive method that will be best for a given individual. This determination should be made by the woman, or couple, in consultation with a physician who can present the advantages and disadvantages, and risks and benefits of all methods available.

—by Marian Segal

Section 13.3

The Pill: 30 Years of Safety Concerns

DHSS Publication No. (FDA) 92-3193, 1992.

When the birth control pill was introduced in 1960, it was a major medical achievement that rewrote the future of women and family life. For the first time in history, it became possible for a woman to safely and effectively control childbearing by taking a pill.

Since its introduction, it has been used by more than 60 million women worldwide. It has proved to be, in the opinion of many, the most socially significant medical advance of the century.

American women were quick to accept the pill. Within two years, approximately 1.2 million women were using it, within five years, 5 million, and by 1973, about 10 million. In the early '80s, following reports of possible harmful side effects, use of the pill dropped to 8.4 million. Today, however, with safer, low-dose versions on the market, use is back up. Approximately 10.7 million American women now use the pill. It is the most popular method of non-surgical contraception.

Concerns about side effects have dogged the pill over the years. And rightly so. Does the pill present society with problems unique in the history of medicine? As an FDA advisory committee on the pill noted in the mid '60s, never would so many people take such a potent drug voluntarily over such a long period for a reason other than to cure disease.

"Since probably no substance, even common table salt, and certainly no effective drug, can be taken over a long period of time without some risk," the advisory committee warned, the pill's potential side effects "must be recognized and kept under continual surveillance."

Oral contraceptives have been kept under surveillance for 30 years. In fact, over the years, more studies have been done on the pill to look for serious side effects than have been done on any other medicine in history, according to FDA.

Fears about blood clots, heart attack, and stroke, which spurred exhaustive research on oral contraceptives in the '60s and '70s, have largely been laid to rest by the safer, low-dose birth control pills on the market today. Current research suggests that healthy, non-smoking women have little if any greater risk of these serious health problems than do women who do not use the pill.

Questions about the pill's association with cancer, however, remain. Some widely reported recent studies support the hypothesis that in certain groups of women the risk of breast cancer increases with oral contraceptive use. A larger number of studies, however, found no significant increased risk. Nor is it definitely known yet whether or not the pill causes cervical cancer in some groups of women. So far, a cause-and-effect relationship has not been established.

But the pill has been found to help *prevent* two major types of cancer—cancer of the ovaries and cancer of the endometrium (the lining of the uterus).

How the Pill Was Developed

It was 1950 when Dr. Gregory Pincus, an American biologist, was invited by the Planned Parenthood Federation of America to develop an ideal contraceptive—one that Planned Parenthood stipulated would be "harmless, entirely reliable, simple, practical, universally applicable and aesthetically satisfactory to both husband and wife."

Planned Parenthood donated $2,100 to the project. Another $20,000 to $30,000 had to be raised from government and private sources before research could get under way.

Within a few years, an oral contraceptive was being clinically tested in 6,000 women in Puerto Rico and Haiti. In 1960, the first commercially produced birth control pill, Enovid-10, was marketed in the United States.

What Dr. Pincus and colleagues developed was a pill containing estrogen and progestin, synthetic hormones similar to those produced naturally in a woman's body. The pill works primarily by suppressing the release of eggs from a woman's ovaries.

The first oral contraceptives contained 100 micrograms (mcg) to 150 mcg of estrogen and as much as 10 milligrams (mg) of progestin—significantly higher levels of both hormones than in today's pill. They were 99 percent effective if taken as directed—the highest rate of contraceptive protection available except sterilization.

Concerns about Side Effects

Although the pill was widely welcomed, it wasn't long before concerns were raised about possible serious side effects.

As early as 1961, suspicions arose in the United States and England that the pill might predispose some women to heart attack and stroke. Evidence of blood clotting had been reported in a few women taking the pill. Blood clots can cause life-threatening heart attacks and strokes.

By 1969, ongoing research had revealed that the risks of blood clots, heart attack, and stroke were directly related to the amount of estrogen in the various versions of the pill. Research also showed that the same rate of contraceptive effectiveness could be maintained with only 50 mcg of estrogen. By that time, 7.5 million women were using oral contraceptives—up from 408,000 women in 1961.

As the 1970s began, FDA issued a bulletin to doctors about the danger of blood clots. It advised using the lowest effective dose of estrogen possible when prescribing oral contraceptives. The agency also revised the product labeling once again to include the "lowest effective dose" recommendation. And, for the first time, FDA required that information for patients about the drug's risks be included in every package of oral contraceptives.

'Mini-Pill' Introduced

In the early 1970s, the "mini-pill," an oral contraceptive containing only progestin, was introduced. Unlike the estrogen-progestin pill, which works primarily by suppressing ovulation, the mini-pill works by creating changes in the cervix and uterus that make it difficult for sperm to unite with an egg. Since mini-pills contain no estrogen, they pose few of the risks associated with the combination pill. However, mini-pills have two drawbacks: they cause irregular bleeding in some women, and they have proven to be less effective in preventing pregnancy. As a result, their use has been limited.

By the mid '70s, most women who used oral contraceptives were taking pills that contained 50 mcg or less of estrogen—a considerable decrease over the 100 to 150 mcg of the '60s. The amount of progestin in the pills had also decreased over the years from the original 10 mg to between 2.5 mg and 0.15 mg.

Between 1973 and 1974, FDA approved several low-dose pills containing as little as 20 to 35 mcg of estrogen. Most pills prescribed today contain 30 to 35 mcg of estrogen and 0.5 mg to 1 mg progestin.

In 1982, a new version of the pill, called the "biphasic" pill, was introduced. Two years later, three "triphasic" pills were introduced. These "multiphasic" oral contraceptives are low-dose pills in which the ratio of progestin to estrogen changes during the 21 days the pill is taken.

By 1986, use of high-dose estrogen pills had been drastically reduced–to 3.4 percent of the oral contraceptive market.

Nevertheless, some 400,000 women were still using high-dose estrogen pills. Most were between 30 and 39 years of age, the age group most at risk of serious side effects.

High-Dose Estrogen Pills Withdrawn

In 1988, at FDA's urging, the three drug companies still manufacturing high-dose estrogen oral contraceptives voluntarily withdrew from the market all remaining products containing over 50 mcg estrogen.

The latest development in the 30-year saga of the pill was its approval in 1989 for use in healthy, non-smoking women over 40. The impact of this move, in terms of the number of women who will choose to continue or start using the pill after they turn 40, remains to be seen. But an estimated 1 million to 1.5 million women between 40 and 54, including the baby boomers could be affected.

Today's Pill Safer

Today's oral contraceptives are considerably safer than the pill of the '60s because they contain less estrogen and progestin. Over the years the amount of estrogen has been reduced to one-third or less of that in the first birth control pills. and the progestin has been decreased to one-tenth or less.

The risks of blood clots, heart attacks and stroke have decreased correspondingly for healthy, non-smoking women. There is a slightly increased risk of cardiovascular disease for women over 40 who use the pill, but the benefits of contraception are considered to outweigh the risk in most women, says Philip Corfman M.D., of FDA's division of metabolism and endocrine drug products.

Most side effects of the pill are not medically serious. The most common are nausea, breakthrough bleeding (bleeding between menstrual periods), and mood changes, including depression. Some women may also experience weight gain, breast tenderness, and difficulty wearing contact lenses due to eye dryness. These side effects, especially nausea, usually subside within the first three months of use.

Health Benefits

In addition to its contraceptive effectiveness, the pill has proven to have significant health benefits. Studies show that the incidence of ovarian and endometrial cancers, benign cysts of the ovaries and breasts, and pelvic inflammatory disease decreases with pill use. The pill also prevents heavy and irregular menstrual periods, a common cause of anemia that leads to surgical procedures, including hysterectomy, in older women.

Whether these benefits will continue with the newer, low-dose pill remains to be seen. The present benefits are associated with oral contraceptives containing 50 mcg of estrogen. As yet, no scientific data are available on the effects of those containing 30 to 35 mcg or less.

Not Safe for All

As safe as today's pill is for most healthy, non-smoking women, it is still not safe for all women. The risk of serious illness and death increases significantly for certain groups:

- Women who smoke—particularly those over 35 who are heavy smokers (more than 14 cigarettes a day)—have a significantly

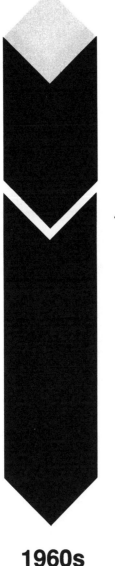

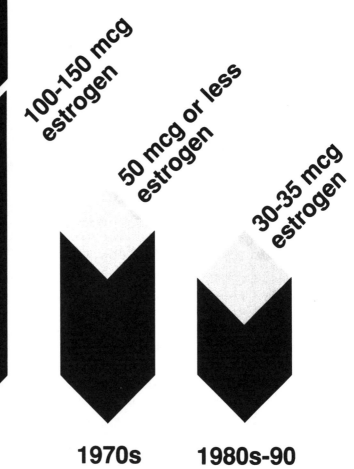

Estrogen Levels of Pill Drop

The amount of estrogen in oral contraceptives has declined significantly over the past 30 years, making today's pill considerably safer than the pill of the 60s.

100-150 mcg estrogen

50 mcg or less estrogen

30-35 mcg estrogen

1960s   **1970s**   **1980s-90**

Figure 13.7.

increased risk of heart attack and stroke. This risk increases with age. Women who use oral contraceptives are strongly advised not to smoke.

- Women who are obese or have underlying health problems, such as diabetes, high blood pressure, or high cholesterol, also have a significantly increased risk of serious side effects from using the pill.

- Women who have a history of blood clots, heart attack, stroke, liver disease, or cancer of the breast or sex organs should not use oral contraceptives.

Women who become pregnant while on the pill should immediately discontinue taking it because of a risk of birth defects in the child.

Uncertainties remain about whether the pill causes breast or cervical cancer in some groups of women. Despite many studies over the years, there is still insufficient evidence to definitely rule out these possibilities.

While there are conflicting results among studies on breast cancer and the pill, most investigations have found that women who have taken the pill have no increased risk of developing breast cancer. However, the product labeling on oral contraceptives recommends that women who use the pill and have a strong family history of breast cancer or who have breast lumps or abnormal mammograms be closely monitored by their doctors.

Some studies have found an increase in the incidence of cervical cancer in women who use the pill, but this may not necessarily be related to the pill, scientists say.

One of the major problems of the studies to date, says Corfman, is that all the data reflect the effects of the higher-dose pills (those containing more than 50 mcg of estrogen). No studies have been done on the low-dose pills, and none are under way. The cancer-pill issue is very complicated and therefore difficult to study, and the research is expensive, he says.

"We really need another breast cancer study on the low-dose pills," Corfman says. "We have the capability of finding out about breast cancer, but no one is doing the research."

Researchers may never find out whether the pill causes cancer of the cervix, Corfman says, because the development of cervical cancer can be affected by numerous other factors, such as the age a woman begins having sex and the number of sexual partners. Corfman says he suspects, however, that such research would show that the risk of getting cervical cancer from the pill is so small as to be outweighed by the benefits of contraception.

Though some safety questions remain unsettled, for most healthy women the pill provides a safe, effective means of birth control with some possible beneficial health effects.

—by Sharon Snider

Section 13.4

Facts about Oral Contraceptives

NIH Publication from the Office of Research Reporting, National Institute of Child Health and Human Development (NICHD).

When oral contraceptives were introduced in the United States in 1960, many women believed they had found the answer to the need for convenient, safe and reliable birth control. By 1965, "the pill" was America's leading contraceptive.

With the 1970's came disillusionment: The pill was not perfect. While it was highly effective and convenient, it had many minor side effects and a few serious ones. Though severe complications were rare, "pill scare" reports created an aura of danger. Pill use dropped in the mid-70's.

Today the pill has been put into perspective. It is not for everyone, but recent studies show it to be safe for most young, healthy, non-smoking users. Despite widespread publicity on the pill's drawbacks, its benefits must be substantial. It is still the most popular reversible birth control method in America, with more than seven million women taking it daily.

Two Decades of Research

Oral contraceptives are probably the most extensively studied medication in history, yet they are not fully understood. Twenty years of research has, however, brought much safer pills and a long list of guidelines to help doctors screen out women most likely to develop serious complications.

The most important outcome of recent research is that groups of women with a high risk of developing pill complications have been identified. These include smokers, older women (the risks start to rise at 30), and those with a history of certain illnesses. While current knowledge is not precise enough to predict exactly which individuals will suffer serious pill complications, it is continually improving.

New studies also show benefits of pill use, besides contraception, such as protection from pelvic inflammatory disease and other conditions. Many doctors today stress that women should be made aware of these benefits, as well as the possible problems, so they can make informed decisions about the pill.

Today's Pills

The most popular oral contraceptives are "combined" pills. These contain two synthetic hormones (an estrogen and a progestogen) similar to the hormones the ovary normally produces.

When studies linked the amount of estrogen in birth control pills with serious side effects—including blood clots, heart attacks, and strokes—researchers developed new pill formulas with less estrogen. They also developed a progestogen-only pill known as the "mini-pill."

Ten years ago, doctors often prescribed combined pills with 100 to 150 micrograms of estrogen. Today the Food and Drug Administration urges physicians to start patients on combined pills with no more than 50 micrograms of estrogen and, if possible, one of the newer "low dose" combined pills with only 30 or 35 micrograms of estrogen.

Major studies have concluded that switching from higher doses to pills with 50 micrograms of estrogen cuts the blood clot risk substantially. Recent research suggests that pills with less than 50 micrograms of estrogen cut the risk even further.

Progestogen levels in pills have also dropped over the years. Mini-pills contain even less progestogen than low-dose combined pills, which may make the mini-pill the safest oral contraceptive known.

How They Work

Combined birth-control pills, including the newer low-dose forms, work by suppressing ovulation, the release of an egg from the ovary. Without a released egg, pregnancy cannot occur. Though rare, it is possible for women using combined pills to ovulate. Then other mechanisms work to prevent pregnancy.

Both kinds of pills make the cervical mucus thick and "in-hospitable" to sperm, discouraging entry to the uterus. In addition, they make it difficult for a fertilized egg to implant, by causing changes in fallopian tube contractions and in the uterine lining. These actions explain why the mini-pill works, as it generally does not suppress ovulation.

Effectiveness

Taken properly, the combined pills are better than 99 percent effective. Some formulas with less estrogen may be slightly less effective, about 98 to 99 percent.

Mini-pills are comparable in effectiveness to the IUD, at around 98 percent. But they must be taken without fail every day—ideally at the same time. Missing just one mini-pill can undo the contraceptive protection. Also, because mini-pills do not generally suppress ovulation, many doctors recommend a backup method, such as a diaphragm or condoms, at midcycle.

Why Pills Fail

If you take oral contraceptives, you should be prepared to use an additional form of birth control, because there are times the pill's effectiveness can be diminished.

1. **Skipping Pills.** This is probably the main reason for reduced effectiveness. Directions for what to do after missing a dose vary with the pill formula and are included in the package insert that comes with all pills. Using a backup method for the rest of the cycle (while continuing to take the pill) will increase protection from pregnancy.

2. **Illness.** If you become sick with vomiting or diarrhea, your oral contraceptives may not be fully absorbed. It is safest to use an additional method for the rest of the cycle.

3. **Drug Interaction.** Some medications can diminish the pill's effectiveness, including certain antibiotics (rifampin, and perhaps ampicillin and tetracycline); epilepsy drugs (Dilantin); anti-inflammatory or antiarthritic drugs (phenylbutazone); and barbiturates (phenobarbital). If you are treated for any ailment, even one that seems totally unrelated to pill use, be sure to inform your physician if you take birth control pills.

Should You Take the Pill?

Many women are attracted by the advantages of the pill but are also concerned by the list of possible complications. Keep in mind that the process of weighing the benefits and risks is a highly individual one. No two women have exactly the same medical history or birth control needs. A doctor will help you make the best decision for *you*.

For some women the pill is ruled out altogether. Using pills with estrogen is too risky for women who have had blood clots, heart attack, or stroke; chest pain caused by angina pectoris; known or suspected breast cancer or cancer of the uterine lining; undiagnosed abnormal vaginal bleeding (which may indicate cancer and must be checked out); liver tumors; or jaundice during pregnancy.

Other health problems may also forbid pill use. These include fibroid uterine growths, diabetes, high cholesterol levels, high blood pressure, obesity, depression, gall bladder disease, and exposure to DES before birth.

In addition, because the pill tends to cause the body to retain water, women with a history of migraine headaches, asthma, epilepsy, or kidney and heart diseases may find the pill worsens their condition. If they choose to take it, they must be monitored closely by their doctors. Cigarette smoking and age also add to the chances of a woman developing serious pill-related complications.

But what about a woman without any of these risk factors? Once a woman's doctor has found that she has no detectable physical reason for avoiding the pill, the decision is in her hands. The pill carries a relatively small risk of serious complications even to the safest group of users—young, healthy nonsmokers. Therefore it is important that the decision be an informed one.

Understanding the Risks

The "patient leaflet" that comes with all pills contains a complete list of potential complications. Women should remember, though:

- The pill affects all body cells, so the potential complications linked with it are many. But the chances of most young, healthy, non-smoking women developing a particular complication are slim.

- The most serious side effects are also the most rare.

- Many of the risks known today were estimated through studies of *older* women using the *higher* dose pills. Therefore some experts believe that these studies may overstate the likelihood of complications in *younger* women using the newer *low-dose* pills or mini-pills.

- Knowledge of the health risks associated with childbirth can help to place in perspective the problems associated with pill use. The chances of dying from a childbirth complication exceed the chances of dying from a pill complication, except for smoking pill users aged 35 and over. As shown in the chart below, in either event, death is very rare. (Many women die each year for other reasons, including accidents and other health problems, as shown by the overall death rate included below for comparison.)

Cause of Death	Ages 15-19	20-24	25-29	30-34	35-39	40-44
Childbirth	5	6	7	13	21	22
Pill complications, smokers	2	4	6	12	31	61
Pill complications, nonsmokers	1	1	2	3	9	18
All causes, including accidents	54	67	74	98	146	237

Table 13.8. Estimated Annual Deaths per 100,000 Women.

193

Other Considerations: Minor Side Effects

The pill also causes many minor side effects. Although they are not life threatening, they are nuisances and many women stop taking the pill because of them.

A minority of women on the pill experience nausea or vomiting (usually only in the first few cycles), weight changes, breast tenderness, abdominal cramps, or skin discoloration. Bladder and vaginal infections may also occur more frequently with pill use. In addition, some women report changes in sex drive (either increased or decreased), a loss of scalp hair, or an intolerance to contact lenses (because of water retention).

Many of these complaints disappear after the first few cycles of pill use. They may occur less often with low-dose pills and mini-pills. The newer formulas, however, are more likely to cause menstrual irregularities, such as spotting, breakthrough bleeding (which should be reported to a doctor), or, rarely, a lack of periods altogether. Menstrual irregularities are much more common with mini-pills than with combined pills, but cycles often become regular with time.

Knowing the Benefits, Too

The combined pill, when taken properly, is unmatched in effectiveness. And the pill in general allows more spontaneity in sexual relations than barrier methods that must be applied at the time of intercourse.

These benefits have long been known. But we are now learning that the pill protects women from some relatively common and potentially serious disorders that have nothing to do with its use as a contraceptive. According to recent estimates, each year, the pill prevents:

- 51,000 cases of pelvic inflammatory disease, 13,300 of which would have required hospitalization,
- 20,000 hospitalizations for certain types of noncancerous breast disease,
- 9,900 hospitalizations for ectopic pregnancy,
- 3,000 hospitalizations for ovarian cysts,
- 27,000 cases of iron deficiency anemia, and
- 2,700 cases of rheumatoid arthritis.

The protection against pelvic inflammatory disease (PID) may be the most important non-contraceptive benefit of the pill. PID—a bacterial infection of the uterus, fallopian tubes, or ovaries—affects an estimated 850,000 U.S. women yearly. It can lead to infertility or, in rare cases, death. Studies have shown that women on the pill have half the chance of developing PID compared to women using no form of birth control. (Women using barrier devices also have half the chance.)

Other advantages of the pill include less menstrual cramping, lighter blood flow, and for those using combined pills, very regular periods. Some women using oral contraceptives also have diminished premenstrual tension. And women with acne often find the pill improves their complexion.

The Major Risk

The most serious side effect of oral contraceptive use is an increased risk of cardiovascular disease—specifically blood clots, heart attacks, and strokes. But even these complications are occurring less frequently, according to Bruce Stadel, M.D. (NICHD), as a result of lower hormone content in pills, better screening of women who might be at high risk, and, perhaps most importantly, the recent drop in pill use among women over 35.

What Are the Odds?

Pill-related heart attacks are very rare. They occur in an estimated one in 14,000 users between the ages of 30 and 39. Between the ages of 40 and 44 the risk rises to about one case in 1,500 women on the pill.

Strokes occur five times more frequently among women taking oral contraceptives. But they are a rare event, too, affecting about one in 2,700 women on the pill.

Although clots in the veins occur more often than heart attacks or strokes, they are still uncommon, affecting about one in 500 previously healthy women on the pill. Hormone changes in pregnancy cause clots far more frequently than pills do.

Who Are the High Risk Women?

The vast majority of heart attacks and strokes among pill users occur in women who smoke, women over 35, and women with other health conditions, such as high blood pressure, that ordinarily contribute to cardiovascular risk. Women with a combination of two or more of these factors carry the greatest risk of all. (See "Compounding the Risks.")

Some research shows that the length of pill use can affect the chances of having a cardiovascular complication. A recent study found that women aged 40 to 49 who had taken the pill for five or more years had twice the average heart attack risk—even years after they stopped taking the pill. Heavy smoking adds far more to the chances of having a heart attack, however.

Perhaps surprisingly, age and smoking habits do not seem to increase the chances of developing blood clots in the veins. But women with certain blood types—A, B, or AB—are twice as likely to develop clots as women with type 0. This is true whether a woman is on the pill or not.

NICHD-funded research has shown that women who experience clotting disorders may lack the ability to produce extra amounts of a certain anti-clotting blood protein that women on the pill need. Unfortunately it is not yet possible to predict who will have this problem. But researchers have found evidence suggesting that women may counteract it through regular exercise, which may spur the body to produce more of the anti-clotting protein.

Because oral contraceptives double the chances of developing blood clots after surgery, doctors advise women taking the pill to stop, if possible, at least four weeks before any scheduled operation. And all women on the pill should know the symptoms that indicate a possible blood clot—sharp pain in the chest, coughing blood, or sudden shortness of breath; pain in the calf; or sudden partial or complete loss of vision—and notify their doctors immediately if they experience any of them.

High Blood Pressure

Although many women experience a mild elevation in blood pressure when they are taking oral contraceptives, it usually remains within the normal range and returns to "pre-pill" levels when they stop. Studies several years ago found that pill users have three to six times the average risk of developing high blood pressure. It has been estimated to occur in one to four percent of women who take the pill and is usually confined to those over 35. Newer studies show that high blood pressure is not a common problem for today's younger pill takers. But all women on the pill should have their blood pressure checked every six to 12 months.

Compounding the Risks

Factors such as smoking, increasing age, or high blood pressure add to the chances of developing cardiovascular disorders—problems in the heart or blood vessels. Combine any of these factors with oral contraceptive use, and the risks multiply. And when a woman has more than one risk factor, her chances of a serious pill complication skyrocket.

Smoking

Most of the women who have a heart attack or stroke while using the pill are smokers. The mechanism is not understood, but the pill somehow intensifies the adverse effects of smoking on the circulatory system.

To illustrate: One study found that either using oral contraceptives or smoking increased the odds of having a stroke by about six times. In women who both smoked and took the pill, the risks did not just add together. Instead, they jumped to 22 times the risk of stroke in women who neither smoked nor took the pill. The

All smokers using the pill are at greater risk than nonsmokers. The likelihood of heart attack or stroke rises sharply for those who smoke more than 15 cigarettes per day. From the standpoint of safety, doctors now advise pill users not to just cut back, but to quit smoking altogether.

Age

The natural aging process also increases the chances of developing cardiovascular disorders, and birth control pills accentuate the risk. An example: In women who don't use the pill, those aged 40 to 44 are about five times as likely to have a heart attack as those aged 30 to 39. But in pill users, the older age group is about nine times as likely to have a heart attack.

The cardiovascular risks of the pill begin to rise substantially around age 30, particularly in smokers. However, there is no definite cutoff age for pill use. Some doctors believe that regardless of smoking habits, women should consider other forms of contraception starting at age 30. Others feel that at age 30, women who smoke and take the pill should choose between the two, while nonsmokers are relatively safe until age 35. Still others hold that the new low-dose pills and mini-pills may be safe options for women over 35 who do not smoke or have other unfavorable health conditions.

Obviously, the final word is not yet in. Over the next few years, NICHD-supported studies should help clarify the pill's risks to women over 30.

Health Conditions

Women at any age with health problems that ordinarily increase the chances of cardiovascular disease are even more at risk when using the pill. The conditions include:

- high blood pressure,
- a history of high blood pressure in pregnancy,
- obesity,
- diabetes mellitus, and
- elevated cholesterol.

Combined Risk Factors

When more than one of the above risk factors are present, the chances of a serious pill complication increase dramatically. A recent study found that the odds of having a heart attack are increased by:

- 3 times among pill users,
- 5 times among smokers,
- 8 times among people with high blood pressure, and
- 170 times among pill users with high blood pressure who smoke.

An expert on oral contraceptives at the Centers for Disease Control (CDC), Dr. Howard Ory, stresses that "the most serious adverse effect of pill use—death from cardiovascular disease—is also the *most preventable.*"

"If women who use the pill would not smoke," he states, "at least *half* of all deaths associated with pill use could be avoided. If in addition, women with other predisposing factors for cardiovascular disease, such as high blood pressure, high cholesterol, and diabetes mellitus would not use the pill, deaths could be further reduced."

The Pill and Cancer

Probably the question women ask most frequently about oral contraceptives is, "Does the pill cause cancer?"

Because most kinds of cancer take so long to develop, the answer must still be tentative, but it is reassuring: There is no firm evidence that the pill causes cancer.

The NICHD and the CDC are currently cosponsoring a long-term project to analyze the pill's relationship to breast cancer and cancer of the reproductive tract. Although final results will not be available until the mid-1980's, the preliminary results are encouraging, showing no association between the pill and breast cancer. Early results also suggest that women who have used the pill for at least one year have *half* the average risk of developing cancer of the ovary and of the endometrium (the lining of the uterus).

No clear cause-and-effect relationship has been established between the pill and cancer of the cervix, but most doctors still feel it is very important for women on the pill to have yearly Pap smears.

One kind of potentially life-threatening cell growth that is linked with the pill is an extremely rare liver tumor known as hepatic adenoma. Although it is not cancerous, it can cause internal bleeding. It occurs in about one in 33,000 pill users per year, mostly women who have taken the pill for about five years or more. Early detection of the condition can make a difference. Make sure that your check-ups include a physical exam of the abdomen.

The Pill and Body Chemistry

Studies of women taking combined pills with at least 50 micrograms of estrogen show changes in the levels of sugars, fats and proteins in the blood, and alterations in the way the body uses certain nutrients. These and other metabolic changes can cause slightly altered thyroid, liver and blood tests, though results usually remain within the normal range.

While it appears that metabolic changes are lessened with the newer formulas, the long-range effects of even small changes in body chemistry in pill users are unknown. Current studies supported by the NICHD are expected to define these changes more precisely and to determine whether they affect the risk of cardiovascular disease in pill users.

Nutritional Changes

Oral contraceptives can affect nutritional status, but studies of this topic often have conflicting results. This is because many variables, such as hormone shifts throughout a menstrual cycle, can also change the body's nutritional needs.

In women taking the combined pill, studies have found increased levels of vitamin A and iron; decreased levels of vitamins B-6, B-12, C, and riboflavin; and both increases and decreases in levels of folic acid and zinc.

A lowered level of vitamin B-6 is the most consistently reported nutritional change in pill users. One NICHD-funded study found that lowered levels of B-6 during pregnancy and lactation were more common in women who used the pill for a long time (more than 30 months), and became pregnant within four months after stopping the pill. Nevertheless, it is uncertain whether pill use is a cause of true vitamin B-6 deficiency, which is linked with depression (see next page). Other symptoms of vitamin deficiency include weakness, lethargy, dizziness, skin and gum irritations, and an increased susceptibility to infection.

Next to vitamin B-6, folic acid is the nutrient most significantly affected by the pill. Changes in folic acid metabolism have been reported in connection with two conditions in pill users. A few women using oral contraceptives have developed a rare but serious anemia which responds to treatment with folic acid supplements. In addition, the pill is linked with changes in folic acid metabolism in cells around the cervix, which may be related to a kind of abnormal cell growth called cervical dysplasia. An NICHD-supported study found that cervical dysplasia sometimes improves with folic acid supplements.

For pill users, a balanced diet is often recommended over routine vitamin and mineral supplements for two reasons. First, overdosing on supplements can be toxic, and second, people taking supplements often do not try as hard to get a balanced diet. Vitamin supplements cannot take the place of a balanced diet; in fact, they need to have proper foods present to work right. But when medical tests show a vitamin deficiency, vitamin supplement therapy may be in order.

Recent studies on oral contraceptives and metabolism found that pill users do not eliminate caffeine or valium as efficiently as nonusers. This means that either substance can accumulate in the body. As a result, women using the pill may be more prone to caffeine side effects such as nervousness and insomnia. Those using valium could become over-sedated if the dosage is not carefully watched.

Depression

Oral contraceptives alleviate depression in some women and worsen it in others. Symptoms of depression related to pill use include pessimism, dissatisfaction, listlessness, tension, crying, and perhaps anxiety or a loss of sex drive. Although many of the reports of pill-related depression came when higher doses of estrogen were widely used, it is not clear whether depression is less common with the newer low-dose pills or mini-pills.

Depression can be a symptom of vitamin B-6 deficiency. The pill can affect the body's use of B-6 and other vitamins and minerals, and studies have found that some depressed pill users are B-6 deficient. These women may respond to vitamin B-6 therapy. Women who become seriously depressed while on the pill should discuss it with their physicians, and consider switching to another form of birth control.

The Pill and Childbearing

Many women taking birth control pills are planning to have children at some time. For them the news is good: There appears to be little risk that use of the pill leads to sterility. In fact, because the pill protects many women from pelvic inflammatory disease, which can damage the fallopian tubes, it guards against a leading cause of infertility.

Fertility

Former pill users may take a few months longer to conceive than other women, but an estimated 80 percent of women resume normal reproductive functions within three months after stopping the pill and more than 95 percent are ovulating within a year.

Women who do not regain normal periods within six months should see a doctor for a complete evaluation. Most women who have menstrual problems after stopping the pill had irregular periods before they started taking it. But some studies suggest that there is a very slim chance that the pill itself causes a condition known as "post-pill amenorrhea"—a lack of periods. Though the cause of the problem is a matter of much debate among researchers, infertility after stopping the pill generally is temporary and responds to treatment.

Pregnancy

Many doctors recommend that women who wish to become pregnant use traditional barrier contraceptives for at least three months after stopping the pill. Usually, a woman's menstrual cycle will become regular during this time, which permits the doctor to accurately date the start of the pregnancy. When former pill users do become pregnant, they have no greater risk of complications than other women.

Although it happens extremely rarely, oral contraceptives can fail even when a woman has been conscientious about taking them every day. In addition to causing an unplanned pregnancy, pill failure can lead to inadvertent exposure of a developing fetus to extra hormones. Some studies show a slight increased risk of birth defects in infants exposed before birth to oral contraceptive hormones; other studies have found no risk. Experts generally agree that the risks, if they exist at all, are very small.

But for absolute safety, if you even suspect you might be pregnant, immediately stop taking the pill, switch to another form of contraception, and have a pregnancy test as soon as possible. Studies have shown no added risk of birth defects when conception occurs one month after stopping the pill.

Breastfeeding

Physicians often recommend methods other than the pill for women who are nursing babies. For one thing, the estrogen in combined pills can suppress milk production. Also, very small quantities of hormones pass from the mother to her nursing infant. Although no long-term effects of this ingestion have been reported, the possibility of risk to the baby has not been extensively studied. For women who want to breastfeed and use an oral contraceptive, doctors frequently suggest the mini-pill, since it does not suppress lactation.

How to Minimize the Risks

Both doctors and the women for whom they prescribe birth control pills have a role in reducing the chances of pill related complications. Doctors must screen patients carefully, follow up conscientiously, and prescribe the lowest possible dose that is compatible with an individual woman's needs. Yet as recently as 1978, one-fourth of the women taking the pill in the United States were still using formulas with more than 50 micrograms of estrogen. Check your prescription: If it contains more than 50 micrograms, you might ask your physician if you can try a lower dose.

Women must be open with their doctors, informing them of any health problems. They must also know the signs that indicate a possibly serious complication of pill use and call their doctors immediately (see next page). In addition, women on the pill should exercise regularly. Above all, they should have medical checkups at least yearly (more frequently if their doctors advise).

Twenty years ago there was hope that the pill would prove to be the perfect form of birth control: effective, convenient, and safe for all women. Ten years ago reports of side effects brought disillusionment. Today we know that the pill, though imperfect, is an option many women can use safely. We now have better formulas, better screening of women, and a better informed public. And as these trends continue we can look forward to even safer use of the pill.

Warning Signals

Women taking oral contraceptives should be alert to any physical or mental change that may warrant a visit to the doctor. If you experience any of the following symptoms, notify your physician at once and remind him or her that you are on the pill.

- Severe abdominal pain
- Chest pain, coughing, shortness of breath
- Pain or tenderness in calf or thigh
- Severe headache, dizziness, or faintness
- Muscle weakness or numbness
- Speech disturbance
- Eye problems: blurred vision, flashing lights, blindness
- Breast lump
- Severe depression
- Yellowing of skin

—by Maureen Gardner

Section 13.5

Depo-Provera: The Quarterly Contraceptive

FDA Consumer Publication No. 93-3206, July 1993.

It may be the birth control compromise many women have been looking for. Falling in between the daily effort of remembering the pill and the once-every-five years appointment for the implant, one injection of Depo-Provera in the muscle of the arm or buttocks protects against pregnancy for three months.

The Food and Drug Administration approved Depo-Provera, manufactured by The Upjohn Co., Kalamazoo, Mich., for contraception in October 1992. The active ingredient in Depo-Provera is a synthetic hormone similar to the natural hormone progesterone.

"I was not happy with other methods," says Becky Schroder, of Jacksonville, Fla. "I was a poor pill taker. I forgot. And I thought that barrier methods were inconvenient and messy."

Schroder, 31, started on Depo-Provera three years ago, when its use as a contraceptive was still investigational. (FDA had previously approved the drug for treating endometrial and renal cancers.)

Depo-Provera inhibits the production of the hormone, gonadotropin, which, in turn, prevents ovulation. Depo-Provera also causes changes in the lining of the uterus that make pregnancy less likely to occur.

Depo-Provera's estimated effectiveness in preventing pregnancy is 99 percent, on a par with Norplant, the contraceptive implant. Norplant contains another synthetic progestin hormone, levonorgestrel.

Mark Your Calendar

The amount of Depo-Provera in the bloodstream is at the highest level just after injection. Over time, the level drops and after three months, the level may no longer offer enough protection against conception.

"Go back on time for the next injection," says Ridgely Bennett, M.D., the FDA medical officer responsible for reviewing the new drug application for Depo-Provera. "That should be made abundantly clear."

He adds that if the time between injections is greater than 14 weeks, the physician should make sure the woman isn't pregnant before giving her the next injection.

Getting Started

A woman should get her first injection of Depo-Provera within five days after the start of her menstrual period. The drug is effective immediately, so no other birth control is necessary.

Because Depo-Provera is not a barrier contraceptive, however, it offers no protection against sexually transmitted diseases such as AIDS, herpes, chlamydia, and gonorrhea. For optimum protection from both disease and pregnancy, couples may choose to use both Depo-Provera and a condom.

A woman who has just had a baby—and wants to wait before having another—should get her shot within five days after the birth if she is not breast-feeding, and six weeks after the baby is born, if she is.

Although numerous studies by the World Health Organization have shown that Depo-Provera does not have any adverse effects on breast milk production or composition, or on the health of the nursing infant, it's best not to expose a newborn to the drug in the first six weeks, according to Philip Corfman, M.D., a supervisory medical officer in FDA's division of metabolism and endocrine drug products. "It's just a precaution," he says.

If a woman decides at the end of three months that she wants to get pregnant, she simply doesn't get the next injection. But, because the length of time between the last injection and becoming pregnant varies widely, any woman starting Depo-Provera should be sure she doesn't want to become pregnant for the next year or two, says Susan Wysocki, executive director of the National Association of Nurse Practitioners in Reproductive Health.

According to the approved physician's label, "the median time to conception for those who do conceive is 10 months following the last injection with a range of four to 31 months." Since Depo-Provera does not accumulate in the body, the return to fertility is independent of the number of injections received, but may be affected by a women's age or weight.

A women should not take Depo-Provera if she has acute liver disease, unexplained vaginal bleeding, breast cancer, or blood clots in the legs, lungs or eyes.

"She also shouldn't have a fear of injections," Wysocki says.

Side Effects

Change in the menstrual cycle is the most common side effect of Depo-Provera. At first there may be irregular bleeding or spotting, but that usually diminishes and eventually disappears after several injections. After a year on Depo-Provera, menstruation will stop completely in approximately half of the women.

Normal menstruation will usually return within a few months once the injections stop.

Women who continue to menstruate while on Depo-Provera may have decreased blood flow, which, in turn, reduces the chance of anemia. There may also be a decrease in menstrual cramps and pain as well as ovulatory pain.

Schroder, who had very painful premenstrual symptoms before starting Depo-Provera, says she thinks of these side effects as benefits.

After menstrual changes, the most common side effect is weight gain. "It's not clear whether the weight gain is due to water retention or a metabolic effect that increases appetite and body fat," says David Grimes, M.D., a professor with the department of obstetrics and gynecology at the University of Southern California School of Medicine. "But it is real, and women should know about it."

In addition, some patients may experience headache, nervousness, abdominal pain, dizziness, weakness, or fatigue.

Breast Cancer Concerns

The possibility of a link between Depo-Provera and breast cancer was first considered in the early 1970s, after breast cancers were found in beagles treated for more than three years with a dose of Depo-Provera equivalent to 25 times that of the human contraceptive dose. However, those studies were eventually discounted at an October 1981 meeting of the World Health Organization. Experts at that meeting concluded, and FDA later agreed, that beagles were not appropriate animal models for determining what the potential effects of Depo-Provera would be on women.

Ten years later, WHO presented the results of a study of over 11,000 women who used Depo-Provera, mainly in Thailand and New Zealand. (The drug has been approved for contraception in about 90 countries.) Based on the study, published in the Oct. 5, 1991, issue of *The Lancet*, WHO concluded that, overall, women on Depo-Provera are not at increased risk of breast cancer. In addition, breast cancer risk did not increase the longer a woman stayed on the injectable contraceptive.

The study did find a slight increase in the risk of breast cancer during the first four years of use, primarily in women under 35. That increase, however, is statistically weak and comparable to the risk associated with oral contraceptives, according to the researchers.

But the National Women's Health Network disagrees with the researchers' conclusion. In testimony presented to FDA's Fertility and Maternal Health Drugs Advisory Committee last June, Cindy Pearson, a representative of the National Women's Health Network, said that the WHO studies were conducted in countries with breast cancer rates less than half that of the United States and therefore can't be accurately applied to women in this country.

She adds that comparing the breast cancer risk to that associated with oral contraceptives is also misleading. "These disturbing data are emerging from much smaller groups of women than was the case with oral contraceptives," she said. "Only three epidemiologic studies have been done on Depo-Provera and breast cancer, and all three raise a red flag."

However, to Grimes, that increased risk in younger women isn't a link to Depo-Provera. Instead, "It suggests to me that women who start taking Depo-Provera may be coming into the health-care system for the first time and having preexisting tumors discovered."

"It should be noted," says FDA's Bennett, "that more data on breast cancer risk is now available for Depo-Provera than has been required for any other drug prior to marketing."

The results of the WHO study also indicated that Depo-Provera use did not increase the overall risk of cancer of the liver, ovaries, endometrium, or cervix.

Osteoporosis Risk?

A study by Tim Cundy and colleagues, published in the July 6, 1991, issue of the *British Medical Journal* found that the bone density in 30 women who had been using Depo-Provera for at least five years was less than the bone density of other women of similar age. Cundy recommends "that women with more than one risk factor for osteoporosis [family history, underweight, cigarette smoking, European or Asian origin] should have bone mineral density measurements undertaken if they are considering Depo-Provera use on a continuing basis, and those in the lower third of the normal range are advised to consider other contraceptive methods."

While FDA's Corfman agrees that a woman considering Depo-Provera needs to discuss the possibility of bone thinning with her doctor, he adds, "[the risk of] osteoporosis is just part of the calculation. There are many other issues involved."

FDA is requiring Upjohn to conduct additional research on the effects of Depo-Provera on bone density.

Best Candidates

"[Depo-Provera] has been a godsend for women who've been unable or unwilling to use other methods." says Grimes.

Becky Schroder's plans to have a baby in the next two or three years made her decide against Norplant. Although the implant can be removed at any time. "It isn't cost effective if it's taken out early," she says.

But Pearson, of the National Women's Health Network, is concerned that Depo-Provera will be forced on poor women. She told FDA's advisory committee that "the women's health movement has already documented many cases of coercion even while Depo-Provera was not approved as a contraceptive."

Wysocki acknowledges Pearson's concern. "That concern stems from some very things that happened back in the 60s, particularly with sterilization, but there's no reason to believe that because the technology is available that it will be abused. The problem itself should be addressed, not the drug."

Wysocki adds that Depo-Provera is a safe, low-cost method of contraception that requires little attention. "No one method of contraception is perfect for all women at all times during their reproductive years," she says. "However, additional options increase the likelihood that a method of contraception that matches each woman's need will be found."

—by Dori Stehlin

208

Section 13.6

Norplant: Birth Control at Arm's Reach

FDA Consumer, May 1991.

Norplant consists of a familiar ingredient in a new package. Six silicone rubber capsules about the size of matchsticks contain a synthetic progestin hormone long used in birth control pills. The flexible tubes are inserted in a fan-like arrangement and can be felt but not easily seen.

Once in place, they steadily release a low dose of hormone into the bloodstream. Effective within 24 hours after insertion, Norplant can continue to prevent pregnancy for up to five years.

The hormone usually inhibits ovulation so that eggs are not produced regularly, and causes the mucus of the cervix to thicken, making it more difficult for sperm to reach the egg. Other ways that Norplant may provide contraceptive effects have been proposed but not proven.

Experimental Attitude

Jennifer Collier, a 28-year-old New York law student, entered a study of Norplant at the Robert Wood Johnson Institute in New Brunswick, N.J., in the spring of 1984 and is now on her second implant, inserted last June.

"It sounded like a really neat invention, so I decided to try it," says Collier. She had been dissatisfied with the weight gain and irritability she experienced using oral contraceptives. With Norplant, she says, she isn't troubled with either of those side effects. Collier describes the implant as visible, "but not terribly obvious. No one has noticed it unless they were looking for it, probably partly because of where it's inserted."

Each Norplant capsule is 2.4 millimeters (about one-tenth of an inch) in diameter and 34 millimeters (just under one-and-a-half inches) long, and holds 36 milligrams of powdered crystals of the progestin levonorgestrel. The tubes are made of Silastic, a silicone material long used in surgical implants such as heart valves and hip joints.

The hormone seeps through the permeable tubes into the bloodstream, initially at a rate of about 85 micrograms a day. The amount declines gradually to about 50 micrograms by nine months, 35 by 18 months, and about 30 micrograms at the end of five years. In comparison, birth control pills that contain levonorgestrel provide about 50 to 150 micrograms of the progestin a day, plus estrogen. (The only progestin-only contraceptive available in the United States contains 75 micrograms of norgestrel, a progestin similar to levonorgestrel.)

When the hormone supply dwindles, usually in about five years, a new implant can be inserted if desired. On the other hand, if a woman wishes to become pregnant earlier, she can have the implants removed at any time, and fertility is restored very soon. Blood levels of the progestin are undetectable within 5 to 14 days.

Population Council Project

Norplant has been marketed in other countries for several years. According to the Population Council, more than half a million women in 46 countries have used the implant since it was first approved in Finland—where it is manufactured—in 1983. It now has regulatory approval in 17 other countries as well, including Sweden, Indonesia, the Dominican Republic, Thailand, China, Peru, and the United States. Norplant's U.S. distributor is the Philadelphia-based pharmaceutical firm Wyeth-Ayerst Laboratories.

"The first implants were tested in 1968," says Population Council vice president Wayne Bardin, M.D., "and then the council began to develop and test implants that released a whole variety of progestins. By 1974, we came up with what is now the Norplant implant, using levonorgestrel. The first clinical trial of that was begun in 1975."

FDA approval of the implant was based on the results of clinical studies involving 2,400 women in the United States, Finland, Sweden, Denmark, Jamaica, Brazil, Chile, and the Dominican Republic.

In the studies, the contraceptive's effectiveness approached that of sterilization in the first year.

Pregnancy rates were slightly higher in heavier women, increasing after the third year of use in those who weighed more than 69 kilograms (153 pounds). Nevertheless, the protection is still quite good. For example, among 100 women of all weights using the implant for five years, it is expected that four would become pregnant during that time. By contrast, of 100 women using the pill for the same time, at least 15 might be expected to become pregnant.

Norplant's effectiveness does not depend on patient compliance—a feature shared by only one other type of reversible contraceptive—the intrauterine device, or IUD. This particularly appeals to Collier for the convenience it affords. "Unlike the pill, you don't have to remember to take it every day, and, unlike the diaphragm, there's no problem with spontaneity," she says.

Because Norplant is not a barrier contraceptive, however, it offers no protection against sexually transmitted diseases such as AIDS, herpes, chlamydia, and gonorrhea. For optimum protection from both disease and pregnancy, couples may choose to use both Norplant and a condom.

The Drawbacks

As with virtually any drug or medical device, Norplant isn't entirely trouble free. Side effects that women have reported with the implant during the first year include irregular menstrual bleeding, headache, nervousness, depression, nausea, dizziness, skin rash, acne, change of appetite, breast tenderness, weight gain, enlargement of the ovaries, and excessive growth of body or facial hair.

Some Norplant users have also reported breast discharge, vaginal discharge, inflammation of the cervix, abdominal discomfort, and muscle and skeletal pain. These effects, however, cannot be linked to use of the implant because the complaints are common among the general population and could stem from many other causes. There is no known biological reason to link the complaints specifically to use of the contraceptive.

By far, the most common side effect is menstrual cycle irregularity. "To give the percentage of women with menstrual irregularities is complex," says Bardin, "because it changes with time." He says that over a five-year period of use, about 45 percent of women will have irregular periods and another 45 percent will have normal periods. The remaining 10 percent will have long periods of time—three to four months—with no bleeding. "That's an average," says Bardin. "Basically what happens is you have more women with irregular periods in the first year and that tends to diminish with continuing use."

The bleeding irregularities result from the continuous hormone release. "With the oral contraceptive pills, estrogen and progestin are taken for three weeks and withdrawn for one week, causing regular bleeding," explains Lisa Rarick, M.D., a medical officer in FDA's division of endocrine and metabolism drug products. "Norplant, on the other hand," says Rarick, "provides no cyclic withdrawal, and thus each individual creates her own bleeding pattern."

In the multi-center trials, more women had increases in their hemoglobin concentrations than decreases, indicating that they lost less menstrual blood when using Norplant. (Hemoglobin is the oxygen-carrying pigment of red blood cells that gives them their red color and serves to transport oxygen to tissues.) Bardin says that this is because, on average, even if the number of bleeding days increases in the first year of use, the total amount of blood lost may be less than would be lost without hormonal contraception.

He says that most women who use Norplant don't perceive bleeding as a problem. "To illustrate," he says, "if you say, 'What is the biggest complaint that women have about Norplant,' it's bleeding irregularities. But if you ask all women if bleeding irregularities bother them, something like 60 percent say 'no.' "

Collier says she has spotting and a lighter flow with Norplant. "Sometimes, I have no discernible cycle at all," she says, but maintains that "although of course I'd rather have regular periods, the effects are not that bad."

Nevertheless, the major reason women give for discontinuing Norplant is bleeding problems, accounting for about 9 percent of those who stop in the first year, according to FDA's Rarick. Another 5 percent stop for other medical reasons, from headaches to dizziness, and perhaps another 5 percent stop for other reasons, including to have a baby. She estimates that about 60 to 65 percent of women continue with the implant longer than two years.

Not for Everyone

More serious complications are possible as well, and Norplant is not recommended for everyone. As with oral contraceptives, women with acute liver disease or liver tumors—whether malignant or benign—unexplained vaginal bleeding, breast cancer, or blood clots in the legs, lungs or eyes should not use the implant.

Norplant contains only progestin, whereas most oral contraceptives contain both progestin and estrogen. Some side effects of the pill, such as eye disorders and increased risk of cardiovascular problems among women who smoke, are believed to be related to the estrogen component.

Nevertheless, FDA advises physicians to "consider the possible increased risks associated with oral contraceptives, including elevated blood pressure, thromboembolic disorders [blood clots obstructing blood vessels], and other vascular problems that might occur with use of the contraceptive implant."

Bardin suggests that Norplant will be most attractive to women who:

- wish to use highly effective low-dose hormone contraception
- want long-term contraception after completing their family, but don't want sterilization
- want to delay childbearing for an extended period of time
- cannot use estrogens
- are unhappy with other forms of contraception.

On the flip side, Bardin expects the implant to be less popular among women who:

- are happy with their present form of contraception
- cannot or do not want to pay the upfront cost of Norplant
- will not tolerate irregular menstrual bleeding if it should occur
- do not want to use a method that requires a visit to a health-care professional to discontinue. ("Some women feel that puts them at the mercy of the clinic and they want to be able to stop it any time they want," says Bardin. "That's why they like pills and barrier methods–it's under their control," he says.)

Surgical Insertion

Successful use of the Norplant system depends on careful insertion of the capsules. Wyeth-Ayerst markets the implant as a kit with detailed instructions for insertion and removal, and, through the Association of Reproductive Health Professionals, offers physician training programs as well.

The firm describes the insertion as a minor, outpatient surgical procedure requiring only 10 to 15 minutes. The area is numbed with a local anesthetic, and a small incision, less than an eighth of an inch long, is made. Using a special instrument called a trocar, the physician places the six capsules just under the skin. The incision is then covered with protective gauze and a small adhesive bandage. Stitches are not required.

When the anesthetic wears off, there may be some tenderness or itching, and perhaps some temporary discoloration, bruising and swelling. Infection at the site of insertion has also been reported.

It takes a bit longer to remove the implant than to insert it—usually from 15 to 20 minutes, according to the distributor. As with insertion, a small incision is made under a local anesthetic. Then the physician removes the capsules and, again, the incision is covered with an adhesive bandage. Sometimes, some capsules may be more difficult to remove than others. When this happens, the woman may have to return a second time, after the area has healed, for removal of the remaining capsules.

The reason for suggesting the second visit, Bardin says, is to let the physician know that "if you have trouble removing, don't cut a big hole in the woman's arm and go fishing around looking for it [the capsule]." If the anesthetic has caused the area to puff up, for example, it may be difficult to feel the implant. "Wait until the next week or whenever she can come in again," says Bardin, "and you'll be able to see it and take it out with minimal trauma."

If desired, a new set of implants can be inserted at the same time the old set is removed, either in the same arm and through the same incision, or in the other arm.

The price to the medical professional for a single Norplant system, which includes all the necessary apparatus for insertion and removal as well as the set of six capsules, has been set at $350. Fees for insertion and related costs, such as counseling and removal, vary, depending on the physician.

Collier says that this will probably be the last Norplant she'll have, at least for a while, as she plans to get pregnant eventually. She's not sure if she would come back to the implant later. "Hormone therapy and the risks associated with it—more with the pill and estrogen than with Norplant—concern me," she says. "I'll just have to see what else might be available when that time comes." For now, Collier is pleased with Norplant and would recommend it to any woman, "especially," she says, "if they're going to be on hormone therapy anyway."

—by Marian Segal

Section 13.7

Your Sterilization Operation

Excerpts from DHSS Publication No. 357-505, revised 1991.

Making Up Your Mind

Sterilization must be considered permanent. For most women, once this operation has been done, it can never be undone. Some doctors try to undo a sterilization with surgery. This is a difficult and expensive operation, and often it doesn't work. Some people call sterilization "tying the tubes." But don't think the tubes can be easily untied! They can't. So it's not a good idea to think your sterilization can be undone.

Make sure you do not want to bear children under any circumstances before you decide to be sterilized. Are you sure you would not want to have children even if one of your present children died? Or your husband died? Or you got divorced and remarried? Be sure of your decision before you decide to be sterilized. Talk it over with your family or others you trust.

No one can force you to be sterilized! Don't let anyone push you into it. If you do not want to be sterilized, no one can take away any of your Federal benefits such as welfare, Social Security, or health care including sterilization at a later date. No one can force you to be sterilized as a condition for delivering your baby or performing an abortion.

To have this operation paid for with Federal funds, you must be at least 21 years old. If you are married, discuss the operation with your husband. However, his consent is not required if Medicaid or any Federal government program is going to pay for your operation. Your consent to sterilization cannot be obtained while you are in the hospital for childbirth or abortion, or if you are under the influence of alcohol or other substances that affect your state of awareness. You must sign the consent form at least 30 days before you plan to have the operation. This is so you will have at least 30 days to think it over and discuss it with your family and others. You may change your mind any time before the operation and cancel your appointment.

When Can a Woman Have a Sterilization Operation?

A sterilization operation can be done at different times. A talk with your doctor or clinic can help you decide what might be most suitable for you.

A woman may choose to have a sterilization operation at any time in her life. It doesn't matter if she is not married or doesn't have children. It is up to her. Sterilization done at too young an age or before a woman has any children may result in regret later. Circumstances can also change in your life which might cause you to regret your decision to be sterilized.

A woman can have a sterilization operation right after having a baby. This means that a woman may want to be sterilized while she is in the hospital for the delivery. A woman should think about this early in her pregnancy because in order for the sterilization to be paid for with Federal funds she must sign the consent form at least 30 days before the baby is due. If the woman delivers prematurely or has emergency abdominal surgery at least 72 hours after she has signed the consent form, she does not need to wait 30 days, and the sterilization may be performed at the same time as the other surgery. She should be sure that she does not want to have children again even if the baby does not live very long after birth.

A woman can have a sterilization operation at the same time she has a baby by cesarean section. A sterilization operation can be done at the same time through the same incision, but the woman must make up her mind at least 30 days before the baby is due.

A woman can have a sterilization operation when she is having another type of surgery if she has signed the consent form at least 30 days previously.

A woman can have a sterilization operation done at any other time as well. The operation need not be done at the time of childbirth, cesarean section or another surgery.

Facts about the Operation

The surgical method of family planning is called a tubal sterilization or tubal ligation.

In this operation the doctor blocks your two tubes to prevent the sperm and egg from uniting. Menstruation (monthly period) continues following sterilization. Tubal sterilization will not cause menopause (change of life). Sterilization does not offer protection against sexually transmitted diseases, including HIV/AIDS.

Is the Operation Guaranteed to Work?

Tubal sterilization works almost all the time. On the average only 4 out of every 1,000 women who have the operation will still get pregnant. Failures occur when sterilization surgery is performed after the woman is already pregnant or when there is incomplete blocking of the woman's tubes. You should use some temporary method of family planning until you have your operation.

The Anesthetic

With any method of sterilization, you will first be given an anesthetic (a drug to keep you from feeling pain during the operation). A medical person who specializes in anesthesia may do this part of the operation.

Sometimes the operation is done under "general" anesthesia. That means you will be asleep during the operation. The drugs used are a gas which you inhale and/or a liquid given to you by injection.

Sometimes the operation is done under "local" anesthesia or "spinal" anesthesia. That means you are awake.

A local anesthetic is given by injection into the skin. It makes your skin numb.

A spinal anesthetic is given by injection low in the spine. This type of injection makes you feel numb from the waist down. With local or spinal anesthesia, you may also be given pills or another injection to help you relax.

You should have a chance to discuss and participate in the decision regarding your type of anesthesia before your operation.

Benefits of Tubal Sterilization

The benefits of tubal sterilization are:

- You never have to use a temporary method of family planning again (such as the pill or the diaphragm).
- You don't have to worry about getting pregnant.

Discomforts and Risks

No matter which type of operation you have, you can expect to feel pain and soreness in your abdomen for a few days. You can take medicine to help relieve the discomfort.

If you had general anesthesia, you may have a sore throat for a day or two from the tube used to keep your airway open while you were asleep. This goes away quickly and is not serious. Spinal anesthesia may give some persons a temporary headache.

Sterilization operations have some risks, including a very small risk of death. This is true of any type of operation. Serious problems rarely happen. Most of the time serious problems can be treated and cured by the doctor without further surgery; however, an operation may be necessary to correct some of these problems.

Some of the medical problems you could have during or after a sterilization operation include:

1. You may bleed from the incision on your skin or in your vagina.

2. You may bleed inside your abdomen. (Another operation may be necessary to stop the bleeding.)

3. You may get an infection on or near the stitches or inside your abdomen.

4. The operation may not make you sterile. The operation cannot be guaranteed 100% to make you sterile. On the average 4 out of 1,000 women get pregnant after the operation. When this happens there is a possibility that the pregnancy may be in the tube. This would require immediate medical or surgical care.

5. As in other operations, the anesthetic drug used to put you to sleep or to make the operation painless may cause problems. You may vomit while under anesthesia and additional complications may result. As with all surgery, complications sometimes lead to death.

6. You may have damage to your internal organs, such as your bowel or bladder. More medical care or another operation may be necessary to repair the damage.

7. Some women have reported irregular periods, increased cramping or changes in their periods after sterilization.

Go back to your doctor at once if you get a fever or severe pain in your abdomen soon after surgery. Either of these could be signs that you have an infection.

Four Types of Tubal Sterilization

The operation you have depends on your health and your doctor. Talk to him or her about which operation you will have.

1. Laparotomy, Mini-laparotomy
2. Laparoscopy
3. Postpartum tubal sterilization
4. Vaginal tubal sterilization

Laparotomy, Mini-Laparotomy

In both of these operations, the doctor makes an incision (cut) in the lower portion of your abdomen. The difference between the two is the length of the incision and the extensiveness of the surgery. In a mini-laparotomy the incision is very short (one or two inches) and leaves only a small scar. In a laparotomy it is much longer (three to five inches) and leaves a longer scar. Ask your doctor which method he or she uses.

Through the incision on the abdomen, the doctor can reach both tubes, one at a time. The doctor can either remove a section and then use surgical thread to tie the tubes shut or seal them with electric current, bands or clips. After the tubes are sealed, the incision on your abdomen is stitched closed.

The operation, including the anesthesia, takes about 30 minutes. With a mini-laparotomy, you will probably stay in the hospital less than 24 hours and be back to normal in two or three days. With a laparotomy, you will probably be in the hospital two or more days, and it may be two weeks before you feel back to normal.

Laparoscopy

Using a special needle, the doctor inflates your abdomen with gas which pushes your intestines away from your uterus and tubes.

The doctor then makes a small incision about one-half inch long near your navel. A "laparoscope," or special instrument, is inserted through this incision. It is a thin metal tube with a light on it which allows the doctor to see your tubes, and through which the doctor can insert the operating instruments. Your tubes are sealed by the use of electric current, bands, or clips. Some doctors make a second small incision near the pubic hair line to insert one of the operating instruments.

After the gas in your abdomen is released, the incision is closed.

The operation, including the anesthesia, takes about 30 minutes. You will probably stay in the hospital less than 24 hours and be back to normal in two or three days. Because of the gas, you may feel a pain in your neck or shoulders, and you may feel bloated after the surgery. This goes away after a day or two.

Postpartum Tubal Ligation

This operation is done in the hospital shortly after a woman has a baby. The doctor makes a small incision below your navel. The doctor then closes off a section of each tube using surgical threads. After the tubes are tied, a small section between the ties is removed. The incision below your navel is stitched closed.

The operation, including the anesthesia, usually takes about 30 minutes. Having the operation may make your hospital stay a day or two longer. How fast you get better will depend on how you feel after having the baby.

Vaginal Tubal Ligation

In this operation, the doctor makes a small incision far back in the vagina. Through this, the doctor finds your tubes, then closes them off with electric current, bands, or clips, or by removing a small section and closing the ends with surgical threads. After the tubes are sealed, the incision in your vagina is stitched closed.

Sometimes the doctor will use a metal tube with a light (called a culdoscope) to find your tubes.

The operation, including the anesthesia, usually takes about 30 minutes. Your stay in the hospital will probably be less than 24 hours. You should be back to normal in two or three days. After this type of operation, you should not have intercourse for three to four weeks so the vagina can heal.

What about Hysterectomy?

Hysterectomy is the removal of the uterus. A hysterectomy should be done only when there is a disease of the woman's uterus or some other problem that is appropriately treated by removal. Hysterectomy should never be performed for sterilization alone.

A hysterectomy is a much more serious operation than a tubal sterilization. A hysterectomy takes much longer to do, and the woman is in the hospital longer. There are more discomforts, and there is a greater chance of serious complications as a result of hysterectomy. For these reasons, neither Medicaid nor any other Federal program will pay for a hysterectomy if you are having it solely to avoid bearing children.

Summary

If you are sure you do not want to bear children and you want to become permanently sterile, then tubal sterilization is a safe, effective option. It requires a short stay in the hospital, and problems are rare.

If You Have Questions

If there is anything that is not clear to you, or anything you are worried about, it is important that you ask these questions. All of your questions should be answered to your satisfaction before the operation. Remember, you may change your mind at any time before the operation. Make sure you do not wish to bear children under any circumstances before you decide to be sterilized.

Rules for Sterilization Operations Funded by the Federal Government

- You must be at least 21 years old.

- You must wait at least 30 days to have the operation after you sign the consent form except in instances of premature delivery or emergency abdominal surgery that take place at least 72 hours after consent is obtained.

- Your consent to sterilization cannot be obtained while you are in the hospital for childbirth or abortion, or under the influence of alcohol or other substances that affect your state of awareness

- You may, if you choose, bring someone with you when you sign the consent form.

- Your consent is effective for 180 days from the date you sign the consent form.

Your consent to sterilization must be documented by signing a consent form.

Chapter 14

Infertility

Chapter Contents

Section 14.1

Trying to Outsmart Infertility

DHSS Publication No. 94-1181, January, 1994.

The human female is born with about a million eggs—all that she will ever have. Beginning with the onset of menstruation in adolescence and continuing until menopause, her hormones prepare one or two of these eggs for possible fertilization each month. The human male, starting at puberty, makes many millions of sperm a day for the next 50 years or more. Biology, it would seem, generously equips both sexes for parenthood. Yet the National Center for Health Statistics reports that roughly 1 out of every 12 American couples that tries to have a baby fails.

Sometimes, the problem is simply impatience. Medically speaking, a couple generally isn't termed infertile unless there is still no baby on the way after at least a year of regular intercourse without using any form of birth control.

The odds are sharply against conception most of the time. A woman has just a 20 to 35 percent chance of conceiving during each menstrual cycle, even at the peak of her fertility, and that starts to decline slightly in her late 20s and early 30s and more steeply after about age 35. For the many members of the baby boom generation in particular who are late in trying to start families, getting pregnant is not necessarily as easy as the proverbial fall off a log.

The other variable in the childbearing equation is male fertility, which, like female fertility, declines with age, although more slowly.

Fertility is impaired in as many men as women. More specifically, according to Robert D. Visscher, M.D., medical director of the American Fertility Society, the problem lies entirely with the man in about a third of infertile couples and entirely with the woman in about another third. In another group of such couples—some 15 to 20 percent of the total—the fertility of both the man and the woman is below par. There are, besides, couples in whom nothing can be found in either partner to explain the reproductive difficulty. Would-be parents can therefore avoid a lot of heartache by thinking of infertility as "our" problem rather than "mine" or"yours."

Health professionals, too, are coming to recognize the importance of this no-fault philosophy. "The realization that the infertile couple is a unit is probably the greatest advance medicine has made in this field," said Elwyn Grimes, M.D., a Kansas City, Mo., reproductive endocrinologist who serves on a Food and Drug Administration obstetrics and gynecology advisory panel. "When a couple is having trouble having a baby and decides to try to do something about it, it makes no sense to evaluate one partner and not the other. Besides, efforts to overcome infertility require the cooperation of both partners and so put both under considerable emotional stress."

Perhaps most stressful of all is the knowledge that those efforts may come to naught. Systematic studies to determine how often treatment results in a successful pregnancy have not been done. But the consensus of the experts, says the American Fertility Society's Visscher, is that the success rate is, typically, in the 50 percent range. Moreover, a pregnancy is no guarantee that a baby will be born. There is always the possibility of a miscarriage or other complication during the nine months of gestation that will leave a couple with a cradle as empty as before.

Identifying Stumbling Blocks

The mishaps that can befall a pregnancy aside, the biology of setting one in motion is itself enormously complex.

Pregnancy cannot occur unless it is preceded by a long series of hormonally controlled interactions that separately prepare sperm and egg for their missions. A woman will not conceive unless her partner is able to deposit semen in her vagina and his sperm are sufficiently vigorous so that at least one can swim into her fallopian tubes to fertilize a waiting egg. (Each of the two ovaries has its own fallopian tube that leads to the uterus. Because the ovaries normally take turns releasing an egg, each of the tubes normally has an egg in it every other month.)

At the same time, the female must be in hormonal readiness to permit egg and sperm to unite when they meet in the tube, and the tube must be open from end to end. In addition, the muscle of the tube and the eyelash-like hairs on its lining (called cilia) must have enough strength and range of motion to sweep the egg into the uterus after it is fertilized. Even then, the fertilized egg will die if it does not implant in the lining of the uterus and if that lining—which is also under hormonal control—is unable to sustain it.

The considerable progress made in identifying the stumbling blocks to conception is the bedrock of advances in treatment, but the solutions are, occasionally, surprisingly simple. It sometimes turns out, for example, that a couple has not realized that a lubricant they have been using also contains a spermicide. Or it may be that unknowingly they have been making love either in a position unconducive to conception or during a time of the month when the woman's egg is not ripe for fertilization. Still another possibility is too frequent intercourse. (It usually takes 48 hours after ejaculation for semen to again have a full complement of sperm.)

Thorough physical examinations, a family health history, and batteries of diagnostic tests are, nonetheless, essential to most infertility

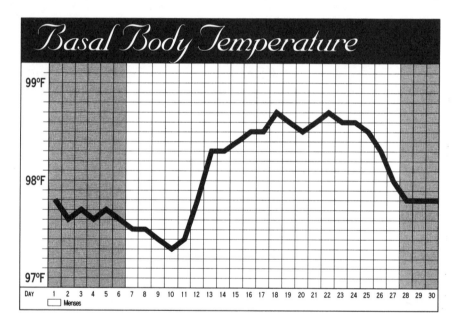

Figure 14.1. *This chart shows an example of how a woman's temperature, as measured before getting out of bed in the morning, varies with her menstrual cycle. Temperature is lower in the first half of the cycle, beginning with onset of menstruation. The substantial sustained rise beginning on day 13 indicates ovulation has probably occurred. Such charts can help couples calculate when conception is most likely.*

evaluations. Some causes of infertility require only lifestyle changes. Some women don't menstruate, for example, because they exercise too vigorously or have anorexia or another eating disorder that has made them far too thin. For them, less activity or a more nutritious diet leading to weight gain may do the trick.

In men, reduced sperm activity may result from wearing clothing that keeps the testes too warm (jockey shorts, for instance, instead of boxer shorts). Sperm quality can sometimes be improved and fertility attained by wearing a water-cooled testicular hypothermia device available by prescription, that FDA has approved for lowering the temperature of the scrotum.

Infertility Tests

Some infertility tests are for women only, others are for men only, and still others cannot be done without the cooperation of both partners.

An initial workup for a woman can take as little as six to eight weeks, or as much as three months or longer because some of the tests may have to be repeated for verification at different specific times in her menstrual cycle.

The initial workup of a man usually can be done faster both because men have no monthly cycles—and because there are fewer tests for men. Diagnostic surgical procedures may be suggested for both men and women to look directly at reproductive structures and to obtain small tissue samples for laboratory analysis.

His Tests

A semen analysis is almost always the first test done on men and is usually repeated several times. After abstaining from intercourse for about 48 hours, the man collects a sperm sample in a container.

The sample is microscopically examined to determine the number, activity and shape of individual spermatozoa (sperm cells) and the characteristics of the fluid part of the semen.

A healthy, potent ejaculate typically contains 1.5 to 5 cubic centimeters (5 cc = 1 teaspoon) of semen and each cc will contain an average of 70 million sperm that look to be of normal size, shape and behavior. If the specimen markedly differs on any of these factors, further tests may be done to determine whether infection, hormonal imbalance, or another problem could be the culprit.

Among these tests may be a testicular biopsy, a minor operation—performed with a local or general anesthetic—in which a small amount of tissue from the testes is removed for laboratory studies. Since even men with sperm counts well below 70 million per cubic centimeter sometimes father children, this test is ordinarily done only when the count is zero.

If damage to one or both of the vas deferens, is known or suspected, an x-ray examination may also be ordered. As an iodine-containing solution has to be injected into the tubes to make them visible on x-rays, the patient is first given local or general anesthesia. If the examination discloses damage, surgical repairs are often attempted at the same time the diagnosis is made.

Other special tests may be ordered if none of the tests already mentioned seems to explain the man's infertility. The most common of these tests are the bovine mucus test and the hamster-oocyte penetration test.

In the first, bovine (cow) mucus (from the cervix, or neck of the uterus where it opens into the vagina) is placed in a special glass column.Samples of the man's semen are applied to the column, and measurements are made of how well the sperm are able to enter and swim through the mucus, giving some indication of their ability to swim through human cervical mucus.

In the hamster-oocyte penetration test, some of the man's semen is mixed with hamster egg cells that have had their outer shells (membranes) removed. If the sperm are functioning normally, they will penetrate the hamster eggs, an indication that they are also capable of fertilizing human eggs. However, failure of the sperm to penetrate the hamster eggs does not always mean that they are incapable of fertilizing human eggs.

Her Tests

Women-only tests, more varied and extensive, generally begin with a determination of if and when the woman is ovulating. One of the most popular techniques for pinpointing ovulation relies on the typically slight rise in resting body temperature midway in the menstrual cycle, signaling that ovulation has recently occurred.

A woman's body temperature fluctuates throughout her menstrual cycle, and she is instructed to record these fluctuations on a chart after taking her temperature each morning before getting out of bed. If the chart—called a basal body temperature, or BBT, chart—indicates that the woman has been ovulating, it can often be used to predict when ovulation will happen during subsequent menstrual cycles. The couple can then use the information to attempt to time conception. Several urine test kits, approved by the Food and Drug Administration for sale over the counter, can be used by consumers to supplement the temperature chart.

Still other methods widely used to predict ovulation rely on examinations of the cervical mucus, which undergoes a series of hormone-induced changes at various times in the menstrual cycle. Some versions of these tests require a health professional's expertise. There are, however, versions of them that some women—with a physician's guidance—can learn to do themselves.

Other methods widely used to diagnose female infertility and to monitor therapy include:

- **Endometrial Biopsy:** A long, hollow tube is passed into the patient's uterus late in her menstrual cycle, and a little of the lining is scraped off and examined with a microscope. The examination helps the physician tell whether the development of the egg and of the lining are in proper phase with each other. In most cases, the scraping is done in a physician's office and because it is only very briefly painful no anesthetic is used.

- **Ultrasound:** This technology relies on sound waves to produce images of internal structures. It is used, often in combination with one or more of the tests already discussed, to find the presence or absence of follicles that contain and release the eggs. Ultrasound is also sometimes used to detect abnormalities in the ovaries or uterus.

- **Hysterosalpingogram:** This is an x-ray study of the uterus and fallopian tubes. It is done just after a woman's menstrual period so there is no danger of her being pregnant and thereby exposing the fertilized egg or embryo to radiation. A dye containing iodine—technically called a contrast medium—is injected through the cervix. It spreads into the uterus and the fallopian tubes, allowing them to be visualized.

  Among other things, this study often enables the physician to determine if the fallopian tubes are open. It is usually done without an anesthetic in the x-ray department of a hospital or clinic.

229

- **Hysteroscopy:** The patient's uterus is filled with a liquid or gas, instilled through the cervix. A thin, lighted tube called a hysteroscope that works like a telescope is then inserted into the uterus through the cervix, enabling the surgeon or physician to look directly inside. Many hysteroscopes have a separate channel through which instruments can be passed, often making it possible to immediately correct any abnormalities. Patients undergoing hysteroscopy are usually given an anesthetic, which may be local or general.

- **Laparoscopy:** A laparoscope, like a hysteroscope, is an instrument with a light that works like a telescope. It is slipped into the abdominal cavity through a small incision in or near the navel. For a clearer view of the woman's reproductive tract, the cavity is filled with gas during the procedure, and a colored solution—usually blue—is injected into the uterus and fallopian tubes. A general anesthetic is required. Advanced operative techniques may allow the repair of defects in the reproductive tract to be made at the same time as the examination.

Tests for Both Partners

Some tests require participation of both partners, as they have to be done after intercourse, which has to take place at the most fertile time in the woman's cycle. During the tests at a doctor's office, 2 to 12 hours after intercourse, several samples of cervical mucus are taken. Laboratory analysis determines whether sperm and mucus have been able to properly interact.

There are also a variety of tests that are used when the doctor suspects that infertility may be due to the man's forming antibodies against his own sperm or the woman's forming antibodies against them. The exact nature of these immunological problems is not yet well understood, but their detection is sometimes helpful in explaining why a couple is having reproductive difficulty. Some of these tests require the participation of both partners; others either one or the other.

A final word about all infertility tests: It is always best to ask in advance why they are being suggested, what they may show, how definitive they are, what the possible remedies are for any problem they may disclose, and what side effects or complications are possible from a given test. Many of these tests have potential risks as well as potential benefits.

Treatment of Infertility

Fertility Drugs

Deciding what to do, if anything, when the evaluation is complete may not be easy. Assuming these problems are treatable—and not all of them are—there is a bewildering array of choices, especially for women, and no guarantee that any of them will work. So it is that specialists in this field speak of "maximizing fertility potential" rather than "curing infertility."

Fertility potential starts in the brain, in an area called the hypothalamus. In both men and women, a hormone made by the hypothalamus travels via the blood to the pituitary gland at the base of the brain. This gland in turn makes hormones of its own that circulate in the blood and act on the reproductive organs.

In males, the message received by the testes causes them to make still another hormone, testosterone, which is their signal to make sperm. In females, an analogous cascade of hormones distributed by the bloodstream plays an equivalent role in ensuring that the right chemical messages get to the right places at the right times to allow women to ovulate and conceive.

When blood and urine tests of an infertility workup suggest some sort of hormone imbalance in one or both partners, corrective therapy with so-called fertility drugs is frequently prescribed. The most popular of these drugs are Clomid and Serophene (both clomiphene citrate in tablet form), which act on the hypothalamus, and Pergonal (human menopausal gonadotropins), which acts on the pituitary gland.

Because these powerful drugs can have a wide range of side effects, patients should always discuss the pros and cons of their use with the physician in advance. Clomid and Serophene, for example, can prolong the menstrual cycle and so make a woman mistakenly think she has conceived. Moreover, there is a risk with some fertility drugs of multiple births. Even if the couple would welcome several babies, multiple births can complicate pregnancy and delivery and endanger infant survival.

Surgery

Surgery is another tool often used to treat infertility in both men and women.

Many men have varicocele, a collection of swollen veins in the scrotum that often looks and feels like a bag of worms, but may be less obvious. Some men with a varicocele easily sire children and so are clearly fertile. For those who seemingly are not and whose sperm are sluggish, surgical repair of the varicocele may better their chances of fatherhood.

However, according to Larry Lipshultz, M.D., professor of urology at the Baylor University College of Medicine in Houston, there is a debate among physicians about when the operation is appropriate. He does not, therefore, usually recommend it to his patients unless he is unable to find other reasons for their infertility.

Another male infertility problem often treated by surgery is damage to the vas deferentia, through which sperm must pass for ejaculation. A common cause of such damage is vasectomy, male sterilization. Though it should be considered irreversible, some men later wish to have it reversed. This is sometimes possible through microsurgery. Other candidates for such surgery are men whose vas deferentia have been blocked by scar tissue caused by earlier unrelated surgery or a sexually transmitted or other infection.

Microsurgery is not a cure-all, however. It cannot help men with extensive damage to these structures, and many with limited damage may not be able to father a child, despite the operation's apparent success.

A sterilization procedure for women, tubal ligation, involves tying, cutting or burning the fallopian tubes and so scarring them. Damage to the tubes by earlier unrelated surgery or infection—again, sometimes sexually transmitted—can also cause female infertility.

In both cases, corrective surgery is sometimes, but not always, a possibility. Nor do seemingly successful surgical repairs of damaged fallopian tubes necessarily mean that any eggs fertilized in them will be able to make their way to the uterus.

Sometimes, instead, an ectopic (literally, out-of-place) pregnancy occurs, in which the fertilized egg gets trapped in the tube where it cannot survive when it grows. Any woman can have an ectopic pregnancy, but those whose tubes have been damaged are at greatest risk, even after corrective surgery. Although surgical repair of the damage lowers the risk of having an ectopic pregnancy, it remains higher than for women with tubes that have never been damaged.

Endometriosis, a common disorder in women, also can cause or contribute to infertility when small pieces of the uterine lining escape and take up residence on the surfaces of organs in the abdominal cavity.

Inflammation and consequent chronic irritation from the misplaced tissue can eventually so badly scar the ovaries, fallopian tubes, inner or outer walls of the uterus, or other nearby structures that the woman cannot conceive.

Both surgery and drug treatments, sometimes combined, are used to treat endometriosis. Success rates in the hands of a physician skilled in treating this disorder are in the 50 to 60 percent range, and depend on several factors, including the patient's age and manifestations of the disease.

Artificial Insemination

Some infertility treatments attempt to get a pregnancy started without intercourse. Artificial insemination, the oldest of these treatments, has been used for more than a century. A hollow, flexible instrument—called a catheter—is used to place the donor's semen into the woman's uterus or vaginal canal.

All inseminations are performed around the time the woman should be ovulating, either naturally or after priming with a fertility drug. The semen may be from the woman's husband ("artificial insemination-husband," or AIH, for short) or from an anonymous donor ("artificial insemination-donor," or AID).

A recent advance in AIH is for men who—because of spinal cord injury, cancer surgery, or other reasons—can't ejaculate normally. Electrical stimulation can be used to help them overcome this problem and the ejaculate collected and inseminated in their wives.

Fresh semen was once used for all inseminations and still is, as a rule, in AIH, but because of concern about AIDS and other sexually transmitted infections, FDA, the Centers for Disease Control, and the American Fertility Society now recommend that anonymous donor semen be frozen for at least 180 days before use. The delay allows the donor semen to be retested for possible infection. Some women become pregnant with one insemination. More often, repeat inseminations over the course of four to five menstrual cycles are required. And there are women who after a year or more of periodic insemination still do not conceive. Depending on the nature of the couple's infertility, studies show success rates between 50 and 65 percent.

In vitro *Fertilization*

Much newer than artificial insemination is *in vitro* fertilization (IVF), made famous by the birth in England in 1978 of Louise Brown, the world's first "test tube" baby. IVF is an option when various other treatments have failed or are inappropriate. It can be used, for example, in women who have a uterus and at least one ovary, but whose fallopian tubes are damaged, missing or diseased.

The woman is prepared for this procedure with fertility drugs that ready several of her eggs for fertilization and the lining of her uterus to support a pregnancy. The eggs are then taken from her by one of several methods and placed in a laboratory dish where they are incubated with her partner's sperm for about 18 hours.

Assuming that some are fertilized and continue to develop normally for two days or so, one or more (as a kind of insurance policy, it is usually several) are transferred by instrument into the woman's uterus. If at least one implants there within about two weeks, the woman is pregnant. Implantation can often be determined at that time by a blood test. However, this chemical assessment is sometimes misleading. Therefore, a conclusive diagnosis cannot be made until a week more or so has passed when—if the pregnancy is real, rather than just chemical—a sac will have formed around the embryo that can be detected by ultrasound.

As with other infertility treatments, couples undergoing IVF should not count their chickens before they hatch. In a study published in 1988, for example, 41 clinics that had treated 3,055 women with one or more cycles of IVF reported that only 485 (15.9 percent) became pregnant and just 311 (10.2 percent) delivered a living infant.

Still Newer Techniques

Newer still than in vitro fertilization are several other techniques that also require the use of fertility drugs. They are:

- **Gamete Intrafallopian Transfer (GIFT):** Similar to IVF except that sperm and eggs are collected and immediately inserted into one or both fallopian tubes, where conception occurs. Unlike IVF, GIFT requires that the woman have at least one healthy fallopian tube. Success rates are similar to those of IVF.

- **Tubal Ovum Transfer:** The woman's eggs are retrieved and put into the fallopian tube close to where it opens into the uterus. The couple then has intercourse or the woman is artificially inseminated. Since this method allows the eggs to be placed beyond the parts of the tube that may be damaged or blocked, it can often be used when GIFT cannot.

- **Embryo Lavage:** A fertile female donor provides the eggs. At the proper time in her menstrual cycle, she is artificially inseminated with the would-be father's sperm. If the donor conceives, the early embryo is washed out of her reproductive tract and transferred to the uterus or a fallopian tube of the woman who is to bear the child. The recipient, meanwhile, has been hormonally treated with fertility drugs to make her uterus receptive to the embryo. This technique allows women who have no eggs of their own to become pregnant—provided they have a uterus.

- **Surrogate Motherhood:** This is an option for women who do not respond to ovulation induction therapies or who have no ovaries or lack a uterus. It also may be an option for those for whom pregnancy might be life threatening or have good reason to worry that they might transmit a serious genetic disorder to the child.

  A healthy, fertile woman agrees to be artificially inseminated and also agrees to let the infertile couple adopt the baby. If the female member of the infertile couple can safely provide eggs of her own, these can be fertilized by the IVF process and then transferred to the surrogate woman who carries the fetus to term. In that case, the surrogate mother takes fertility drugs to prepare her uterus. Surrogate motherhood is controversial and has resulted in court cases about custody and parentage, which is rare with other forms of fertility treatment.

When to Stop?

If efforts to have a baby are unsuccessful, the question ultimately arises, "When do we stop trying?" Though it may not be easy, giving up the effort can have a happy ending, as is clear from the stories of two couples who met through a small social group in a distant suburb of Washington, D.C., and learned about their mutual interest during casual conversation.

The first couple had tried almost everything, including IVF, and, after 10 years of getting nowhere, gave up medical interventions. Two cycles later the woman conceived and—after a difficult pregnancy—bore a healthy baby girl. The other couple took a different route that is available to many couples who abandon hope for a child of their own. They adopted a newborn baby and now wish they had done it a lot sooner.

Preventing Reproductive Problems

Many infertile couples wonder why something so easy for most people is so hard for them. Although science cannot fully answer that question, it does know that some reproductive problems are preventable.

Heading the list is damage to the structures that allow sperm and egg to meet, caused by gonorrhea, chlamydia, and other sexually transmitted diseases (STDs). This damage accounts for about 20 percent of all infertility in men and women alike. Use of barrier methods of contraception—condoms for men, diaphragms (with spermicide), or contraceptive sponges for women—can stop many of these infections before they start.

Both women and men who are sexually active should be regularly checked for the possible presence of STDs as these infections often have no symptoms. The longer the delay before antibiotic treatment is started, the greater the risk of impaired fertility. This risk rises the more sexual partners a person has and with the number of times he or she has these infections.

Tobacco, alcohol, and the use of illicit drugs can also diminish the reproductive potential of both sexes, as can the use of steroid drugs for body-building purposes and for enhancing sports performance. So can poor nutrition, rapid weight loss, and either too much or too little body fat. The same goes for excessive rigorous exercise, meaning more than an hour a day. While too much exercise is more likely to impair female than male fertility, neither sex can count on escaping its reproductive effects.

Childhood immunizations also have a bearing on future fertility. Immunization against mumps and rubella (German measles) is particularly important because the male who gets mumps in adolescence or later runs a high risk of becoming permanently sterile, and the female who gets rubella while pregnant particularly early in pregnancy—is at high risk of miscarriage or having a baby with birth defects.

In addition, boys who are born with an undescended testicle, which is fairly common, are more likely than other boys to later have reproductive problems. They are also at a somewhat higher risk for later developing testicular cancer. Undescended testicles can be surgically corrected during childhood.

Girls who don't menstruate by age 16 or are plagued with menstrual problems need to be evaluated by a physician. Neither condition is necessarily an indication of impaired fertility, but it is also true that delaying needed treatment can sometimes make the situation worse.

Choosing a Doctor

Rather than relying on advertisements or affiliations, when choosing a physician for infertility services, it is wise to check on his or her qualifications. The local medical society can usually provide background information on the doctor you are considering consulting.

For women, the right physician will probably be a board-certified obstetrician-gynecologist and may well be one who, besides, has had two years of further training in reproductive endocrinology.

For men, the right doctor will likely be a board-certified urologist with a special interest in infertility. Often, such a urologist has had a fellowship in male reproductive problems in addition to his basic training in urology.

For More Information

Resolve, Inc., a nonprofit organization, has a nationwide list of specialists for both men and women and information about all aspects of infertility care. Write:

Resolve, Inc.
5 Water St.
Arlington, Mass. 02174
phone (1-800) 662-1016.

Many communities have Resolve chapters listed in local telephone books.

—by Judith Randal

Section 14.2

Infertility Services

Federal Trade Commission Publication No. F027640, October 1993.

About one in six U.S. couples is infertile. If you are among them, you may have considered contacting a health care provider that offers advanced infertility services.

Most infertility service providers will tell you what their record has been in helping couples. But in talking with or writing to different providers, you may find that success rates are calculated differently—making it confusing to select among the more than 200 programs offering these advanced services.

In addition, a particular infertility service may have a lower success rate than others, but specialize in more difficult cases. Or, a service may have a very good overall success rate, but not be the best one to treat your particular problem. Infertility experts emphasize that your chances for success depend on many factors, such as age and cause of infertility.

The staff at the Federal Trade Commission has reviewed how success-rate claims are calculated by infertility services. The following information may help in evaluating these claims and selecting the best program for your specific needs.

How Success Rates Are Advertised

As you contact infertility service providers, consider carefully how success rates are calculated. Make sure to ask for the success rate for people who fit your particular patient profile, such as your age and cause of infertility.

Ask which specific procedures are included or omitted in the figures. This information can be difficult to understand, so ask for it in "plain English."

Included here are explanations of some frequently used success-rate calculations.

Live Birth Rate per Egg Stimulation

This figure tells how many births occurred in relation to the number of egg-stimulation procedures performed. Experts say this figure is the most meaningful overall success-rate statistic, because it includes live births as well as all procedures performed, including those that failed.

Live Birth Rate per Embryo Transfer

This figure refers to the percentage of births from all embryo transfer procedures. Although this number reflects live births—which may be the most meaningful figure—it does not include those instances where the attempt at egg stimulation, egg retrieval, and fertilization did not succeed.

Pregnancy Rate per Attempted Egg Stimulation

This rate refers to the number of clinical pregnancies resulting from all egg-stimulation attempts. This figure does not tell you whether these pregnancies resulted in live births, but does include the women who received multiple treatments.

Pregnancy Rate per Woman in the Program

This rate refers to how many clinical pregnancies occurred per woman in the program. Excluded from this figure are the number of births and the number of times an individual woman may have undergone the procedure prior to achieving a pregnancy.

Pregnancy Rate per Attempted Egg Retrieval

This rate reflects the number of clinical pregnancies resulting from all egg-retrieval attempts. This statistic does not tell whether these pregnancies resulted in live births and does not include instances where egg stimulation did not produce an egg to retrieve.

Pregnancy Rate per Embryo Transfer

This usually refers to how many clinical pregnancies occurred in relation to the number of embryo-transfer procedures performed. This figure does not say how many births occurred or how successful the program was in stimulating egg production, in obtaining egg retrieval, and in fertilizing eggs retrieved.

It takes time for new infertility service providers to establish success rates based on live births. For this reason, some providers cite only national statistics in discussing success rates.

Be wary of any claims not based on a provider's own experience. Experts say it is fair for new providers to report anticipated births by including those pregnancies that have progressed beyond 26 weeks at which point the pregnancy is highly likely to continue to term.

Some providers also favor reporting "cumulative" pregnancy and birth rate claims. Cumulative rates suggest the overall probability of a pregnancy or birth occurring based on women undergoing several successive procedures. You may want to ask how such calculations are made and what percentage of patients were able to go through multiple treatments. Evaluate all claims of success carefully.

How to Select an Infertility Service

You may want to begin your search for fertility specialists by asking your gynecologist, obstetrician, family doctor, or friends and relatives for recommendations. Ask your local hospital or medical society for names. In addition, you may want to contact local infertility support groups, which can provide you with both information and emotional support.

Plan to talk with several providers of infertility services before taking any particular course of action. By doing so, you can compare programs, gain more information about the field, and learn about different treatments applicable to your situation.

You may want to contact infertility programs first by telephone, study any literature sent to you and, then, visit those that most interest you. Try to select an infertility provider that you feel comfortable with and is convenient for you. Here are some questions to ask providers.

1. What is your infertility service's success rate and how is it calculated?

2. For established programs: What is your live birth rate per egg stimulation attempted?

3. For new programs: What is your live birth rate plus ongoing pregnancies past 26 weeks per egg stimulation?

You will want to examine how each infertility service tabulates its success rate and consider how meaningful these figures are.

4. What is your success rate with couples who have problems similar to ours?

    Most importantly, find out how successful an infertility service has been in helping couples with your specific problems. Tell the staff your individual circumstances. Then ask: "Given our particular medical history, what are our chances of having a baby after undergoing a single egg-stimulation procedure?"

5. How long has your infertility service been in existence? How many patients have you treated? What is the specific training of your medical personnel?

    You probably will want to select a program that is well-established, has worked with many patients, and has a highly-trained medical staff.

6. Is your infertility service associated with a medical board specializing in infertility?

    You may wish to determine whether the infertility service has a doctor who is board certified by the American Board of Obstetrics and Gynecology in the sub-specialty of Reproductive Endocrinology. This board certification provides recognition of tested expertise in IVF and GIFT procedures.

7. Can you send me written material about the particular procedure you are recommending?

    It is helpful to get written information about any medical procedures you may undergo. IVF and GIFT treatments should be explained to you in detail so that you fully understand the nature of these procedures.

8. What are the fees for these procedures? How much will drugs cost? What is typically covered by insurance?

    Costs for infertility procedures are relatively expensive, and coverage by health insurance plans varies. Ask the cost of each step in the IVF or GIFT procedure. Most infertility services charge you as you advance through each step of the procedure rather than require a payment-in-full prior to the start of a treatment. You should review your health insurance to see which parts, if any, of the IVF or GIFT procedures are covered and discuss the matter with the provider of your choice.

9. Can we talk with several former or current patients who have had problems similar to ours?

Talking with a provider's patients can help confirm your impressions of an infertility program, particularly the way in which patients are treated. You frequently can get an idea of a program's strengths and weaknesses from those who have participated in it.

Terms You Need to Know

In Vitro Fertilization (IVF)

In this procedure, a woman's eggs are retrieved and combined with sperm to fertilize in the laboratory. Any fertilized eggs, called embryos, are returned to the uterus.

The steps involved in IVF are:

Step 1 Egg Stimulation
Step 2 Egg Retrieval
Step 3 Fertilization
Step 4 Embryo Transfer

If all goes well, the next two steps are:

Step 5 Clinical Pregnancy
Step 6 Live Birth

Gamete intrafallopian transfer (GIFT)

This procedure differs from IVF in that retrieved eggs and sperm are injected into a woman's fallopian tubes where fertilization can take place.

Because fertilization does not take place outside the body, there is no embryo transfer step in GIFT.

Egg Stimulation

This refers to the administration of fertility drugs to a woman to "stimulate" and increase egg production.

Egg Retrieval

This process involves the removal of an egg or eggs from the ovaries and follicles for subsequent fertilization through IVF or GIFT.

Fertilization

The retrieved egg is mixed with sperm, after which the egg becomes fertilized and forms what then becomes an embryo.

Embryo Transfer

After an egg and sperm fertilize in the laboratory, the newly formed embryo is transferred to the uterus.

Clinical Pregnancy

This is a pregnancy which has been confirmed by ultrasound or other clinical means. Prior to this point, a blood test or a urinary pregnancy test may indicate a pregnancy. Such tests look for human chorionic gonadotropin or hCG. If the blood or urinary tests indicate a positive reading, then the pregnancy is referred to as a "chemical pregnancy." Infertility service providers generally do not accept chemical pregnancies as anything more than an indicator because conditions other than pregnancy can account for a positive reading.

Live Birth

This refers to the actual live birth of one or more babies. In determining success-rate data using live births, the industry standard is to count a "live birth" as a single delivery, regardless of how many babies were born.

Where to Go for More Information

For help in researching or checking possible complaints about particular infertility programs, you may want to contact the state medical board or county medical society. For more information about infertility, write:

American Fertility Society,
2140 Eleventh Avenue South, Suite 200,
Birmingham, AL 35205.

Section 14.3

Laser Scalpels Cut Path to Parenthood

NCRR Reporter, January/February 1995.

More than 2 million American couples have fertility problems that can stymie their plans for parenthood. To overcome difficulties such as sparse or weak-swimming sperm, many couples seek help at in vitro fertilization (IVF) clinics. But this time-consuming, expensive approach is often unsuccessful. At the NCRR-supported Laser Microbeam Biotechnology Resource, located at the Beckman Laser Institute and Medical Clinic, University of California, Irvine, researchers use lasers to study sperm and egg physiology to improve fertilization and pregnancy rates.

In cases of poor sperm motility or low sperm count, attempts to fertilize a woman's eggs combining them with her husband's sperm outside the body frequently fail. The egg's thick outer coating called the zona pellucida blocks the aspiring sperm. Although scientists can snare an egg with a micropipette and puncture the zona with tiny needles that inject sperm, this technique requires delicate, expensive equipment and special training.

Enter the laser, which can he used as a "light scalpel" to gently slice into the egg's zona pellucida. The laser's narrow, high-intensity stream of light can drill tiny holes into the zona prior to conception. This opens a path for easier sperm entry, and the rate of fertilization improves.

But in many cases it is not fertilization but failure of fertilized eggs to attach to the uterine wall that poses the greatest challenge to the IVF clinicians. In laser-assisted hatching, a technique designed to boost the chances that the fertilized egg will implant in the uterus, researchers make laser cuts after sperm has entered the egg and cell divisions have begun. "We know that about 60 to 80 percent of eggs will be fertilized when exposed to normal sperm, but only 10 to 20 percent of the embryos transferred to the uterus will implant and grow to viable pregnancies," says Dr. Yona Tadir, medical director of the

Beckman Laser Institute and professor of obstetrics and gynecology at the University of California, Irvine. "And this major gap between 60 to 80 percent and 10 to 20 percent is the gap that people are trying to narrow. One of the ways of doing that is manipulating the zona pellucida".

"With lasers we can manipulate gametes (egg and sperm) in a non-contact mode, and we don't need a micromanipulator or direct contact with the eggs," explains Dr. Tadir. "The advantage is that it's faster and cheaper because you don't have to have any disposable equipment, which is very expensive and time-consuming to prepare. With the laser, there's nothing to sterilize. The beam of light is sterile."

Fertility researchers have set up a system that uses a variety of lasers that can be reflected down the objective of a microscope. A video camera peers down the microscope's objective to record the image, which is then projected onto a video monitor. Instead of moving the eggs or sperm around with micropipettes or other tiny tools, scientists move the motorized stage to bring the gametes in contact with the laser beam. Since the zona pellucida is tenfold to fifteenfold thicker than the width of the laser beam, researchers can make precision slices through the edge of the zona. This technique is far more precise than other methods of zona opening, such as mechanical dissection or chemical drilling.

Dr. Tadir says clinical application of laser-assisted hatching is bearing fruit. In a recent study, researchers used the technique to help women with implantation resistance who had failed to conceive after three or more attempts at implanting embryos. The researchers used a laser to slice a wide gash in the zona. The results were dramatic: about 37 percent of the women became pregnant, which is almost double the pregnancy rate seen in even their standard IVF patients.

Laser-assisted hatching can significantly reduce IVF's cost. In the United States one IVF treatment cycle costs about $8,000, only some of which is covered by insurance. Dr. Tadir and his colleagues at the institute aim to provide a simple technique for assisted conception and hatching that reduces costs of traditional labor-intensive IVF treatments, while improving the success rate of each treatment cycle.

The Beckman Institute researchers use lasers not only as scalpels but also as tweezers, in a process known as optical trapping. When laser light enters and subsequently leaves a cell, it generates forces that draw the cell toward the focal point of the laser beam. Once caught, the sperm behaves like a stick caught in an eddy of a stream: it stays put. Transfixed in this optical trap, the sperm can then be manipulated at will by moving the microscope stage.

In one study, researchers used the optical trap to check the motility of previously frozen sperm. Although scientists have long observed that previously frozen sperm are far less capable of fertilizing an egg, the exact causes are not known. First, scientists trapped the sperm with a laser. They then reduced the laser power until the sperm broke free. The energy needed to trap the sperm, which reflects their swimming strength, was converted into a measure called the relative escape force (REF) of the individual sperm. The researchers found that freezing kills many sperm, but those that survive swim just as strongly as fresh sperm. The scientists are now using the trap, in combination with laser fluorescent techniques, to learn what other factors may affect the ability of frozen sperm to fertilize an egg.

—by Scott Veggeberg

Chapter 15

Abortion

Questions and Answers

What is abortion?

Abortion ends a pregnancy before birth takes place. When an embryo or fetus dies in the womb and is expelled by the body, it is called a spontaneous abortion or "miscarriage." When a woman decides to end her pregnancy voluntarily, she has an induced abortion. When a fetus is dead at birth, it is called a "stillbirth."

When are abortions performed?

More than 90 percent of all induced abortions are performed during the first trimester—the first three months of pregnancy. In fact, more than half are performed within the first two months of pregnancy. These abortions are usually performed at a clinic, health center, or in a doctor's office, and the women go home an hour or so later.

Fewer than nine percent of abortions take place in the second trimester—14 through 24 weeks of pregnancy. Abortions in the second trimester are more complicated procedures but are safer than childbirth.

Reprinted with permission from Abortion: Commonly Asked Questions by Planned Parenthood Federation of America, Inc. Revised Version, 1996 PPFA. All rights reserved.

Abortion in the last three months of pregnancy is extremely rare. Only one out of 10,000 abortions takes place after 24 weeks. It is more complicated and is performed only when the pregnancy seriously threatens a woman's health or life or when the fetus is severely deformed.

Who has abortion?

Approximately 1.5 million U.S. women with unwanted pregnancies choose abortion each year. Most are under 25 years old and unmarried. Women who are separated from their husbands and poor women are more likely to choose abortion than other women. More than two-thirds of the women who seek abortions have jobs. Nearly one-third are in school. More than two-thirds plan to have a child in the future.

Approximately six million women in the U.S. become pregnant every year. About half of those pregnancies are unintended. Either the woman or her partner did not use contraception or the contraceptive method failed.

Why do women choose abortion?

A recent survey showed that in most cases a woman who chooses abortion has at least three reasons. The most common of these reasons are:

- She is not ready for the way becoming a parent will change her life—it would be hard to keep her job, continue her education, and/or care for her other children.

- She cannot afford a baby now.

- She doesn't want to be a single parent, she doesn't want to marry her partner, he can't or won't marry her—or she isn't in a relationship.

- She is not ready for the responsibility.

- She doesn't want anyone to know she has had sex or is pregnant.

- She is too young or too immature to have a child.

- She has all the children she wants.

- Her husband, partner, or parent wants her to have an abortion.

- She or the fetus has a health problem.

- She was a victim of rape or incest.

Whatever your situation may be, it is important to consider all of your options and make your own decision.

Who will help me decide if abortion is right for me?

Abortion is not always the best solution to an unwanted pregnancy. You have to decide for yourself if abortion is your best choice. However, most women look to their husbands, partners, families, health care providers, religious leaders, and friends for support and guidance as they make their decisions.

Family planning and abortion clinics also have specially trained counselors to talk with you about your choices when you face an unwanted pregnancy. You may bring your partner or your parents to the counseling session if you wish. All options— adoption, parenting, and abortion—will be discussed.

Your counselor will describe the abortion procedure and try to make sure that you are not being pressured into having an abortion by your husband, partner, family, or friends. The counselor should not try to influence your decision. If you want to have a child and are being pressured to have an abortion, call Planned Parenthood for help. The Planned Parenthood policy is to provide counselors who will listen objectively, provide accurate information, and support your decision—whatever it is.

If abortion is chosen, the counselor or other clinic staff person may be with you during your pelvic exam and during the abortion. Some clinics may allow a supportive partner, husband, friend, or family member to be with you during the abortion.

Does my partner, my husband, or a parent need to know?

Up to half of all women who have abortions go to the clinic with their partners. However, you do not have to notify your partner or husband to have an abortion. The clinic will ensure complete confidentiality.

More than half of all teenagers who have abortions have already talked with at least one parent. However, telling a parent is not required in many states.

But 26 states do require a woman under 18 to tell a parent or get a parent's permission before she can have an abortion. If she cannot talk with her parents, or chooses not to, she can appear before a judge who will decide whether she is mature enough to make her own decision about abortion. If she is not mature, the judge must decide whether an abortion is in her best interests.

If you are a minor considering abortion, you must find out about the laws in your state. Your local Planned Parenthood health center can provide this information.

Is abortion safe?

Yes. Today, abortion is about twice as safe as having your tonsils out and is safer than childbirth. In fact, abortion is 11 times safer than giving birth up to the 18th week of pregnancy. However, the risk of rare, serious complications or death from abortion increases the longer a pregnancy goes on.

Does abortion hurt?

Most women say the discomfort of early abortion with local anesthetic is like menstrual cramps. For some women, abortion is very uncomfortable. Others feel very little. Abortion with local anesthetic after 24 weeks of pregnancy is about as painful as labor during birth. With a local anesthetic, a woman's pain is relieved, but she remains awake. Some clinics offer general anesthesia so the woman sleeps and feels nothing. General anesthesia, however, increases the medical risks and the length of time a woman must remain at the clinic.

What tests, exams, and counseling must I have before I can have an abortion?

You must be tested for pregnancy. You must be counseled about your pregnancy options. And you must have a physical examination before an abortion can take place.

The usual tests include:

- a urine or blood test for pregnancy

- a test for the Rh factor in your blood
- a blood test to screen for anemia
- a pelvic exam.

Sometimes a sonogram (see glossary) is needed to help determine how long you've been pregnant. Depending on your circumstances, testing for sexually transmitted infections such as gonorrhea or chlamydia may also be helpful.

During the physical:

- your medical history will be taken
- your weight, temperature, and blood pressure will be measured.

Depending on your circumstances, the physical exam may be more comprehensive.

Your counselor will answer any questions you have about your pregnancy and provide information about your choices, which are:

- having a baby and keeping it
- having a baby and giving it up for adoption
- abortion.

Depending on your needs, your counselor will review:

- prenatal care and where it is provided
- adoption and the location of adoption agencies
- abortion and where it is provided
- birth control and how to get it
- insurance coverage or other reimbursement for abortion, prenatal care, and delivery
- psychological counseling services available in the community.

Will I have to sign anything?

You will need to sign a form requesting abortion services. This assures the clinician performing the abortion that you:

- have been informed about all your options
- have been counseled about the procedure, its risks, and how to care for yourself afterward
- have chosen abortion of your own free will.

How is abortion performed?

The procedure used for an abortion depends on how long a woman has been pregnant.

How is a very early abortion performed?

In very early abortion, the uterus is emptied with the gentle suction of a syringe. It can be done up to 49 days after the last menstrual period.

In some clinics, women can choose to use a combination of drugs to end their pregnancies. This is called medical abortion.

The U.S. Food and Drug Administration is expected to approve methods for medical abortion in the near future. Medical abortion uses medication prescribed by a doctor and does not require surgery. Medical abortion must take place within the first six weeks of pregnancy. Two combinations of medication are used for medical abortion:

- **The methotrexate-misoprostol method**-a woman receives an injection of methotrexate from her clinician. From five to seven days later she returns and inserts suppositories of misoprostol into her vagina. The pregnancy usually ends at home within a day or two. The embryo and other tissue that develops during pregnancy are passed out through the vagina.

- **The mifepristone-misoprostol method**-a woman swallows a dose of mifepristone under the guidance of her clinician. She returns in several days and inserts suppositories of misoprostol into her vagina. The pregnancy usually ends at home within four hours. The embryo and other tissue that develops during pregnancy are passed out through the vagina.

From 5 to 10 percent of medical abortions fail. In these cases, surgical procedures are required to end the pregnancy.

Medical abortion may not be available from all abortion providers even after it is approved.

How is early abortion performed?

The usual method of early abortion is suction curettage. It is performed from six to 14 weeks after your last period. The procedure takes about 10 minutes.

- The vagina is washed with an antiseptic.

- Usually, a local anesthetic is injected into or near the cervix.

- The opening of the cervix is gradually stretched. One after the other, a series of increasingly thick rods (dilators) are inserted into the opening. The thickest may be the width of a fountain pen.

- After the opening is stretched, a tube is inserted into the uterus. This tube is attached to a suction machine.

- The suction machine is turned on. The uterus is emptied by gentle suction.

- After the suction tube has been removed, a curette (narrow metal loop) may be used to gently scrape the walls of the uterus to be sure that it has been completely emptied.

How are early second-trimester abortions performed?

Abortions performed early in the second trimester are performed in two steps—dilation and evacuation (D&E). Second-trimester abortions are available in some clinics, as well as certain hospitals, up to the 25th week of pregnancy.

During the first step of a D&E:

- The vagina is washed with an antiseptic.

- Absorbent dilators may be put into the cervix, where they remain for several hours, often overnight. The dilators absorb fluids from the cervical area and stretch the opening of the cervix as they thicken.

- If you are to go home with the dilators in place, you will be given instructions for your care until you return for the abortion. You may be given antibiotics to prevent infection. If the dilators are left in overnight, you will also be given a 24-hour telephone number so you can contact the clinic staff should any problem arise. Gradual dilation is safer than having it done all at once. However, you may feel pressure or cramping while the dilator is in place.

During the second step of a D&E:

- You may be given intravenous medications to ease pain and/or prevent infection.

- A local anesthetic is injected into or near the cervix.

- The dilators are removed from the cervix.

- The fetus and other products of conception are removed from the uterus with instruments and suction curettage. This procedure takes about 10-20 minutes.

How is abortion after 24 weeks of pregnancy performed?

Only one out of every 10,000 women who have abortions have them after 24 weeks. These are performed only when there is a serious threat to a woman's life or health or if the fetus is severely deformed.

One of the procedures is called the induction method. The doctor injects urea or salt solution into the uterus to induce contractions (labor) and cause a stillbirth. Or the doctor may insert prostaglandin into the vagina to induce labor and expel the fetus. Labor pains, which usually last from six to 24 hours, can be relieved with medication.

The induction method is usually done in a hospital and usually means staying overnight or longer. The chance of complications is greater than with early abortion or D&E—abortion after 24 weeks is about as risky as carrying the pregnancy to term.

Some providers use a three-step D&E procedure instead of the induction method for abortions after 24 weeks. In the first two steps, the cervix is dilated several times until it is wide enough to allow removal of the fetus with grasping instruments.

What are the health risks of abortion?

Complications can occur with any kind of medical procedure. Fewer than five out of 1,000 women who have early abortion will have serious complications. Women giving birth are much more likely than women having abortions to need major abdominal surgery, such as cesarean section, as a result of complications.

Complications from early abortion include:

- Allergic reactions to specific anesthetics or other medications. Women taking medications or drugs, including street drugs, may experience serious reactions to anesthesia. Be sure to tell your clinician what medications or recreational drugs you take. What you say will be strictly confidential.

- Incomplete abortion. This occurs in fewer than one out of 100 abortions. Incomplete D&E abortion occurs in one out of 200 of those performed. In such cases it may be necessary to repeat the suction and remove the tissue. Incomplete abortion may lead to infection, heavy bleeding, or both. In rare instances, more surgery is required.

- Blood clots in the uterus. Clots that may cause severe cramping occur in about one out of 100 abortions. The clots are usually removed by a repeated suction curettage.

- Infection by germs from the vagina or cervix that get into the uterus. In many cases, the infection is a flareup of a preexisting sexually transmitted infection. Fewer than one out of 100 women who have abortion become infected. Usually antibiotics clear up the infection. In rare cases, a repeat suction, hospitalization, or surgery is needed.

- Heavy bleeding that requires medical treatment. This is rare. Such bleeding may require medication, a repeat suction or dilation and curettage, or, rarely, surgery. Fewer than one in 1,000 cases require blood transfusions.

- A cut or torn cervix. This occurs in fewer than one out of 100 early abortions. Stitches are rarely needed to repair the injury.

- Perforation of the wall of the uterus. In about one of 1,000 early abortions, an instrument goes through the wall of the uterus. In even fewer cases, perforation leads to infection, heavy vaginal or abdominal bleeding, or both. In D&E the number of perforations rises to three in 1,000 abortions. Surgery may be necessary to repair the uterine tissue. Very rarely, hysterectomy is required.

- Very rarely, in about six out of one million cases, a woman dies of complications from legal abortion.

Is abortion always 100 percent effective?

Abortion is almost always effective. It fails to end the pregnancy in only two out of 1,000 cases. This usually happens if there is more than one embryo or fetus or if an ectopic pregnancy has developed outside the uterus where suction curettage does not reach. Ectopic pregnancy threatens the life of the woman and requires surgery.

In cases when abortion fails, curettage is usually repeated. Otherwise, the pregnancy may develop abnormally.

What happens after an abortion?

After an abortion up to the 25th week, you will rest in a medically supervised recovery room for as long as necessary, usually about an hour. You will be able to rest until you feel ready to leave. During that time, you will be observed to make sure there are no complications.

If you have an Rh negative blood type, you will receive an injection to prevent the development of antibodies that could endanger any future pregnancy.

The clinic will give you written instructions for after-care and a 24-hour emergency phone number to use if complications arise. You will be able to discuss birth control with your counselor, and an appointment will be made for a follow-up examination in two to four weeks.

Can I leave the clinic alone?

You may need to have a companion with you when you leave the clinic. Depending on which procedure you have, you may be weak or disoriented from the medication or anesthetic. Your health care providers will tell you what to do. They want to be sure you get home safely. You should not drive after general anesthetic or sedation.

How long will it take to recover from an abortion?

Usually you can return to work or your normal activities the day after early abortion—depending on how strenuous your normal activities are. The day of the abortion, you may want to relax for the rest of the day. You may shower as soon as you wish. Do not take tub baths, douche, use vaginal medications, or have vaginal intercourse until after your follow-up exam—from two to four weeks after the abortion. Recovery after later abortions may take longer.

Will I bleed after abortion?

Very often there is a dark, menstrual-like flow that occurs off and on for a couple of weeks after the abortion. Some women will have cramps and pass a few large clots of blood up to 10 days after the abortion. Some will have little or no bleeding. After an abortion, use sanitary pads—do not use tampons—until bleeding stops.

Your next regular period may come at any time within six weeks after the abortion. Be sure to contact your clinician if you do not have a period in six weeks.

Are heavy bleeding, pain, and fever normal after an abortion?

No. If you experience any of these after an abortion, contact your clinician immediately.

How soon may I have intercourse after abortion?

Wait until after your follow-up exam or until three weeks after bleeding has stopped. Abstaining from vaginal intercourse will allow time for the cervix to close and protect you from infection. If you choose not to abstain, use a condom to reduce your risk of infection, but having vaginal intercourse before the cervix has closed is not a good idea.

How soon might I get pregnant again after an abortion?

It is possible to get pregnant again within two weeks after an abortion. That is why it is important to use birth control when you begin to have sexual intercourse again.

How soon should I see a health care provider after an abortion?

Follow-up should take place within two to four weeks after a suction curettage. After a D&E, see your clinician within four weeks.

What are the emotional effects of abortion?

The emotion most women experience after an abortion is relief. Because of the abrupt hormonal changes caused by abortion, some women experience short-term anger, regret, guilt, or sadness. After abortion most women who feel a brief sadness or other negative feeling recover very quickly.

Serious, long-term emotional problems after abortion are rare and less frequent than those following childbirth. They are more likely if:

- the pregnancy was wanted but the health of the fetus or the woman was jeopardized by its continuation

- having an abortion is related to serious problems in a relationship or other disturbing life events.

In spite of these facts, some people who are opposed to abortion claim that most women who have an abortion suffer severe and long-lasting emotional problems. They call these problems "post-abortion syndrome." This "syndrome" is not recognized by the American Psychological Association, the American Psychiatric Association, or the National Association of Social Workers.

If a woman does have prolonged feelings of sadness, guilt, or depression it is important for her to talk about her feelings with a counselor. Her abortion provider may be able to offer follow-up counseling or refer her to a counselor in the community.

What about future pregnancies?

Will an early abortion affect my ability to have a child? No. Safe, uncomplicated, legal abortion should not affect fertility.

Does an early abortion make miscarriage more likely in future pregnancies? No.

Does an early abortion make ectopic pregnancy more likely in the future? Not unless infection occurs after an abortion. Ectopic pregnancies usually result from sexually transmitted infections. Infection occurs in only one out of 100 first-trimester abortions.

Does an early abortion cause premature birth in future pregnancies? No.

Does an early abortion cause birth defects in future pregnancies? No.

Does an early abortion lead to low infant birth-weight in the future? No.

Does an early abortion increase the chance of infant death in the future? No.

Does having several abortions affect future pregnancies? Early abortions done by experienced clinicians that are not followed by complications like infection do not cause infertility. Neither do they make it more difficult to carry a later pregnancy to term. It is unclear whether several abortions in later pregnancy result in a greater risk of miscarriage or premature birth.

Does abortion cause breast cancer? No, but abortion does not offer the protection against breast cancer that having several full-term pregnancies does.

How much does abortion cost?

Fees vary depending on how long you've been pregnant and where you go for the abortion. In most cases, the fees cover one examination and laboratory tests, the anesthetic, the procedure, the follow-up exam, and a birth control method. At clinics the cost ranges from about $250 to $450 for abortion in the first trimester. Costs at hospitals will be higher, depending on how long you stay and what anesthetics are used. There may be additional charges if extra tests or medications are needed.

Ask beforehand about payment. Some places want to be paid in advance. Some accept credit cards. An installment plan or other special arrangement can sometimes be worked out. Some health insurance policies will cover some or all of the cost. In all states, Medicaid will pay for an abortion when the life of the woman is in danger. In some states, Medicaid will pay for abortions under other circumstances as well. Check with your local Planned Parenthood health center or your state or local health or welfare department for the kind of Medicaid coverage in your state.

Glossary

Anesthetic. Medication that is injected or inhaled to reduce or eliminate the feeling of pain.

Cervix. The lower part of the uterus, with an opening connecting the uterus to the vagina.

Ectopic Pregnancy. Abnormal pregnancy that develops outside the uterus, usually in a fallopian tube.

Embryo. The organism that develops from the pre-embryo and begins to share the woman's blood supply about nine days after fertilization—after eight weeks of pregnancy the embryo becomes a fetus.

Fallopian Tubes. Two narrow tubes that carry eggs from the ovaries to the uterus.

Fetus. The organism that develops from the embryo at the end of eight weeks of pregnancy and receives nourishment through the placenta—the fetus continues to develop until pregnancy ends.

Hysterectomy. The total or partial removal of the uterus.

Intravenous. Within a vein or veins, a way of giving medication so that it acts more rapidly than if taken orally.

Methotrexate. A medication that inhibits the growth of tissue, used to end ectopic pregnancy and, more commonly, to treat cancer, arthritis, and psoriasis.

Mifepristone. Formerly known as RU 486, a drug that blocks the effects of progesterone, the hormone that sustains pregnancy. It is also used to prevent pregnancy and to treat several forms of cancer.

Misoprostol. A medication, commonly used to treat stomach ulcers, that can stimulate contractions of the uterus.

Placenta. The organ that unites the fetus with the uterus and through which nourishment passes from the woman to her fetus.

Pre-Embryo. The ball of cells that develops from the fertilized egg until about nine days after fertilization, when implantation is completed and pregnancy begins.

Prostaglandins. Chemicals produced by the body to stimulate contractions of the smooth muscles, including those that form the uterus.

Rh Factor. Genetic material found on the surface of red blood cells. If a woman and her fetus have different Rh factors, the woman must receive medication in order to prevent the development of antibodies that would endanger the fetus in future pregnancies.

Sonogram. A picture shown on a video display terminal that is obtained by bouncing sound waves off an object. This harmless procedure shows the fetus in the uterus. It is frequently performed by inserting a probe into the vagina.

Trimester. One of three periods during pregnancy that are each three months long.

Uterus. The pear-shaped reproductive organ from which women menstruate, and where normal pregnancy develops (womb).

Vagina. The stretchable passage between a woman's vulva (outer sex organs) and the cervix and uterus.

Part Four

Other Common
Physical Health Concerns
Prevalent in Women

Chapter 16

Breast Care

Chapter Contents

Section 16.1

Breast Self-Exam

NIH Pub No. 91-2151.

If you menstruate, the best time to do Breast Self-Exam (BSE) is 2 or 3 days after your period ends, when your breast is least likely to be tender or swollen. If you no longer menstruate, pick a day, such as the first day of the month, to do BSE. Here is how to do BSE:

1. Stand before a mirror. Inspect your breast for anything unusual, such as any discharge from the nipple, or puckering, dimpling, or scaling of the skin.

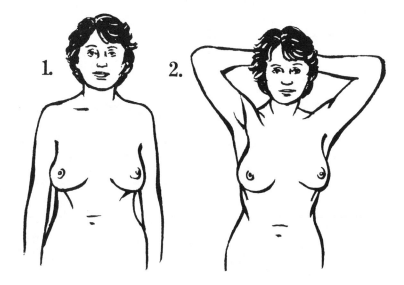

Figure 16.1.

266

The next two steps are designed to emphasize any change in the shape or contour of your breast. As you do them, you should be able to feel your chest muscles tighten.

2. Watching closely in the mirror, clasp your hands behind your head and press your hands forward.

3. Next, press your hands firmly on your hips and bow slightly toward your mirror as you pull your shoulders and elbows forward.

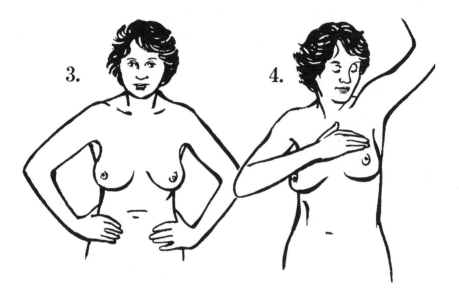

Figure 16.2.

The next part of the exam is done while standing. Some women do it in the shower because fingers glide over soapy skin, making it easy to concentrate on the texture underneath.

4. Raise your arm on one side. Using three or four fingers of your other hand, explore your breast firmly, carefully, and thoroughly. Beginning at the outer edge, press the flat part of your fingers in small circles, moving the circles slowly around

the breast. Gradually work toward the nipple. Be sure to cover the entire breast. Pay special attention to the area between the breast and the underarm, including the underarm itself. Feel for any unusual lump or mass under the skin.

5. Gently squeeze the nipple and look for a discharge. Raise your other arm. Use three or four fingers of your opposite hand. Press gently, using small circular motions. Look for thickenings, lumps, and hard places.

6. Steps 4 and 5 should be repeated lying down. Lie flat on your back, raise your arm side over your head, and place a pillow or folded towel under your shoulder. This position flattens the breast and makes it easier to examine. Use the same circular motion described earlier.

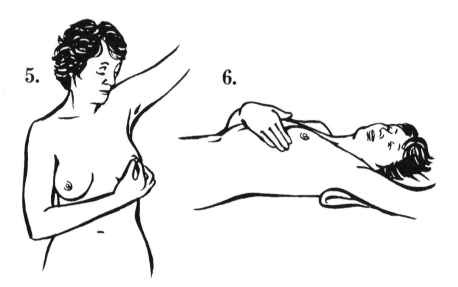

Figure 16.3.

Section 16.2

Breast Cancer

Source: NIH Pub. No. 94-1556.

What Is Cancer?

Cancer is a group of diseases. It occurs when cells become abnormal and divide without control or order.

Every organ in the body is made up of various kinds of cells. Cells normally divide in an orderly way to produce more cells only when they are needed. This process helps keep the body healthy.

If cells divide when new cells are not needed, they form too much tissue. The mass of extra tissue. called a tumor, can be benign or malignant.

- Benign tumors are not cancer. They can usually be removed, and in most cases, they don't come back. Most important, the cells in benign tumors do not invade other tissues and do not spread to other parts of the body. Benign breast tumors are not a threat to life.

- Malignant tumors are cancer. They can invade and damage nearby tissues and organs. Also, cancer cells can break away from a malignant tumor and enter the bloodstream or lymphatic system. That is how breast cancer spreads and forms secondary tumors in other parts of the body. The spread of cancer is called metastasis.

The Breasts

Each breast has 15 to 20 sections, called lobes, that are arranged like the petals of a daisy. Each lobe has many smaller lobules, which end in dozens of tiny bulbs that can produce milk. The lobes, lobules, and bulbs are all linked by thin tubes called ducts. These ducts lead to the nipple in the center of a dark area of skin called the areola. Fat fills the spaces between lobules and ducts. There are no muscles in the breast, but muscles lie under each breast and cover the ribs.

Each breast also contains blood vessels and vessels that carry lymph. The lymph vessels lead to small bean-shaped organs called lymph nodes. Clusters of lymph nodes are found under the arm, above the collarbone, and in the chest. Lymph nodes are also found in many other parts of the body.

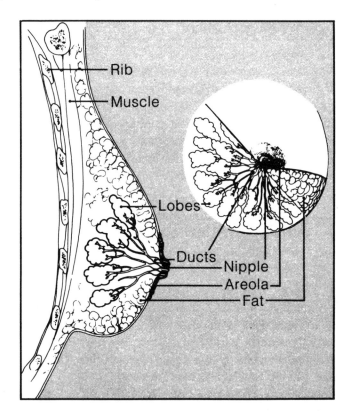

Figure 16.4.

Types of Breast Cancer

There are more than 100 different types of cancer, including several types of breast cancer. The most common type of breast cancer begins in the lining of the ducts and is called ductal carcinoma. Another type, called lobular carcinoma, arises in the lobules. Cancers that begin in other tissues in the breast are rare and are not discussed in this section.

When breast cancer spreads outside the breast, cancer cells are often found in the lymph nodes under the arm. If the cancer has reached these nodes, it may mean that cancer cells have spread to other parts of the body, other lymph nodes and other organs, such as the bones, liver, or lungs.

Cancer that spreads is the same disease and has the same name as the original (primary) cancer. When breast cancer spreads, it is called metastatic breast cancer, even though the secondary tumor is in another organ. Doctors may call this problem "distant" disease.

Early Detection

When breast cancer is found and treated early, a woman has more treatment choices and a good chance of complete recovery. So it is important to detect breast cancer as early as possible. The National Cancer Institute encourages women to take an active part in early detection. They should talk with their doctor about this disease, the symptoms to watch for, and an appropriate schedule of checkups. The doctor's advice will be based on the woman's age, medical history, and other factors. Women should ask the doctor about:

- Mammograms (x-rays of the breast);
- Breast exams by a doctor or nurse; and
- Breast self-examination (BSE).

A mammogram is a special kind of x-ray. It is different from a chest x-ray or x-rays of other parts of the body.

Mammography involves two x-rays of each breast, one taken from the side and one from the top. The breast must be squeezed between two plates for the pictures to be clear. While this squeezing may be a bit uncomfortable, it lasts only a few seconds. In many cases, mammograms can show breast tumors before they cause symptoms or can be felt. A mammogram can also show small deposits of calcium in the breast. A cluster of very tiny specks of calcium (called micro-calcifications) may be an early sign of cancer.

Mammography should be done only by specially trained people using machines designed just for taking x-rays of the breast. The pictures should be checked by a qualified radiologist. Women should talk with their doctor or call the Cancer Information Service for help in finding out where to get a mammogram.

Mammography is an excellent tool, but we know that it cannot find every abnormal area in the breast. So another important step in early detection is for women to have their breasts examined regularly by a doctor or nurse.

Between visits to the doctor, women should examine their breasts every month. It's important to remember that every woman's breasts are different. And each woman's breasts change because of age, the menstrual cycle, pregnancy, menopause, or taking birth control pills or other hormones. It is normal for the breasts to feel lumpy and uneven. Also, it's common for a woman's breasts to be swollen and tender right before or during her menstrual period. These are some of the reasons why many women are not certain what their breasts are supposed to feel like. By doing monthly BSE, a woman learns what is normal for her breasts, and she is more likely to detect a change. Any changes should be reported to the doctor.

Symptoms

Early breast cancer usually does not cause pain. In fact, when it first develops, breast cancer may cause no symptoms at all. But as the cancer grows, it can cause changes that women should watch for:

- A lump or thickening in or near the breast or in the underarm area;
- A change in the size or shape of the breast;
- A discharge from the nipple; or
- A change in the color or feel of the skin of the breast, areola, or nipple (dimpled, puckered, or scaly).

A woman should see her doctor if she notices any of these changes. Most often, they are not cancer, but only a doctor can tell for sure.

Diagnosis

An abnormal area on a mammogram, a lump, or other changes in the breast can be caused by cancer or by other, less serious problems. To find out the cause of any of these signs or symptoms, a woman's doctor does a careful physical exam and asks about her personal and family medical history. In addition to checking general signs of health, the doctor may do one or more of the breast exams described below to help make a diagnosis.

Palpation. The doctor can tell a lot about a lump by palpation (carefully feeling the lump and the tissue around it): its size, its texture, and whether it moves easily. Benign lumps often feel different from cancerous ones.

Mammography. X-rays of the breast can give the doctor important information about a breast lump. If an area on the mammogram looks suspicious or is not clear, additional views may be needed.

Ultrasonography. Sometimes the doctor orders ultrasonography, which can often show whether a lump is solid or filled with fluid. This exam uses high-frequency sound waves, which cannot be heard by humans. The sound waves enter the breast and bounce back. The pattern of their echoes produces a picture called a sonogram, which is displayed on a screen. This exam is often used along with mammography.

Based on these exams, the doctor may decide that no further tests are needed and no treatment is necessary. In such cases, the doctor may want to check the woman regularly to watch for any changes. Often, however, the doctor must remove fluid or tissue from the breast to make a diagnosis.

Aspiration or needle biopsy. The doctor uses a needle to remove fluid or a small amount of tissue from a breast lump. This procedure may show whether the lump is a fluid-filled cyst (not cancer) or a solid mass (which may or may not be cancer). The material removed in a needle biopsy goes to a lab to be checked for cancer cells.

Surgical biopsy. The doctor cuts out part or all of a lump or suspicious area. A pathologist examines the tissue under a microscope to check for cancer cells.

When a woman needs a biopsy, these are some questions she may want to ask her doctor:

- What type of biopsy will I have? Why?
- How long will the biopsy or aspiration take? Will I be awake? Will it hurt?
- How soon will I know the results?
- If I do have cancer, who will talk with me about treatment? When?

When Cancer Is Found

When cancer is present, the pathologist can tell what kind of cancer it is (whether it began in a duct or a lobule) and whether it is invasive (has invaded nearby tissues in the breast).

Special laboratory tests of the tissue help the doctor learn more about the cancer. For example, hormone receptor tests (estrogen and progesterone receptor tests) can show whether the cancer is sensitive to hormones. Positive test results mean hormones help the cancer grow and the cancer is likely to respond to hormone treatment. Other lab tests are sometimes done to help the doctor predict whether the cancer is likely to grow slowly or quickly. If the diagnosis is cancer, the patient may want to ask these questions:

- What kind of breast cancer do I have? Is it invasive?
- What did the hormone receptor test show? What other lab tests were done on the tumor tissue, and what did they show?
- How will this information help the doctor decide what type of treatment or further tests to recommend?

The patient's doctor may refer her to doctors who specialize in treating breast cancer. Treatment generally follows within a few weeks after the diagnosis. The woman will have time to talk with the doctor about her treatment choices, to consider getting a second opinion, and to prepare herself and her loved ones.

Treatment

Many treatment methods are used for breast cancer. Treatment depends on the size and location of the tumor in the breast, the results of lab tests (including hormone receptor tests) done on the cancer cells, and the stage (or extent) of the disease. The patient may have further tests to find out whether the cancer has spread. For example, the doctor usually orders x-rays of the lungs and blood tests to check the liver. In some cases, the doctor orders other special exams of the liver, lungs, or bones because breast cancer tends to spread to these areas. To develop a treatment plan to fit each patient's needs, the doctor also considers the woman's age and general health as well as her feelings about the treatment options. Women with breast cancer are likely to have many questions and concerns about their treatment plan. They want to learn all they can about their disease and their treatment choices so they can take an active part in decisions about their medical care. The doctor is the best person to answer questions about how the disease can be treated, how successful the treatment is expected to be, and how much it is likely to cost. Also, the patient may want to talk with her doctor about taking part in a research study of new treatment methods.

Many patients find it helps to make a list of questions before seeing the doctor. Taking notes during talks with the doctor can make it easier to remember what the doctor says. Some patients also find that it helps to have a family member or friend with them when they see the doctor, to take part in the discussion, to take notes, or just to listen.

Here are some questions a woman may want to ask the doctor before treatment begins:

- What is the stage of the disease?
- What are my treatment choices? Which do you recommend for me? Why?
- What are the expected benefits of each kind of treatment?
- What are the risks and possible side effects of each treatment?
- Would a clinical trial be appropriate for me?

Most patients also want to know how they will look after treatment and whether they will have to change their normal activities. There's a lot to learn about breast cancer and its treatment. Patients should not feel that they need to ask all their questions or understand all the answers at once. They will have many other chances to ask the doctor to explain things that are not clear and to ask for more information.

Planning Treatment

Before starting treatment, the patient might want a second opinion about the diagnosis and the treatment plan. It may take a week or two to arrange to see another doctor. Studies show that a brief delay between biopsy and treatment does not make breast cancer treatment less effective. There are a number of ways to find a doctor for a second opinion:

- The patient's doctor may refer her to a specialist. Specialists who treat breast cancer include surgeons. medical oncologists, and radiation oncologists. Sometimes these doctors work together at cancer centers or special centers for breast diseases.

- The Cancer Information Service, at 1-800-4-CANCER, can tell callers about cancer centers and other NCI-supported programs in their area.

- Patients can get the names of specialists from their local medical society, a nearby hospital, or a medical school.

Methods of Treatment

Methods of treatment for breast cancer are local or systemic. Local treatments are used to remove, destroy, or control the cancer cells in a specific area. Surgery and radiation therapy are local treatments. Systemic treatments are used to destroy or control cancer cells all over the body. Chemotherapy and hormone therapy are systemic treatments. A patient may have just one form of treatment or a combination, depending on her needs.

Surgery. Surgery is the most common treatment for breast cancer. An operation to remove the breast is a mastectomy; an operation to remove the cancer but not the breast is called breast-sparing surgery. Breast-sparing surgery usually is followed by radiation therapy to destroy any cancer cells that may remain in the area. In most cases, the surgeon also removes lymph nodes under the arm to help determine the stage of the disease.

Several types of surgery are used to treat breast cancer. The doctor can explain them in detail and can tell the patient how each will affect her appearance.

- In lumpectomy, the surgeon removes just the breast lump and a margin of normal tissue around it. In partial (segmental) mastectomy, the tumor, some of the normal breast tissue around it, and the lining over the chest muscles below the tumor are removed.

- In total (simple) mastectomy, the whole breast is removed.

- In modified radical mastectomy, the surgeon removes the breast, some of the lymph nodes under the arm, and the lining over the chest muscles. Sometimes the smaller of the two chest muscles is removed.

- In radical mastectomy (also called Halsted radical mastectomy), the surgeon removes the breast, the chest muscles, all of the lymph nodes under the arm, and some additional fat and skin. This operation was the standard one for many years, but it is seldom used now.

These are some questions a woman may want to ask her doctor before surgery:

- What kind of operation will it be?
- How will I feel after the operation? If I have pain, how will you help me?
- Where will the scars be? What will they look like?
- If I decide to have plastic surgery to rebuild my breast, when can that be done?
- Will I have to do special exercises?
- When can I get back to my normal activities?

Radiation Therapy or Radiotherapy. In radiation therapy (also called radiotherapy), high-energy rays are used to damage cancer cells and stop them from growing. Radiation may come from a machine outside the body (external radiation). It can also come from radioactive materials placed directly in the breast in thin plastic tubes (implant radiation). Sometimes the patient receives both kinds of radiation therapy.

Patients go to the hospital or clinic each day for external radiation treatments. When this therapy follows breast-sparing surgery, the treatments are given 5 days a week for 5 to 6 weeks. At the end of that time, an extra "boost" of radiation is often given to the tumor site. The boost may be either external or internal (using an implant). Patients stay in the hospital for a short time for implant radiation.

Before radiation therapy, a patient may want to ask her doctor these questions:

- Why do I need this treatment?
- When will the treatments begin? When will they end?
- How will I feel during therapy?
- What can I do to take care of myself during therapy?
- Can I continue my normal activities?
- How will my breast look afterward?

Chemotherapy. Chemotherapy is the use of drugs to kill cancer cells. In most cases, breast cancer is treated with a combination of drugs. The drugs may be given by mouth or by injection into a vein or muscle. Either way, chemotherapy is a systemic therapy, because the drugs enter the bloodstream and travel through the body. Chemotherapy is given in cycles: a treatment period followed by a recovery period, then another treatment, and so on. Most patients have chemotherapy in an outpatient part of the hospital, at the doctor's office, or at home. Depending on which drugs are given and the woman's general health, however, she may need to stay in the hospital during her treatment.

Hormone Therapy. Hormone therapy is used to keep cancer cells from getting the hormones they need to grow. This treatment may include the use of drugs that change the way hormones work or surgery to remove the ovaries, which make hormones. Like chemotherapy, hormone therapy is a systemic treatment; it can affect cancer cells throughout the body.

Patients may want to ask these questions about chemotherapy or hormone therapy:

- Why do I need this treatment?
- If I need hormone treatment, which would be better for me — drugs or an operation?
- What drugs will I be taking? What will they do?
- Will I have side effects? What can I do about them?
- How long will I be on this treatment?

Treatment Choices

Treatment decisions are complex. These decisions are affected by the experience and judgment of the doctor and by the desires of the patient. The choices available for a particular patient depend on a number of factors. These include the woman's age and menopausal status, her general health, the location of the tumor, and the size of her breast. Certain features of the cancer cells (such as whether they depend on hormones and how fast they are growing) are also considered. The most important factor is the stage of the cancer. The stage is based on the size of the tumor and whether the cancer is only in the breast or has spread to other organs. On the following pages are brief descriptions of the treatments most often used for each stage of breast cancer.

Carcinoma *in situ*. Carcinoma *in situ* is very early breast cancer. Cancer cells are found in only a few layers of cells. Because it has not invaded nearby tissue, the cancer is called non-invasive.

Patients with carcinoma *in situ* may have breast-sparing surgery or mastectomy. The type of surgery depends mainly on whether the cancer developed in a duct (intraductal carcinoma) or a lobule (lobular carcinoma *in situ*). In some cases, some of the underarm lymph nodes are removed, and radiation therapy may be recommended.

Stage I and Stage II Cancers. Stage I and stage II are early stages of breast cancer, but the cancer has invaded nearby tissue. Stage I means that cancer cells have not spread beyond the breast and the tumor is no more than about an inch across. Stage II means that cancer has spread to underarm lymph nodes and/or the tumor in the breast is 1 to 2 inches across.

Women with early stage breast cancer may have breast-sparing surgery followed by radiation therapy as their primary local treatment, or they may have a mastectomy. These treatments are equally effective. With either approach, lymph nodes under the arm generally are removed.

In addition, some women with stage I and most with stage II breast cancer have chemotherapy and/or hormone therapy in addition to their local treatment. This added treatment is called adjuvant therapy. It is given to prevent the cancer from recurring by killing undetected cancer cells that may have begun to spread.

Stage III Cancers. Stage III means the tumor in the breast is more than 2 inches across, the cancer is more extensive in the underarm lymph nodes, or it has spread to other lymph node areas or to other tissues near the breast. This stage of breast cancer is also called locally advanced cancer.

Patients with stage III breast cancer usually have both local treatment to remove or destroy the cancer in the breast and systemic treatment to stop the disease from spreading. The local treatment may be mastectomy and/or radiation therapy to the breast; also, the lymph nodes under the arm may be removed or treated with radiation. The systemic treatment may be chemotherapy, hormone therapy, or both; it may be given before local treatment.

Stage IV or Metastatic Cancers. Stage IV is metastatic cancer. The cancer has spread from the breast to other organs of the body.

Women who have stage IV breast cancer receive chemotherapy and/ or hormone therapy to shrink the tumor or destroy cancer cells. They may have surgery or radiation therapy to control the cancer in the breast. Radiation may also be useful to control tumors in other parts of the body.

Recurrent Cancers. Recurrent cancer means the disease has reappeared, even though the patient's treatment has seemed to be successful. Even when a tumor in the breast seems to have been completely removed or destroyed, the disease sometimes returns because undetected cancer cells have remained in the area after treatment or because the disease had already spread before treatment.

When the cancer returns only in the breast area, it is called a local recurrence. If the disease returns in another part of the body, it is called metastatic breast cancer (or distant disease). The doctor will choose one type of treatment or a combination of treatments to meet the woman's needs.

Side Effects of Treatment

It is hard to limit the effects of cancer treatment so that only cancer cells are removed or destroyed. Because healthy cells and tissues may also be damaged, treatment often causes unpleasant side effects.

Removal of a breast can cause a woman's weight to shift and be out of balance, especially if she has large breasts. This imbalance can also cause discomfort in a woman's neck and back. Also, the skin in the breast area may be tight, and the muscles of the arm and shoulder may feel stiff. After a mastectomy, a few women have some permanent loss of strength in these muscles, but for most women, reduced strength and limited movement are temporary. The doctor, nurse, or physical therapist can recommend exercises to help a woman regain movement and strength in her arm and shoulder.

Because nerves are injured or cut during surgery, a woman may have numbness and tingling in the chest, underarm, shoulder, and arm. These feelings usually go away within a few weeks or months, but some numbness may be permanent.

Removing the lymph nodes under the arm slows the flow of lymph. In some women, lymph builds up in the arm and hand and causes swelling (lymphedema). Also, it is harder for the body to fight infection after the lymph nodes have been removed, so women need to protect the arm and hand on the treated side from injury, for the rest of their lives. They should ask the doctor how to handle any cuts, scratches, insect bites, or other injuries that may occur. Also, they should contact the doctor if an infection develops. The radiation oncologist will explain the possible side effects of radiation therapy for breast cancer, including uncommon side effects that may involve the heart, lungs, and ribs, before treatment begins. Some of the more common side effects are described here. For example, during radiation therapy, patients may become very tired, especially in the later weeks of treatment. Resting is important, but doctors usually advise their patients to try to stay reasonably active. Women should match their activities to their energy level. It's common for radiation to cause the skin in the treated area to become red and dry, tender, and itchy. Toward the end of treatment, the skin may become moist and "weepy." This area should be exposed to the air as much as possible. Patients should avoid wearing a bra or clothes that may rub; loose-fitting cotton clothes are usually best. Good skin care is important at this time, but patients should not use any lotions or creams without the doctor's advice, and they should not use any deodorant on the treated side. The effects of radiation therapy on the skin are temporary. The area will heal when the treatment is over.

Following radiation therapy, the treated breast may be firmer. Also, it may be larger (due to fluid buildup) or smaller (because of tissue changes) than before. For some women, the breast skin is more sensitive after radiation treatment; for others, it is less sensitive.

The side effects of chemotherapy depend mainly on the drugs the patient receives. In addition, as with other types of treatment, side effects vary from person to person. In general, anticancer drugs affect rapidly dividing cells. These include blood cells, which fight infection, cause the blood to clot, and carry oxygen to all parts of the body. When blood cells are affected by anticancer drugs, patients are more likely to get infections, bruise or bleed easily, and have less energy. Cells in hair follicles and cells that line the digestive tract also divide rapidly. As a result of chemotherapy, patients may lose their hair and may have other side effects, such as loss of appetite, nausea, vomiting, or mouth sores. These generally are short-term side effects. They gradually go away during the recovery part of the chemotherapy cycle or after the treatment is over.

Some anticancer drugs can damage the ovaries. If the ovaries fail to produce hormones, the woman may have symptoms of menopause, such as hot flashes and vaginal dryness. Her periods may become irregular or may stop, and she may not be able to become pregnant. In women over the age of 35 or 40, some of these effects, such as infertility, are likely to be permanent.

Hormone therapy can cause a number of side effects. They depend largely on the specific drug or type of treatment, and they vary from patient to patient. Tamoxifen is the most commonly used form of hormone treatment. This drug blocks the body's use of estrogen but does not stop estrogen production. Its side effects usually are not severe. Tamoxifen may cause hot flashes, vaginal discharge or irritation, and irregular periods, but it does not cause menopause or infertility. Young women whose ovaries are removed to deprive the cancer cells of estrogen experience menopause immediately. The side effects they have, including hot flashes and vaginal dryness, are likely to be more severe than those of natural menopause.

Loss of appetite can be a problem for cancer patients. They may not feel hungry when they are uncomfortable or tired. Also, some of the common side effects of cancer treatment, such as nausea and vomiting, can make it hard to eat. The doctor may suggest medicine to help with these problems because good nutrition is important. Patients who eat well often feel better and have more energy. They also may be better able to withstand the side effects of their treatment. Eating well means getting enough calories and protein to help prevent weight loss, regain strength, and rebuild normal tissues. Many patients find that eating several small meals and snacks during the day works better than trying to have three large meals.

The side effects of cancer treatment are different for each person, and they may even be different from one treatment to the next. Doctors try to plan treatment to keep problems to a minimum. They also watch patients carefully so they can help with any problems that occur. Doctors, nurses, and dietitians can explain the side effects of treatment and can suggest ways to deal with them. The NCI booklets *Radiation Therapy and You*, *Chemotherapy and You*, and *Eating Hints* have helpful information about cancer treatment and coping with side effects.

After Treatment

Rehabilitation is a very important part of breast cancer treatment. The medical team makes every effort to help women return to their normal activities as soon as possible. Recovery will be different for each woman, depending on the extent of the disease, the treatment she had, and other factors.

Exercising after surgery can help a woman regain motion and strength in her arm and shoulder. It can also reduce pain and stiffness in her neck and back. Carefully planned exercises should be started as soon as the doctor says the woman is ready, often within a day or so after surgery. Exercising begins slowly and gently and can even be done in bed. Gradually, exercising can be more active, and regular exercise should become part of a woman's normal routine. (Women who have a mastectomy and immediate breast reconstruction-plastic surgery to rebuild the breast-need special exercises, which the doctor or nurse will explain.)

Lymphedema after surgery can be reduced or prevented with certain exercises and by resting with the arm propped up on a pillow. If lymphedema occurs later on, the doctor may suggest exercises and other ways to deal with this problem. For example, some women with lymphedema wear an elastic sleeve or use an elastic cuff to improve lymph circulation. The doctor also may suggest other approaches, such as medication or use of a machine that compresses the arm.

After a mastectomy, some women decide to wear a breast form (prosthesis). Others prefer to have breast reconstruction, either at the same time as the mastectomy or later on. Each plan has its pros and cons, and what is right for one woman may not be right for another. What's important is that nearly every woman treated for breast cancer has a choice. It may be helpful to talk with a plastic surgeon before the mastectomy, but reconstruction is still possible years later.

Various procedures are used to reconstruct the breast. Some use artificial implants; others use tissue moved from another part of the woman's body. The woman should ask the plastic surgeon to explain the risks and benefits of each type of reconstruction. The Cancer Information Service can suggest sources of printed information about breast reconstruction and can tell callers about breast cancer support groups. Members of such groups are often willing to share their personal experiences with breast reconstruction.

Follow-up Care

Regular follow-up exams are very important after breast cancer treatment. The doctor will continue to check the woman closely to be sure that the cancer has not returned. Regular checkups usually include exams of the chest, underarm, and neck. From time to time, the woman has a complete physical exam, blood and urine tests, mammography, and a chest x-ray. The doctor sometimes orders scans (special x-rays) and other exams as well. A woman who has had cancer in one breast has a higher-than-average risk of developing cancer in her other breast. She should continue to practice breast self-examination, checking both the treated area and her other breast each month. She should report any changes to her doctor right away.

Also, a woman who has had breast cancer should tell her doctor about other physical problems if they come up, such as pain, loss of appetite or weight, changes in menstrual periods, or blurred vision. She should also report dizziness, coughing or hoarseness, headaches, or digestive problems that seem unusual or that don't go away. These symptoms may be a sign that the cancer has returned, but they can also be signs of many other problems. Only the doctor can tell for sure.

Living With Cancer

The diagnosis of breast cancer can change a woman's life and the lives of those close to her. These changes can be hard to handle. It's common for the woman and her family and friends to have many different and sometimes confusing emotions.

At times, patients and their loved ones may be frightened, angry, or depressed. These are normal reactions when people face a serious health problem. Most people find it helps to share their thoughts and feelings with loved ones. Sharing can help everyone feel more at ease and can open the way for others to show their concern and offer their support.

Sometimes women who have had breast cancer are afraid that changes to their body will affect not only how they look but how other people feel about them. They may be concerned that breast cancer and its treatment will affect their sexual relationships. Most couples find that talking about these concerns helps them find ways to express their love during and after treatment.

Cancer patients may worry about holding a job, caring for their families, or starting new relationships. Worries about tests, treatments, hospital stays, and medical bills are also common. Doctors, nurses, or other members of the health care team can help calm fears and ease confusion about treatment, working, or daily activities. Also, meeting with a nurse, social worker, counselor, or member of the clergy can be helpful to patients who want to talk about their feelings or discuss their concerns about the future or about personal relationships.

Members of the health care team can provide information and suggest other resources. In addition, the public library is a good source of books and articles on living with cancer.

Support for Breast Cancer Patients

Finding the strength to deal with the changes brought about by breast cancer can be easier for patients and those who love them when they have appropriate support services.

Many patients find it helpful to talk with others who are facing problems like theirs. Cancer patients often get together in self-help and support groups, where they can share what they have learned about cancer and its treatment and about coping with the disease. Often a social worker or nurse meets with the group.

The American Cancer Society's Reach to Recovery program offers special help for breast cancer patients. Trained volunteers, who have had breast cancer themselves, visit patients at the doctor's request and lend emotional support to women before and after treatment. They share their experiences with breast cancer treatment and rehabilitation and with breast reconstruction.

Friends and relatives, especially those who have had cancer themselves, can also be very supportive. It's important to keep in mind, however, that each patient is different. Treatments and ways of dealing with cancer that work for one person may not be right for another even if they both have the same kind of cancer. It is always a good idea to discuss the advice of friends and family members with the doctor.

Often, the doctor's staff or a social worker at the hospital or clinic can suggest local and national groups that can help with emotional support, rehabilitation, financial aid, transportation, or home care. Information about programs and services for breast cancer patients and their families is also available through the Cancer Information Service.

What the Future Holds

Researchers are finding better ways to detect and treat breast cancer, and the chances of recovery keep improving. Still, it is natural for patients to be concerned about their future.

Sometimes patients use statistics they have heard to try to figure out their own chances of being cured. It is important to remember, however, that statistics are averages based on large numbers of patients. They can't be used to predict what will happen to a particular woman because no two cancer patients are alike. The doctor who takes care of the patient and knows her medical history is in the best position to talk with her about the chance of recovery (prognosis). Women should feel free to ask the doctor about their prognosis, but they should keep in mind that not even the doctor knows exactly what will happen. Doctors often talk about surviving cancer, or they may use the term remission. Doctors use these terms because, although many breast cancer patients are cured, the disease can recur.

The Promise of Cancer Research

Scientists at hospitals and medical centers all across the country are studying breast cancer. They are trying to learn more about what causes this disease and how to prevent it. They are also looking for better ways to diagnose and treat it.

Causes and Prevention

Each year, more than 180,000 women in the United States find out they have breast cancer. Although this disease also occurs in about 1,000 men in this country each year, more than 99 percent of all breast cancer patients are women.

Scientists do not know what causes breast cancer, and doctors can seldom explain why one person gets this disease and another doesn't. It is clear, however, that breast cancer is not caused by bumping, bruising, or touching the breast. And this disease is not contagious; no one can "catch" breast cancer from another person.

By studying large numbers of women all over the world, researchers have found certain risk factors that increase a woman's chance of developing breast cancer. Women with these risk factors have a higher-than-average chance of getting this disease. However, studies also show that most women with these risk factors do not get breast cancer. And many women who get breast cancer have none of the risk factors we know about: The following are some of the known risk factors for this disease:

- **Age.** The risk of breast cancer increases as a woman gets older. Most breast cancers occur in women over the age of 50; the risk is especially high for women over 60. This disease is uncommon in women under the age of 35.

- **Family history.** The risk of getting breast cancer increases for a woman whose mother, sister, or daughter has had the disease. The woman's risk increases more if her relative's cancer developed before menopause or if it affected both breasts.

- **Personal history.** Women who have had breast cancer face an increased risk of getting breast cancer again. About 15 percent of women treated for breast cancer get a second breast cancer later on. The risk is greater for women who have had lobular carcinoma in situ.

Other risk factors for breast cancer include starting to menstruate at an early age (before 12) or having a late menopause (after 55). The risk is also greater in women who had their first child after the age of 30 and those who never had children. Because these factors are all related to a woman's natural hormones, many people are concerned about medicines that contain hormones (either for birth control or as estrogen replacement therapy to control symptoms of menopause), especially if women take them for many years. At this time, no one knows for sure whether taking hormones affects the risk of breast cancer.

Scientists hope to find the answer to this important question by studying a large number of women taking part in hormone-related research.

Research suggests that a person's diet may affect the chances of getting some types of cancer. Breast cancer appears to be more likely to develop in women whose diet is high in fat. Older women who are overweight also seem to have a greater risk. Although the possible link between diet and breast cancer is still under study, some scientists believe that choosing a low-fat diet, eating well-balanced meals with plenty of fruits and vegetables, and maintaining ideal weight can lower a woman's risk.

Some studies suggest a slightly higher risk of breast cancer among women who drink alcohol. The risk appears to go up with the amount of alcohol consumed, so women who drink should do so only in moderation.

Many women are concerned about benign breast conditions. For most women, the ordinary "lumpiness" they feel in their breasts does not increase their risk of breast cancer. However, women who have had breast biopsies that show certain benign changes in breast tissues, such as atypical hyperplasia, do have an increased risk of breast cancer.

Women who are at high risk for breast cancer are taking part in a study of the drug tamoxifen, which is often used to treat breast cancer patients. This nationwide study is designed to help doctors learn whether tamoxifen can prevent breast cancer in these women. The Cancer Information Service can provide information about this study.

Detection

When breast cancer is found early, patients have more treatment choices and their chance of complete recovery is better. Because breast cancer often occurs in women with none of the known risk factors, it is important for all women to ask their doctor about mammography, breast exams by a doctor or nurse, and breast self-examination.

Unfortunately, the tests we have now cannot reveal every breast cancer at an early stage. Scientists are trying to find better ways to detect breast cancers when they are very small. For example, they are looking for ways to make mammography more accurate. They are also exploring new techniques to produce detailed pictures of the tissues in the breast.

In addition, researchers are studying tumor markers, substances that may be present in abnormal amounts in the blood or urine of a woman who has breast cancer. Several markers have been studied, and this research is continuing. At this time, however, no blood or urine test is reliable enough to reveal early breast cancer.

Treatment

Researchers also are looking for more effective ways to treat breast cancer. In addition, they are exploring ways to reduce the side effects of treatment and improve the quality of patients' lives. When laboratory research shows that a new treatment method has promise, cancer patients receive the treatment in clinical trials. These trials are designed to answer scientific questions and to find out whether the new approach is both safe and effective. Often, clinical trials compare a new treatment with a standard approach. Patients who take part in clinical trials make an important contribution to medical science and may have the first chance to benefit from improved treatment methods.

Trials to study new treatments for patients with all stages of breast cancer are under way. Researchers are testing new treatment methods, new doses and treatment schedules, and new ways of combining treatments. They are working with various anticancer drugs and drug combinations as well as several types of hormone therapy. They are also exploring new ways to combine chemotherapy with hormone therapy and radiation therapy. Some trials include biological therapy, treatment with substances that boost the immune system's response to cancer.

In a number of trials, doctors are trying to learn whether very high doses of anticancer drugs are more effective than the usual doses in destroying breast cancer cells. Because these higher doses seriously damage the patient's bone marrow, where blood cells are formed, researchers are testing ways to replace the bone marrow or to help it recover.

[There are] possible benefits and risks of treatment studies. Those who are interested in taking part in a trial should discuss this option with their doctor.

One way to learn about clinical trials is through PDQ, a computerized resource developed by NCI. PDQ contains information about cancer treatment and an up-to-date list of trials all over the country. Doctors can obtain an access code and use a personal computer to get PDQ information. Also, the Cancer Information Service can provide PDQ information to doctors, patients, and the public.

Section 16.3

Breast Implant Safety

FDA Consumer, November 1995 and excerpts from
DHSS Publication No. 94-1181, January 1994.

Recently published studies have shown that women with silicone
gel-filled breast implants do not have a greatly increased risk of some
well-defined autoimmune diseases, which were among the serious
health concerns surrounding the devices. These include potentially
fatal connective tissue diseases such as scleroderma and lupus
erythematosus.

Widespread reports of adverse reactions to silicone gel-filled implants and a lack of evidence supporting their safety led the Food and
Drug Administration to order the devices off the market in April 1992.
They remained available only to women in clinical studies, mostly
women seeking breast reconstruction after breast cancer surgery. Saline-
filled implants were allowed to remain on the market for all uses.

The new studies do not, however, rule out the possibility that a
subset of women with implants may have a small increased risk of
these conditions, or that some women might develop other immune-
related symptoms that don't conform to "classic" disease descriptions.

Nor did the studies address other important safety questions, including implant rupture rates and the incidence of capsular
contracture (shrinking of scar tissue around the implant, which can
cause painful hardening of the breast or distort its appearance). Answers to these and other questions await the results of new or ongoing studies.

Reasons for New Studies

Breast implants had been marketed since the early 1960s—several years before the first medical device law was enacted in 1976,
charging FDA with regulation of medical devices. Every year, thousands of American women had had implant surgery for augmentation

(to enlarge or reshape their breasts) or for reconstruction following mastectomy (removal of the breast) to treat breast cancer. Most of the implants consisted of a rubber silicone envelope filled with silicone gel; about 10 percent were filled with saline (salt water).

Under the 1976 law, implants and many other devices already in use were allowed to remain on the market, with the understanding that the agency would at some time ask manufacturers to submit scientific data showing these "grandfathered" products were safe and effective.

FDA requested this information for silicone gel-filled implants in April 1991 in response to a growing number of adverse reaction reports that raised safety concerns about the devices. The data submitted did not prove the devices safe, as required by law, so the agency restricted their use to clinical trials designed to resolve the safety questions.

Between Jan. 1, 1985, and March 16, 1995, FDA received 91,322 adverse reaction reports associated with silicone breast implants and 19,296 reports involving the saline implants. These reports included risks clearly associated with the devices, as well as adverse effects attributed to the implants, but not proved to be linked to them.

Silicone Implant Studies

Some recent studies comparing the rates of immune-related diseases in women with implants versus those without implants have provided reassurance that women with implants are not at a greatly increased risk of these disorders.

The largest of these retrospective, or "look-back," studies is the Harvard Nurses' Health Study. The study used data from 87,501 nurses followed for other research purposes from 1976 through May 31, 1990, before there was widespread media coverage of the possible association between breast implants and connective tissue disease. None of the women had connective tissue disease at the start of the study.

In an article published in the June 22, 1995, *New England Journal of Medicine*, the researchers reported that 516 of the nurses had developed definite connective tissue diseases. Women with breast implants numbered 1,183. The types of implants included 876 silicone gel-filled, 170 saline-filled, 67 double lumen (silicone gel-filled implants with a saline-filled outer envelope), 14 polyurethane-coated, and 56 of unknown type. Only three of the 516 women with definite connective tissue disease had implants (one silicone-gel filled, one saline, and one double lumen).

The authors reported they "did not find an association between silicone breast implants and connective tissue disease, defined according to a variety of standardized criteria, or signs and symptoms of these diseases."

Similarly, a 1994 study conducted at the Mayo Clinic found no increased risk of connective tissue diseases among implant recipients. The investigators based their conclusion on comparison of the medical histories of 749 women with breast implants in Olmsted County, Minn., with a similar group of women who did not have implants.

"Because of the limitations in the size and type of the studies, however, the true risk of these diseases is not known," says S. Lori Brown, Ph.D., a research scientist officer in the epidemiology branch of the agency's Center for Devices and Radiological Health. "Although the criteria others may be using to assess those studies show that some concerns are eliminated," Brown says, "unfortunately, they don't rule out a small, but significant, increased risk."

An immunology and epidemiology expert, Brown explains that an inherent problem in the studies is that some connective tissue diseases are extremely rare. "If you have a disease that has an incidence of 1 in 100,000 in the general population, for example, and you do a study of 750 women with implants, like the Mayo Clinic Study, then you wouldn't really expect to see even a single case of that disease," she says, "unless there's an exceedingly high—more than a hundred-fold—increase in risk."

Small studies like these can rule out huge risks, but not smaller, yet significant risk increases that would only show up in studies that include several thousand women with implants, Brown says. Nor do the studies fully examine or answer whether the implants might in some women lead to symptoms not typical of classical disease manifestations.

Other Concerns

Brown also stresses that connective tissue diseases are not the only issue of concern, especially since they may affect a much smaller proportion of women with implants. The larger issue, she says, is the local complications that are clearly related to breast implants, such as rupture and migration of the silicone gel, capsular contracture, and infection.

"Of the two groups of women who consider getting implants—for breast reconstruction or for augmentation," Brown says, "the larger group wants them for cosmetic purposes. These are healthy women who may go out and get implants without a clear picture of what the possible risks are. They may end up going back in for surgery time and again and never be happy with the cosmetic effect."

In testimony before a congressional subcommittee in August 1995, FDA Commissioner David A. Kessler, M.D., stated that "Published studies to date suggest a rupture rate between 5 and 51 percent—an enormous range—and unfortunately, we do not know with any confidence where within that range the real rupture rate lies." He also cited two studies that indicate the risk of rupture increases as the implants age.

Another concern—increased risk of breast cancer—has not been borne out by studies. Several studies have indicated there is no increased risk of breast cancer in women with implants," Brown says. However, she adds, these women are not yet in the age group that is more prone to breast cancer, and it remains to be seen whether they will eventually have a higher incidence of breast cancer than women without implants. Longterm studies to look at this are underway.

Manufacturers' Studies

The events that led to removal of silicone implants from the market made it clear that prospective, or forward-looking, studies were also needed to answer important safety questions. Implant manufacturers agreed to conduct human trials in three phases: urgent need, adjunct, and core studies.

"The purpose of the first phase [urgent need] actually was simply to quickly provide implants to women who were already in the process of getting them for breast reconstruction or for another medical reason, and to bridge the time until the adjunct studies were begun," says Sahar M. Dawisha, M.D., a rheumatologist and medical officer who joined FDA's division of general and restorative devices in April 1993.

The women did, however, have to sign an informed consent form that summarized the risks and benefits of the implants. This form had not previously been required.

"The second phase, or adjunct, studies were intended to follow reconstruction patients for five years to assess short-term safety data, including rates of capsular contracture, rupture, and complications such as infection and hematoma [collection of blood that may cause swelling, pain and bruising]," Dawisha says. "These studies are open to all women wanting breast reconstruction with implants because of mastectomy, traumatic injury to the breast, or a disease or congenital disorder causing a severe breast abnormality. They do not include augmentation patients."

Mentor Corporation of Santa Barbara, Calif., began adjunct studies in 1992. According to Pamela Powell of the company's Clinical Programs Department, as of July 5, 1995, 12,125 patients were enrolled in the studies.

The third phase, or core studies, Dawisha says, were intended to determine the full safety and effectiveness profile of the device, including rupture rates, quality-of-life benefits, extent of interference with mammography, and many more safety concerns—including rheumatologic assessments—that would need a large number of women. They were also to include augmentation patients. The sponsors, however, have not initiated these studies.

Saline Implants

Although many of the local complications of gel-filled implants are also associated with saline implants, the latter were permitted to remain on the market unrestricted for both reconstruction and augmentation. FDA considers saline filled implants less risky, because although they have the same silicone rubber envelope as gel-filled implants, leakage or rupture would release only salt water, not silicone gel, into the body.

Nevertheless, FDA is requiring manufacturers to collect data on the saline implants as well, because the incidence of known risks (for example, deflation and capsular contracture) is not well defined. When the Medical Device Amendments were passed, it was determined that these devices would also eventually require pre-market approval. In January 1993, FDA notified saline implant manufacturers that they would have to submit safety and effectiveness data for their products. In December 1994, the agency told them what type of safety and effectiveness data were needed, and delineated objectives and time frames for the trials.

Saline implants will stay on the market while the studies are conducted, but the companies must report the laboratory, animal and clinical data in stages, and must provide written information on the known and possible risks of their products.

"Women considering saline implants should ask their doctor for a copy of the manufacturer's information sheet, a copy of the product insert sheet for the specific implant to be used, and a copy of the hospital informed consent form," says Barbara Stellar, FDA's breast implant information and outreach coordinator.

Stellar recommends women be given these documents at least a month before surgery is planned, if possible, so they can thoroughly discuss benefits and possible risks with surgeons, radiologists, and other women. These women should also ask their physicians about participating in the saline breast implant trials.

Brown hopes that further studies will more clearly define risks associated with all types of implants.

"We need to be able to tell women considering breast implants—whether for augmentation or reconstruction—the specific risks on which they can base their decision," she says. "It should be made clear that implants do not last forever, that they may break, and in what time period it is thought they might break. Most women have no idea implants break and there's very little information about rupture rates.

"The same is true for other complications, some of which may require further surgery or may cause the woman to be displeased with the cosmetic effect, which, of course, is the reason she got them," Brown says. "For a product that a person is putting in her body presumably for 20 years or more, we should have this information."

Polyurethane-Coated Implants

About 110,000 women have silicone gel-filled implants with a polyurethane coating, intended to reduce the risk of capsular contracture. In April 1991, an FDA analysis showed that polyurethane foam could break down under human body conditions to form a chemical called TDA, which can cause cancer in animals. As a result, the manufacturer immediately stopped selling the product.

Recently, however, a study to measure TDA in women with polyurethane implants found that a woman's risk of cancer from exposure to TDA released by the implant is negligible—about one in a million over a lifetime. FDA considers it unlikely that even one woman would develop cancer from these implants. The study supports the agency's original recommendation that women who are not having problems should not have the implants removed solely because of concern about cancer from TDA exposure.

Immunology Tests

Several laboratories are offering tests that claim to detect levels of antibodies to silicone that presumably indicate a leaking or ruptured implant.

FDA has not cleared or approved these tests for such purposes, and the agency has sent letters to several companies, warning of future regulatory action if they continue to promote the devices without a pre-market approval application.

"There are important unresolved issues with these tests," says Peter Maxim, Ph.D., chief of the Center for Devices and Radiological Health's immunology branch of the division of clinical laboratory devices. "For one thing, the very existence of silicone antibodies has not been proven to the satisfaction of all scientists," he says. "Secondly, if antibodies are detected, is there in fact a correlation with the presence or the status of implants, or do they reflect prior environmental exposure? Silicone is in a myriad of products, including foods, medicines, and antiperspirants absorbed by the skin, to name a few."

The next problem, Maxim says, is that there are claims that extremely high antibody levels may indicate a leaking or ruptured implant. This, then, raises the question of what medical intervention, if any, should be taken.

Sahar M. Dawisha, M.D., a rheumatologist in FDA's division of general and restorative devices, adds that no one really knows what the clinical significance of an antibody to silicone means or at what level it is harmful.

"Furthermore," she says, "in autoimmune or connective tissue disease—where antibody tests are generally used—the presence of antibodies doesn't define the disease. A disease is defined by clinical signs and symptoms, and antibodies are used as supporting evidence."

Finally, John Nagle, consumer safety officer in the Center for Devices and Radiological Health's diagnostic devices branch, says, "The tests themselves may be harmless, but they sure are expensive, somewhere between $500 and $1,000," adding that "a lot of them are being done for litigation purposes rather than to help the patient medically."

Known Risks of Breast Implants

Surgical Risks

- possible complications of general anesthesia, as well as nausea, vomiting and fever
- infection
- hematoma (collection of blood that may cause swelling, pain and bruising, perhaps requiring surgical draining)

- hemorrhage (abnormal bleeding)
- thrombosis (abnormal clotting)
- skin necrosis–skin tissue death resulting from insufficient blood flow to the skin. The chance of skin necrosis may be increased by radiation treatments, cortisone-like drugs, an implant too large for the available space, or smoking.

Implant Risks

- capsular contracture (hardening of the breast due to scar tissue)

- leak or rupture–silicone implants may leak or rupture slowly, releasing silicone gel into surrounding tissue; saline implants may rupture suddenly and deflate, usually requiring immediate removal or replacement

- temporary or permanent change or loss of sensation in the nipple or breast tissue

- formation of calcium deposits in surrounding tissue, possibly causing pain and hardening

- shifting from the original placement, giving the breast an unnatural look

- interference with mammography readings, possibly delaying breast cancer detection by "hiding" a suspicious lesion. Also, it may be difficult to distinguish calcium deposits formed in the scar tissue from a tumor when interpreting the mammogram. *When making an appointment for a mammogram the woman should tell the scheduler she has implants to make sure qualified personnel are on-site. At the time of the mammogram she should also remind the technician she has implants before the procedure is done so the technician can use special techniques to obtain the best mammogram and to avoid rupturing the implant.*

Possible Risks of Breast Implants

- Autoimmune-like disorders—signs include joint pain and swelling; skin tightness, redness or swelling; swelling of hands and feet; rash; swollen glands or lymph nodes; unusual fatigue; general aching; greater chance of getting colds, viruses and flu; unusual hair loss; memory problems; headaches; muscle weakness or burning; nausea or vomiting; and irritable bowel syndrome.

Recent studies have shown, however, that there is not a large increased risk of traditional autoimmune, or connective tissue disease, from silicone gel implants.

- Fibrositis/fibromyalgia-like disorders (pain, tenderness and stiffness of muscles, tendons and ligaments).

Reporting Problems

To report a problem with an implant, write to

The Problem Reporting Program,
12601 Twinbrook Parkway
Rockville, MD 20852

A copy of your report will be forwarded to the manufacturer and to FDA. If you have documentation you feel would be helpful, please enclose it with your report. Include the following information, if known:

- manufacturer's name
- product brand name
- style, size, and lot number
- dates of all implant surgeries
- patient's age at time of first implant
- whether the procedure was done for augmentation or reconstruction
- date of problem
- nature of problem
- time between implant and onset of symptoms
- name and address of surgeon and facility where surgery was performed
- your name, address, and telephone numbers (optional).

For information about what kind of implants you have, ask your surgeon or contact the facility where you had the surgery.

If You Have Implants....

Most women with silicone gel-filled breast implants do not experience serious problems. *If you are not having problems there is no need to have your implants removed.* But you should have regular checkups by a physician or plastic surgeon. If you have any breast discomfort, changes in size or shape of your breast, or any symptoms you think may be related to your implants, see your doctor.

Regarding specific concerns, the agency advises the following:

- **You should be checked periodically by your physician for as long as you have implants.**

Implants can last from a very short time to many years, depending on the patient and the implant. In any case, they should not be expected to last a lifetime.

- **A ruptured implant should be removed.**

The percentage of implants that rupture is not certain. An FDA advisory panel concluded that the rupture rate may be higher than previously thought. Manufacturers' reports suggest a range between 0.2 and 1.1 percent; the medical literature contains figures ranging between 0 and 25 percent; and individual doctors have said the implants fail in as many as 32 percent of their patients.

The panel also noted that rupture may go undetected in some patients. In some undetected ruptures, the gel may be contained within the fibrous tissue that forms around the implant. Also, the implants "bleed," or leak, silicone, but the significance of the leakage is uncertain.

Routine mammograms are not recommended to detect such "silent" ruptures. Other methods of detection, such as ultrasound, computed axial tomography (CAT) scans, and magnetic resonance imaging (MRI), are being studied, but are not now recommended on a routine basis.

The chance for rupture may increase the longer the implant is in the body. Injury to the breast may also increase the chance of rupture, as may capsular contracture (shrinking of scar tissue around the implant that makes the breast feel hard). Closed capsulotomy—a nonsurgical technique sometimes used to reduce the contracture—may also increase the likelihood of rupture.

- **The value of tests to detect silicone in the blood and urine is uncertain.**

Since small amounts of silicone "bleed" even from intact implants, these tests cannot tell whether your implant has ruptured. Also, silicone is found in many products, including commonly used medicines and cosmetics, so the source of silicone detected may not be clear.

- **If you have symptoms of connective tissue or immune-related disorders, see your doctor.**

It is not known whether implants can cause or contribute to the development of connective tissue and immune-related disorders. But you should be aware of symptoms that can occur with these disorders. They include:

- joint pain and swelling
- skin tightness, redness or swelling
- swollen glands or lymph nodes
- unusual and unexplained fatigue
- swollen hands and feet
- unusual hair loss

People who have immune-related disorders generally have a combination of these and other symptoms. These symptoms can also occur with a variety of other health problems, however, and a doctor's evaluation can rule out other possible causes.

- **Although the possibility cannot be ruled out, there is currently no evidence that silicone gel-filled implants increase the risk of cancer in humans.**

Studies now under way should shed more light on this matter in the next few years.

About 10 percent of women have silicone gel-filled implants coated with polyurethane foam, intended to reduce the risk of capsular contracture. These implants have not been used since April 1991, because studies showed the polyurethane coating could break down to release very small amounts of TDA, a substance that can cause cancer in animals. It is not known whether women with this type of implant have an increased risk of cancer. However, based on current evidence, FDA does not recommend removing polyurethane-coated implants because of cancer concerns. The agency is requiring the manufacturer of these implants to conduct studies analyzing blood, urine, and breast milk for TDA.

- **It is not known whether the silicone that "bleeds" from an implant gets into breast milk and, if so, whether it could affect a nursing child.**

Research is being planned to resolve these concerns.

- **As is recommended for all women, you should have regular breast examinations by a trained health professional, and you should do monthly self-exams.**

To examine your breasts, stand in front of a mirror and look for anything unusual, such as changes in the shape or appearance of your breasts or nipples. Then, with your right arm raised above your head, use the flat surface of your fingertips on your left hand to feel for any unusual lump, swelling, or mass under the skin of the right breast. Also feel for swollen glands or lumps in the armpit. Using your right hand, follow the same procedure to examine the left breast. Repeat the procedure lying down.

Pay particular attention to changes in the firmness size or shape of the breasts. Also note pain tenderness or color changes in the breast area or any discharge or unusual sensation around the nipple. Report them, or any other concerns about your breasts, to your doctor.

- **You should have screening mammography at the same intervals recommended for all women in your age group.**

Good quality mammograms are essential to detect cancer in any woman—with or without breast implants. (If you have had breast cancer surgery, ask your doctor whether mammograms are still necessary.) Mammography is not recommended to detect implant rupture. The radiation exposure to younger women is not justified for this purpose.

Mammographic examination of women with breast implants requires special expertise, however, because implants can often obscure breast tissue, impairing the ability to detect cancer. By taking extra views of the breast and pushing the implant backward and breast tissue forward, visibility is improved. Be sure the mammography facility you go to has personnel trained and experienced in the special techniques needed for women with implants.

Tell the radiologist and the technician that you have implants before they take the mammograms so they know to use special techniques and can take extra care when compressing the breasts to avoid rupturing the implant.

Facilities accredited by the American College of Radiology (ACR) are likely to have appropriately trained staff. For names and locations of ACR-accredited facilities, call the Cancer Information Service (toll-free 1-800-4-CANCER) or your local American Cancer Society chapter. Then double-check with the facility to make sure it can perform the needed techniques.

For Further Information

Additional information and support are available from the agencies listed below.

To obtain a comprehensive packet of information on breast implant issues, request FDA's publication, "Breast Implants, An Information Update," by calling the agency's breast implant information line at (1-800) 532-4440, or For written information on breast implants, write:

FDA, Breast Implant Information
HFE-88
5600 Fishers Lane
Rockville, MD 20857
or call (301) 443-3170

For breast cancer information, including brochures, treatment information, and local resources.

National Cancer Institute
Call 1-800-4-CANCER

A breast cancer support group that provides information and counseling. Write:

Y-Me
18220 Harwood Ave.
Homewood, IL 60430
or call (1-800) 221-2141

An advocacy organization for support and information about breast implants and breast implant surgery. For information, send $1 and a self-addressed, stamped envelope to:

Command Trust Network, Inc.
P.O. Box 17082
Covington, KY 41017

—by Marian Segal

Chapter 17

Osteoporosis

Chapter Contents

Section 17.1

Osteoporosis:
Medicine for the Layman

NIH Publication No. 89-2893, April 1989.

A major health problem, osteoporosis or "porous bone," affects an estimated 20 million Americans. This bone loss disease is most common in the elderly and in postmenopausal women. The loss of bone mass places extra stress on the thin, fragile bone structure that remains causing bones to be susceptible to fracture. Osteoporosis is estimated to cause 1.3 million bone fractures a year in people over 45 years of age. Moreover, in 1985, the national estimated cost of osteoporotic fractures was estimated to be $7 billion a year.

Osteoporosis-related fractures can occur in any of the bones, but the main fractures occur in the vertebral spinal column, the wrist, and the hip. In the spinal column, loss of bone mass starts in women during their 50s and 60s. A simple action like bending forward can be enough to cause a "crush fracture," or spinal compression fracture. These vertebral fractures cause loss of height and a humped back, or a "dowager's hump."

Wrist fractures called a "Colles fracture" also commonly occur among women with osteoporosis. Typically, the fracture occurs when a woman falls and uses her hand to break the fall; this results in a broken wrist.

Fractures of the hip are the most severe. They are associated with more death, more disability, and higher medical costs than all other osteoporotic fractures combined. Twelve to 20 percent of older people with hip fractures die within a year after the fracture. Of the survivors, only a few return to the full level of activities that they enjoyed before the hip fracture.

Risk Factors for Osteoporosis

Many risk factors for osteoporosis have been identified. They include:

- *age.* The chief risk factor for this disease is age; the likelihood of developing osteoporosis increases progressively as we grow older.

- *being a woman.* Osteoporosis is estimated to be six to eight times more common in women than in men. In early adult life women develop less bone mass than men do. Even more critical is that for years after menopause, women lose bone mass much more rapidly because of a reduction in their production of estrogen.

- *early menopause.* The chances of developing osteoporosis increase during early menopause or surgical menopause (after removal of the ovaries), which causes a sudden significant drop in estrogen.

- *being caucasian.* White women are at higher risk than black women, and white men are at higher risk than black men. In general, blacks have 10 percent greater bone mass than whites do.

- *consistently low calcium intake.*

- *lack of weight-bearing exercise.* The significant loss of bone mass in our astronauts who spend considerable time in the weightless environment of outer space dramatically demonstrates the importance of weight-bearing exercise.

- *being underweight.*

- *a family history of osteoporosis.*

- *smoking cigarettes.* The concentration of estrogen in the bloodstream is lowered by cigarette smoking.

- *excessive use of cortisone-like drugs such as prednisone.*

Symptoms of Osteoporosis

Osteoporosis is a silent disease. Usually, it develops for many years until the bones become so weak that a minor injury can cause the bones to fracture. Detection of bone loss with ordinary x-rays does not show up until a person has lost 30 percent of their bone density.

Several techniques for early detection of bone loss have been developed in recent years. In one technique, photon absorptiometry, a machine measures how much the rays like x-rays penetrate the bone (measuring how dense the bones are). Another very useful technique is computerized tomography (CT), which uses x-rays that yield a three-dimensional image.

Bone Growth and Loss

Bone continues to grow and develop throughout childhood and adolescence. During a person's twenties, bone growth increases by 15 percent. Peak bone mass, when the bones are most dense and strong, occurs at 30 to 35 years of age. After this time bone mass gradually diminishes and the bones become less dense.

There is a great need to understand how bone grows and diminishes. By studying the cellular processes responsible for bone growth, researchers hope to discover new treatments for osteoporosis. There is much active and promising research in this area.

Treatment and Prevention

Hormone Replacement Therapy

Scientists now know that a leading cause of osteoporosis in women is postmenopausal estrogen deficiency. They have discovered that estrogen not only slows bone loss but also prevents bone fractures if given when a woman's production of estrogen drops. It is important that the hormone be given during or shortly after menopause because estrogen given years later is of less value. Women who have gone through menopause, and especially those with an early or surgical menopause, should discuss the benefits and risks of estrogen replacement therapy with their physicians.

Another benefit of estrogen therapy is its positive effect on the cardiovascular system. Estrogen reduces cholesterol and the concentration of other lipids (fats) in the bloodstream associated with heart disease. For women on estrogen therapy, the risk of developing endometrial cancer increases from one per 1,000 women to about four per 1,000 women. Fortunately, endometrial cancer is easy to detect and is highly curable. In fact, the death rate from endometrial cancer is lower than the death rate from osteoporotic hip fracture.

One side effect women on estrogen replacement therapy may experience is periodic bleeding. This is because estrogen therapy causes the lining of the uterus to build up. Estrogen usually is prescribed for 20 days, then the hormone is stopped for the remaining 10 days. The lining of the uterus is shed during the days off estrogen.

Progestogen, another female hormone, given in combination with estrogen may help reduce the risk of endometrial cancer. Women in the menopausal period are encouraged to discuss estrogen or progestogen therapy with their doctors.

Calcium Intake

The average American consumes about 450 to 550 milligrams of calcium a day. Experts recommend that both men and women take at least 1,000 milligrams of calcium daily. This is the amount of calcium contained in three eight-ounce glasses of milk. Other sources of calcium include yogurt, cheese, salmon, canned sardines, oysters, shrimp, dried beans, and dark green vegetables such as broccoli, turnip greens, and kale.

People who do not meet their daily requirements of calcium through their diet are encouraged to take a daily supplement of calcium such as calcium carbonate, calcium lactate, calcium gluconate, or calcium citrate. Older men and women should increase their calcium intake up to 1,200 to 1,500 milligrams a day, or about four to five glasses of milk, because calcium absorption from the digestive tract is reduced in the elderly.

Exercise

Research has shown clearly that inactivity leads to bone loss. Studies revealed that astronauts in space lost a great deal of bone from lack of exercise against gravity. A program of moderate weight-bearing exercise three to four hours a week, such as brisk walking, running, tennis, or aerobic dance, is recommended. Swimming is not as valuable because it is not a weight-bearing exercise.

Experimental Treatments

Several promising treatments for osteoporosis are being investigated. Calcitonin, a new drug approved by the Food and Drug Administration in 1984, slows the breakdown of bone. Calcitonin, produced naturally in the body, is a hormone produced by the thyroid gland. The synthetic form is given by daily injection and is expensive. Recently, a less expensive nasal spray of calcitonin has been developed.

Scientists also are studying fluoride combined with calcium for osteoporosis. Still experimental, fluoride is promising in that it has been shown to increase bone mass. Some people experience side effects including nausea, vomiting, diarrhea, and pain in their lower extremities. Fluoride compounds currently are available for treatment in Germany and France. However, more research is needed before this treatment can be proven to be both safe and effective.

Research Directions

This section has described the steps to be taken to protect the bones. Recent studies on nutrition is one new area of new research. Clinicians know that by taking calcium at the right time in life there is hope of preventing bone loss. Researchers also know more about exercise as a method of preventing osteoporosis.

Until recently, there were no clues as to how the hormone, estrogen, prevented osteoporosis. Now investigators have reported the discovery of estrogen receptors on bone. New methods might be harnessed to treat osteoporosis. Through continued research, there is hope for future treatments of osteoporosis.

Section 17.2

Osteoporosis: NIH Consensus Statement

Excerpts from NIH Consensus Statement, April 2-4 1984.

Introduction

Osteoporosis is a major underlying cause of bone fractures in post-menopausal women and older persons in general. It is a condition in which bone mass decreases, causing bones to be more susceptible to fracture. A fall, blow, or lifting action that would not bruise or strain the average person can easily cause one or more bones to break in a person with severe osteoporosis.

Medical practitioners and patients alike are concerned with the optimum approach to the treatment and prevention of osteoporosis. The appropriate timing and proper use of agents, such as calcium, vitamin D, estrogens, and fluorides, as well as the role of exercise are issues that have generated major research efforts and considerable controversy.

In an effort to resolve some of the questions surrounding these issues, the National Institutes of Health convened a Consensus Development Conference on Osteoporosis on April 2-4, 1984. After a day and a half of presentations by experts in the field, a consensus panel including representatives of orthopaedics, endocrinology, gynecology, rheumatology, epidemiology, nutrition, biochemistry, family medicine, and the general public considered the evidence and agreed on answers to the following key questions:

- What is osteoporosis?
- What are the clinical features of osteoporosis, and how is it detected?
- Who is at risk for developing osteoporosis?
- What are the possible causes of osteoporosis?
- How can osteoporosis be prevented and treated?
- What are the directions for future research?

Osteoporosis is a major public health problem. Although all bones are affected, fractures of the spine, wrist, and hip are typical and most common. The risk of developing osteoporosis increases with age and is higher in women than in men and in whites than in blacks. Its cause appears to reside in the mechanisms underlying an accentuation of the normal loss of bone, which follows the menopause in women and occurs in all individuals with advancing age. There are no laboratory tests for defining individuals at risk or those with mild osteoporosis. The diagnosis of primary osteoporosis is established by documentation of reduced bone density or mass in a patient with a typical fracture syndrome after exclusion of known causes of excessive bone loss.

Prevention of fracture in susceptible patients is the primary goal of intervention. Strategies include assuring estrogen replacement in postmenopausal women, adequate nutrition including an elemental calcium intake of 1,000-1,500 mg a day, and a program of modest weight-bearing exercise. There is great need for additional research on understanding the biology of human bone, defining individuals at special risk, and developing safe, effective, low-cost strategies for fracture prevention.

What Is Osteoporosis?

Primary osteoporosis is an age-related disorder characterized by decreased bone mass and by increased susceptibility to fractures in the absence of other recognizable causes of bone loss.

Osteoporosis is a common condition affecting as many as 15-20 million individuals in the United States. About 1.3 million fractures attributable to osteoporosis occur annually in people age 45 and older. Among those who live to be age 90, 32 percent of women and 17 percent of men will suffer a hip fracture, most due to osteoporosis. The cost of osteoporosis in the United States has been estimated at $3.8 billion annually.

Bone is composed of a collagen-rich organic matrix impregnated with mineral—largely calcium and phosphate. Two major forms of bone exist. Compact cortical bone forms the external envelopes of the skeleton; trabecular or medullary bone forms plates that traverse the internal cavities of the skeleton. The proportions of cortical and trabecular bone vary at different sites. Vertebral bodies contain predominantly trabecular bone, while the proximal femur contains predominantly cortical bone. The responses of the two forms of bone to metabolic influences and their susceptibility to fracture differ.

312

Bone undergoes continuous remodeling (turnover) throughout life. Osteoclasts resorb bone in microscopic cavities; osteoblasts then reform the bone surfaces, filling the cavities. Normally, bone resorption and formation are linked closely in space, time, and degree. Mechanical and electrical forces, hormones, and local regulatory factors influence remodeling.

Peak bone mass is achieved at about 35 years of age for cortical bone and earlier for trabecular bone. Sex, race, nutrition, exercise, and overall health influence peak mass. Bone mass is approximately 30 percent higher in men than in women and approximately 10 percent higher in blacks than in whites. In each group, bone mass varies among individuals.

After reaching its peak, bone mass declines throughout life due to an imbalance in remodeling. Bones lose both mineral and organic matrix but retain their basic organization. In women, bone mass decreases rapidly for 3 to 7 years after menopause. Bone loss also is enhanced in a variety of diseases.

Women have more fractures than men, and whites have more fractures than blacks. Three factors determine the likelihood of fractures:

1. The magnitude, direction, and duration of the applied force.

2. The dissipation of that force by muscle contraction and soft tissue absorption

3. Bone strength.

Injuries are more frequent and energy dissipation diminishes with advancing age. Reduction in bone mass is the most important reason for the increased frequency of bone fractures in postmenopausal women and in the elderly.

Classifying primary osteoporosis into clinical, histological, or biochemical subsets may be useful from the standpoints of etiology, prevention, and treatment. There is clinical and histological evidence for different subsets. Vertebral fractures occur most frequently in women aged 55 to 75 with accelerated loss of trabecular bone. Hip fractures occur most frequently in older men and women who slowly have lost both cortical and trabecular mass. Bone biopsies from some individuals with primary osteoporosis show high turnover rates; biopsies from others show low or intermediate rates of turnover.

What Are the Clinical Features of Osteoporosis, and How Is It Detected?

The clinical manifestations of osteoporosis include fractures of the vertebral bodies, the neck and intertrochanteric regions of the femur, and the distal radius. Osteoporotic individuals may fracture any bone more easily than their non-osteoporotic counterparts.

Vertebral Fractures

Vertebral compression fractures occur more frequently in women than in men, and typically affect T8-L3. These fractures may develop during routine activities, such as bending, lifting, or rising from a chair or bed. Immediate, severe, local back pain often results. Pain usually subsides within several months. Some individuals experience persistent pain due to altered spinal mechanics. In contrast, some vertebral fractures do not cause pain. Gradual asymptomatic vertebral compression may be detected only upon radiographic examination. Loss of body height and/or the development of kyphosis may be the only signs of multiple vertebral fractures. Discomfort, debility, and, rarely, pulmonary dysfunction may accompany thoracic shortening. Abdominal symptoms may include early satiety, bloating, and constipation.

Hip Fractures

Hip fractures are another important manifestation of osteoporosis. The affected population tends to be older and the sex distribution more even than is the case in vertebral fracture. Acute complications—hospitalization, depression, and mechanical failure of the surgical procedure—are common. Most patients fail to recover normal activity, and mortality within 1 year approaches 20 percent. Distal radial fractures limit use of the extremity for 4 to 8 weeks, although long-term disability is uncommon. These fractures promote fear of loss of independent living, fear of additional falls and fractures, and depression.

Detection of low skeletal mass and/or a fracture after minor trauma should alert the physician to the presence of metabolic bone disease. The physician should evaluate further to exclude osteomalacia, hyperparathyroidism, hyperthyroidism, multiple myeloma, metastatic disease, syndromes of glucocorticoid excess, and other causes of secondary osteoporosis. No blood or urine test establishes specifically the diagnosis of primary osteoporosis, but such tests may exclude secondary causes.

Evaluating Bone Density

Several non-invasive methods are available to evaluate bone density. These vary widely in cost, availability, and radiation dose. Standard radiographs of the spine are most widely available. Roentgenograms are, however, insensitive indicators of bone loss, since bone density must be decreased by at least 20 to 30 percent before the reduction can be appreciated. Characteristic abnormalities on standard roentgenograms are sufficient for establishing the diagnosis of osteoporosis if secondary causes are excluded clinically or radiographically. If the spine film is not diagnostic but clinical suspicion is high, a variety of other procedures may be indicated. These include radiogrammetry for measurement of cortical thickness, photodensitometry, the Singh Index of femoral trabecular pattern, single and dual photon absorptiometry, neutron activation, Compton scattering, and single and dual energy computed tomography. Use of these techniques will depend on their availability, cost, and further studies of their discriminatory capabilities and sensitivity.

With histomorphometry, usually performed on a bone biopsy from the iliac crest, bone mass can be evaluated and osteomalacia and certain forms of secondary osteoporosis excluded. Bone biopsy is safe but requires specialized equipment and expert analysis that are not widely available.

Who Is at Risk for Developing Osteoporosis

The correlation of osteoporosis with the following factors is well documented. Bone mass declines with age in all people and is related to sex, race, menopause, and body weight-for-height.

Women are at higher risk than men in that they have less bone mass and, for several years following natural or induced menopause, the rate of bone mass decline is accelerated. Early menopause is one of the strongest predictors for the development of osteoporosis. White women are at much higher risk than black women, and white men are at higher risk than black men. Women who are underweight also have osteoporosis more often than overweight women. Cigarette smoking may be an additional predictor of risk. Calcium deficiency has been implicated in the pathogenesis of this disease.

Immobilization and prolonged bed rest produce rapid bone loss, while exercise involving weight bearing has been shown both to reduce bone loss and to increase bone mass. The optimal type and amount of physical activity that will prevent osteoporosis have not been established. Exercise sufficient to induce amenorrhea in young women may lead to decreased bone mass.

The relationship of osteoporosis to hereditary and dietary factors, such as alcohol, vitamins A and C, magnesium, and protein, is less firmly established. Some of these factors may act indirectly through their effect on calcium metabolism or body weight.

What Are the Possible Causes of Osteoporosis?

Because primary osteoporosis is characterized by decreased bone mass, the causes of the disorder must be sought among the factors that determine the quantity and quality of bone, including the magnitude of maximum bone mass at maturity and the rate of bone loss with aging.

Complex cellular, physiologic, and metabolic factors may underlie the pathogenesis of osteoporosis. Discrete cell types, anatomically and functionally connected, are continually renewed and maintain the complex skeletal tissue. Several systemic hormones and an increasingly recognized number of local (paracrine) factors regulate bone cell activity. Diet, as well as intestinal and renal function, influences mineral ion homeostasis needed to maintain the skeleton. The formation and resorption of bone and their coupling also are modified by external physical forces such as those generated by body weight and exercise.

Osteoporosis is histologically, biochemically, and kinetically heterogeneous; rapid bone turnover or reduced rates of bone formation have been documented in patients with primary osteoporosis. Multiple etiologies would not be surprising, considering the complex factors regulating normal bone metabolism. Among the many possible etiologies of primary osteoporosis, current data point to two probable causes: deficiency of estrogen and deficiency of calcium. Rapid bone loss often accompanies menopause, and premature osteoporosis follows bilateral oophorectomy. Estrogen replacement prevents bone loss in both conditions. The following observations support a causal relationship between calcium deficiency and osteoporosis: Calcium deficiency in experimental animals causes osteoporosis; a low calcium intake is common among the elderly in the United States; and calcium supplementation reduces bone loss.

How Can Osteoporosis Be Prevented and Treated?

Physicians must emphasize measures that retard or halt the progress of osteoporosis before irreversible structural defects occur. The mainstays of prevention and management of osteoporosis are estrogen and calcium; exercise and nutrition may be important adjuncts.

Estrogen Therapy

Estrogen replacement therapy is highly effective for preventing osteoporosis in women. Estrogen reduces bone resorption and retards or halts postmenopausal bone loss. Case-controlled studies have shown a substantial reduction in hip and wrist fractures in women whose estrogen replacement was begun within a few years of menopause. Studies also suggest that estrogen reduces the rate of vertebral fractures. Even when started as late as 6 years after menopause, estrogen prevents further loss of bone mass but does not restore it to premenopausal levels. Oral estrogen protects at low doses, such as 0.625 mg of conjugated equine estrogen, (25 micrograms of mestranol and 2 mg of estradiol valcrate daily exemplify other protective regimens reviewed by the panel).

All of the above data on efficacy are based almost exclusively on studies in white women. Therefore, the following recommendations on therapy for osteoporosis pertain to that group. Cyclic estrogen therapy should be given to women whose ovaries are removed before age 50 in whom there are no specific contraindications. Women who have had a natural menopause also should be considered for cyclic estrogen replacement if they have no contraindications and if they understand the risks and agree to regular medical evaluations. The duration of estrogen therapy need not be limited. There is no convincing evidence that initiating estrogen therapy in elderly women will prevent osteoporosis. The decision to treat women of other racial backgrounds should be determined on a case-by-case basis.

Estrogen-associated endometrial cancer is usually manifested at an early stage and is rarely fatal when managed appropriately. The bulk of evidence indicates that estrogen use is not associated with an increased risk of breast cancer. Adding a progestogen probably reduces the risk of endometrial cancer, but there is little information about the safety of long-term combined estrogen and progestogen treatment in postmenopausal women. Younger patients receiving progestogens in oral contraceptives experienced an increased risk of hypertension and cardiovascular disease. Some progestogens may blunt or elimi-nate the favorable effects of estrogen on lipoproteins.

Until more data on risks and benefits are available, physicians and patients may prefer to reserve estrogen (with or without progestogen) therapy for conditions that confer a high risk of osteoporosis, such as the occurrence of premature menopause.

Calcium Intake

The usual daily intake of elemental calcium in the United States, 450 mg to 550 mg, falls well below the National Research Council's (NRC) recommended dietary allowance (RDA) of 800 mg; the RDA is designed to meet the needs of approximately 95 percent or more of the population. Calcium metabolic balance studies indicate a daily requirement of about 1,000 mg of calcium for premenopausal and estrogen-treated women. Postmenopausal women who are not treated with estrogen require about 1,500 mg daily for calcium balance. There-fore, the RDA for calcium is evidently too low, particularly for post-menopausal women and may well be too low in elderly men. In some studies, high dietary calcium suppresses age-related bone loss and reduces the fracture rate in patients with osteoporosis. It seems likely that an increase in calcium intake to 1,000 to 1,500 mg a day begin-ning well before the menopause will reduce the incidence of osteoporo-sis in postmenopausal women. Increased calcium intake may prevent age-related bone loss in men as well.

The major sources of calcium in the U.S. diet are milk and dairy products. Each 8 ounce glass (240 ml) of milk contains 275-300 mg calcium. Skim or low fat milk is preferred to minimize fat intake. For those unable to take 1,000 to 1,500 mg calcium by diet, supplemen-tation with calcium tablets is recommended, with special attention to their elemental calcium content.

Levels of calcium intake greater than those recommended herein could cause urinary tract stones in susceptible people. Anyone with a history of kidney stones should only undertake calcium supplemen-tation with the guidance of a physician.

Normal levels of vitamin D are required for optimal calcium ab-sorption. The requirement for vitamin D increases with age. Persons who do not receive adequate daily sunlight exposure, such as those confined to home or to a nursing facility, are at special risk for vita-min D deficiency. Vitamin D has dangerous effects at high doses. Al-though the toxic dose varies among individuals, toxicity has occurred at levels as low as 2,000-5,000 international units [I.U.] daily. No one should consume more than 15 to 20 micrograms (600 to 800 units, twice the daily RDA) without a doctor's recommendation.

Other Treatments

Inactivity leads to bone loss. Some recent studies suggest that weight-bearing exercise may reduce bone loss. Modest weight-bearing exercise, such as walking, is recommended.

Several agents and modalities of treatment are currently under investigation, but their efficacy and/or safety have not been established. These include sodium fluoride, calcitriol, calcitonin, weakly androgenic anabolic steroids, thiazides, bisphosphonates, the 1-34 fragment of parathyroid, and "ADFR", a complex system of several drugs. Sodium fluoride, in association with a high calcium intake, may have a role to play in patients afflicted with severe osteoporosis, but its efficacy and safety are unproven; prospective studies are now under way.

Strategies to prevent falls are important in elderly patients who may fall frequently for a variety of reasons, such as from effects of drugs. Specific environmental interventions can minimize home hazards that increase the chances of falling.

Physicians treating fractures in osteoporotic patients should recognize the benefits of rapid return to function and avoidance of prolonged immobilization.

What Are the Directions for Future Research?

Future research in osteoporosis should approach the currently unanswered basic research questions concerning the development and maintenance of bone as a tissue. At the same time, there is great need for clinical and epidemiological research to further explore and extend the current potential for practical prevention and treatment of the disease. A deeper knowledge of factors controlling bone cell activity and regulation of bone mineral and matrix formation and remodeling should contribute ultimately to our understanding of the etiology of osteoporosis. This understanding will permit a more rational choice and evaluation of therapies, even as current treatments are evaluated clinically.

The panel recommends:

1. Observational and epidemiological studies to determine the impact of multiple demographic and behavioral factors on

bone mass and fracture frequency. Such studies could be conducted by appropriate additions to existing population-based studies.

2. Clinical studies to determine whether the observed age, sex, and skeletal distribution differences in osteoporosis reflect different mechanisms and predict different responses to intervention.

3. Studies to develop accurate, safe, inexpensive methods for determining the level of risk for osteoporosis in an individual, to establish early diagnosis, and to assess the clinical course of the disease.

4. Studies to develop safe, effective, low-cost strategies which might be applicable to populations at large for maximizing peak bone mass, minimizing bone loss, and preventing fractures.

5. Studies to determine the optimal regimen of gonadal hormones for prevention of bone loss and fracture.

6. Studies to elucidate further the mechanisms of bone growth and remodeling, their local and systemic regulation, and their alteration in osteoporosis.

7. Studies to understand alterations in the structure and biomechanical properties of bone in osteoporosis and the relationship of these alterations to the mechanisms and management of fractures.

Section 17.3

Osteoporosis Treatment Advances

DHSS Publication No. 94-1181, January 1994.

While its cause remains a mystery, scientists are learning more about treating and preventing osteoporosis, the most common disease affecting bone. Characterized by loss of bone density and strength, osteoporosis is associated with debilitating fractures, especially in people aged 45 and older.

As many as 24 million Americans, 80 percent of them women, now suffer from the condition, with more than 1.3 million osteoporosis-related fractures occurring annually.

With the "graying of America" as baby boomers age, the incidence of broken wrists and hips could skyrocket within the next couple of decades. Fortunately, research to identify treatments not only to arrest bone loss, but to reverse it, is starting to pay off.

Bone Basics

Although bones seem to be as lifeless as rocks, they are, in fact, composed of living tissue that is continually being broken down (or resorbed) and rebuilt, in a process called remodeling.

Bone is made from a protein framework—the osteoid matrix—into which calcium is deposited. About 99 percent of the calcium in the body is stored in the bones and teeth. Calcium not only makes bone hard, but also is involved in other essential functions, such as enabling the heart and other muscles to contract. Whenever dietary intake of calcium is insufficient to meet the body's needs, increased amounts are drawn from the bones to maintain a relatively constant supply in the bloodstream.

Complex chemical signals prompt bone cells known as osteoclasts to break down bone and others called osteoblasts to deposit bone. Calcitriol (a form of vitamin D), calcitonin (a thyroid hormone),

321

parathyroid hormone, growth factors, and prostaglandins are among the substances that orchestrate bone remodeling.

It takes about 90 days for old bone to be resorbed and replaced by new bone; then the cycle begins anew. Bones continue to grow in strength and size until a person's mid-30s, when peak bone mass is attained.

After that, the rate of bone resorption exceeds the rate of deposition, resulting in decreased bone mass and density (osteoporosis is Latin for "porous bones").

"There are many factors involved, and it's hard to pinpoint why this imbalance occurs," says Chanda Dutta, Ph.D., a pharmacologist with FDA's division of metabolism and endocrine drug products.

Who's at Risk?

According to one hypothesis, there are two types of primary osteoporosis. Type I occurs only in women, typically in the years immediately following menopause, from age 50 to 70. Dutta explains that Type I is related to decreased estrogen, and is characterized by rapid bone loss, especially in trabecular bones (vertebrae and flat bones, such as the pelvis). At greatest risk are thin, small-boned Caucasian or Asian women who have had a hysterectomy or reached natural menopause before age 45 and have a family history of the condition.

"Heredity is probably the most important factor," says Mona Calvo, Ph.D., a nutritionist in FDA's Center for Food Safety and Applied Nutrition. Thus, someone whose parents or grandparents have had the tell-tale signs, such as fracturing a hip after a minor fall, may be at greater risk of developing this type of osteoporosis.

Lifestyle factors that may contribute to or worsen Type I osteoporosis include low calcium intake, a sedentary lifestyle (weight-bearing exercise promotes bone deposition), cigarette smoking (heavy smokers have lower blood levels of estrogen), and excessive alcohol consumption (alcohol inhibits calcium absorption).

"While you don't have any control over heredity, you can attenuate your genetic legacy by focusing on those lifestyle risk factors you can do something about," advises Calvo.

Type II primary osteoporosis affects nearly half of all people over the age of 75. It's the only type of primary osteoporosis that men get; however, it's twice as common in women. According to Dutta, Type II is characterized by reduced osteoblast cell activity and decreased formation of bone. Loss occurs in both trabecular and cortical bones (hip and long bones such as those in the leg). Over the expected lifespan, women typically lose as much as 35 percent of cortical bone and up to half of trabecular bone; men, who have denser bones to begin with, lose only about 23 percent of cortical bone and 33 percent of trabecular bone. Experts say that everyone who lives long enough will develop Type II primary osteoporosis. But the extent of its severity is very individual. The same lifestyle factors that play a role in Type I primary osteoporosis can also cause an acceleration of bone loss in those with Type II.

Secondary osteoporosis may occur as a side effect of such drugs as corticosteroids and heparin. Hyperthyroidism, rheumatoid arthritis, kidney disease, and certain cancers such as lymphoma and leukemia are among the disorders that also contribute to secondary osteoporosis.

Diagnosis Important

Bone loss develops over the span of many years and is largely symptomless, though some women may experience chronic pain along the spine or muscle spasms in the back. Often, the first indication that a person has osteoporosis is a wrist or hip fracture or a compression fracture that causes the vertebrae in the upper back to collapse, curving the spine into the dowager's hump that has come to symbolize osteoporosis.

All told, 20 to 25 percent of postmenopausal women in this country are at risk of suffering an osteoporotic fracture. Such fractures cost some $10 billion each year in direct medical expenses such as hospitalization and home nursing care, as well as an incalculable amount in lost earnings. Hip fractures, in particular, can have dire consequences: Up to 20 percent of victims will die, within a year of fracture, from such complications as pneumonia, blood clots in the lungs, and heart failure. Fewer than half of those who survive can walk unaided or return to their former level of activity. Some 300,000 Americans suffer osteoporosis-related hip fractures each year.

Medical technology has developed several methods to detect osteoporosis before fractures occur. With the non-invasive radiologic imaging techniques photon absorptiometry and computed tomography, doctors can measure bone mass in the spine, wrist and hip.

"A fracture is the endpoint of the disease. If you can prevent a fracture by taking preventive measures, you can slow down progression of osteoporosis," explains Dutta. However, since scans to measure bone density are not currently reimbursed by most insurance companies and are not covered by Medicare, testing is currently reserved only for women at risk for osteoporosis rather than as a mass screening tool.

Prevention Through Diet

Osteoporosis is a complex condition, and researchers have been investigating a number of treatment approaches. However, prevention remains paramount.

"Calcium intake over lifetime really seems to matter, especially during periods of bone growth," says Linda Golden, M.D., a medical officer in FDA's division of metabolism endocrine drug products. "Starting in childhood, a diet adequate in calcium can maximize peak bone mass," she says.

Calvo agrees: "The more bone mass you have at maturity, the more you can lose before you will succumb to an osteoporotic fracture."

Health experts are divided over how much calcium is enough, and whether supplements are necessary. A consensus statement issued in October 1990 by a panel of experts at the Third International Symposium on Osteoporosis held in Copenhagen, Denmark, recommended a minimum intake of 800 milligrams of calcium daily for all adults. The year before, the U.S. National Academy of Sciences set the Recommended Dietary Allowances (RDA) for calcium at 1,200 mg daily for females from age 11 to 24 (the peak bone-forming years), dropping to 800 mg thereafter. Previously, the 1984 National Institutes of Health Consensus Development Conference on Osteoporosis had concluded that all women should get 1,000 to 1,500 mg of calcium daily.

Why the discrepancies in recommendations? For a while, "everyone was gung-ho about calcium; the more calcium you could get in a woman, the better," says Calvo. "But enthusiasm waned when subsequent research showed that raising calcium intake was not effective in slowing bone loss in pre-menopausal women," she explains, citing a study of 25- to 34-year-old women showing that highest bone density was achieved with a daily calcium intake of 800 to 1,000 mg, and that exceeding this range did not appear to result in any additional benefit to bone. But older women may need to take in greater amounts of calcium because as a person ages, the body's ability to absorb calcium diminishes.

While nutritionists and medical experts recommend eating a calcium-rich diet during the crucial bone-forming years between adolescence and young adulthood, new evidence suggests that dietary intervention may be more effective in menopausal women than was previously thought. Increasing daily calcium intake to 800 mg can slow or prevent bone loss in post-menopausal women, according to a study reported in the September 1990 issue of *The New England Journal of Medicine.* In the study by researchers at Tufts University in Boston, 361 women aged 40 to 70 were divided according to whether their diets were high or low in calcium (400 mg daily was the dividing line). The subjects were given either a placebo or 500-mg doses of calcium supplements daily. Supplementation significantly retarded bone loss in those who had undergone menopause at least six years earlier and whose diets were very low in calcium.

Allowing that "this research shows that people with low calcium intake in their late menopausal years can benefit from taking supplements," Calvo nonetheless recommends that calcium intake come from dairy foods. "I'll bet that if the subjects in the Tufts study had received their calcium from dairy foods, they would have done even better because milk and milk products are naturally rich in vitamin D, which enhances calcium absorption. Dairy products also provide vitamins A and D, protein, magnesium, and phosphorus, which are also building blocks for bone."

Surprising Sources of Calcium

While the Tufts study indicates that older women whose diets are low in calcium can benefit from increasing their intake of the mineral American women at any age do not seem eager to eat more calcium-rich foods. Many worry about the caloric and saturated fat content of dairy foods. To address this concern, food manufacturers have introduced low-fat—and, in some cases, nonfat—versions of just about every dairy food, from cottage cheese to ice cream.

But being good to your bones doesn't necessarily mean eating yogurt every day for the rest of your life. Many products contain calcium-based food additives, and the tap water in some parts of the country contains a fair amount of calcium. In addition, a lot of foods contain some calcium and, depending on the quantities eaten, they can be a significant source of the mineral. For example, several slices of bread can provide a healthy dose of calcium.

If you read labels carefully, you'll spot some unexpected sources of calcium. See for Figure 17.1. for some examples.

Food	Serving Size	Calcium	Calories	Fat
Sardines (in oil, with bones)	3 medium (3 oz)	370 mg	175	9 g
Cheese pizza	1 slice (1/8th of 15" pie)	220 mg	290	9 g
Macaroni & cheese	1 cup	200 mg	230	10 g
Oatmeal (instant, fortified)	1 packet	160 mg	105	4 g
Tomato soup (made w/milk)	1 cup	160 mg	160	6 g
Baked beans (w/pork & tomato sauce)	1 cup	140 mg	310	7 g
Tofu	1 piece (1 1/2" x 2 3/4" x 1")	100 mg	85	5 g
Hot cocoa	6 oz	90 mg	100	1 g
Pancakes (from mix)	1 4" pancake	30 mg	60	2 g
Wheat bread (enriched)	1 slice (18 per loaf)	30 mg	65	1 g

Source: Adapted from the "USDA Nutritive Value of Foods," *Home and Garden Bulletin,* No. 72.

Figure 17.1. Surprising Sources of Calcium.

The Tufts study also found that bone loss was more rapid during the first five years following menopause, and then slowed to a constant rate. This finding is consistent with other studies showing that dietary calcium had little effect in moderating the rate of bone loss immediately following menopause. Recognizing this, the consensus statement developed at the Third International Symposium on Osteoporosis termed estrogen therapy "the drug of choice for preventing bone loss in women after the menopause or in women with impaired ovarian function."

Estrogen Replacement

It has been known for some time that estrogen prevents osteoporosis-related fractures. Conjugated estrogens—a mixture of estrogens from natural sources—received FDA approval as a treatment for osteoporosis in 1988. More recently, a Swedish study reported in the *Annals of Internal Medicine* in September 1990 found that combined estrogen-progestin therapy may also have a protective effect in preserving bone and preventing fractures. The study reported that taking a combination of the female sex hormones estrogen and progestin at or soon after menopause can lower the risk of a broken hip during the next 10 years by 60 percent.

These new findings are encouraging because a debate has been raging for years about the safety of taking estrogen after menopause. While the hormone decreases the risk of osteoporosis and heart disease, with long-term use it may also increase the risk of breast and endometrial cancers. Recent research indicates that added progestin can lower the uterine cancer risk, but may also slightly increase a woman's chances of developing breast cancer.

"For post-menopausal women who have no contraindications, estrogen is the first line of treatment," says Golden. However, "estrogen only works for as long as you take it, and the protective effects wear off when you discontinue use—but the longer you're on it, the higher the cancer risk." Golden adds that each woman's profile of risk and benefit depends on individual circumstances, and that the decision whether to begin hormone replacement therapy rests with a women and her doctor.

Other Possible Therapies

In clinical studies, calcitonin, a thyroid hormone that inhibits the breakdown of bone, has been reported to reduce back pain from compression fractures; however, the hormone has not yet been proven to prevent fractures. With long-term use, some women develop antibodies to calcitonin, rendering the drug ineffective. FDA has approved an injectable form of calcitonin for treating osteoporosis. The effectiveness of a nasal spray version is being studied.

Researchers are also investigating several non-hormonal therapies. Currently, the most promising is etidronate, a drug used in treating Paget's disease of bone (a condition characterized by an excessive bone turnover that results in new bone being dense but fragile).

In a study by the Emory University School of Medicine in Atlanta, and reported in the July 1990 issue of *The New England Journal of Medicine,* 429 postmenopausal women who had suffered one to four spinal fractures took either a placebo or etidronate for 14 days, followed by calcium supplementation for 76 days (to match the body's 90-day bone turnover cycle). Etidronate slowed the loss of bone resorption while the calcium helped build bone mass, resulting in a 4 to 5 percent increase in spinal bone density. The women on the drug-and-supplement regimen also suffered less than half the vertebral fractures as the group receiving the placebo. On the minus side, the study found neither evidence of improved bone mass in the wrist and hip, nor any indication that fractures at those sites could be prevented.

Sodium fluoride, another experimental treatment for osteoporosis-related spinal fractures, increased bone mass but did not prevent fractures in a Mayo Clinic study of 202 women 50 to 75 years old, reported in *The New England Journal of Medicine* in March 1990. The group treated with a combination of sodium fluoride and calcium had a 35 percent increase in spinal bone density. The new bone was structurally abnormal and weak, however. The number of spinal fractures was not significantly different between the treated and placebo groups. Furthermore, the treated group sustained more broken hips.

Although treatments being developed aim to stop bone loss and rebuild weak and brittle bones, none of them can undo the damage caused by hip or spinal compression fractures. Thus, while researchers are getting a better understanding of the factors that increase bone resorption—and can mitigate their action to some degree—a true cure for osteoporosis remains as elusive as the origins of the condition.

—by Ruth Papazian

Section 17.4

Optimal Calcium Intake

Excerpts from NIH Consensus Development Statement, June 6-8 1994.

The National Institutes of Health Consensus Development Conference on Optimal Calcium Intake brought together experts from many different fields including osteoporosis and bone and dental health, nursing, dietetics, epidemiology, endocrinology, gastroenterology, nephrology, rheumatology, oncology, hypertension, nutrition and public education, and biostatistics, as well as the public to address the following questions:

1. What is the optimal amount of calcium intake?
2. What are the important cofactors for achieving optimal calcium intake?
3. What are the risks associated with increased levels of calcium intake?
4. What are the best ways to attain optimal calcium intake?
5. What public health strategies are available and needed to implement optimal calcium intake recommendations?
6. What are the recommendations for future research on calcium intake?

The panel concluded that:

- A large percentage of Americans fail to meet currently recommended guidelines for optimal calcium intake.

- On the basis of the most current information available, optimal calcium intake is estimated to be 400 mg/day (birth-6 months) to 600 mg/day (6-12 months) in infants; 800 mg/day in young children (1-5 years) and 800 1,200 mg/day for older children (6-10 years); 1,200 1,500 mg/day for adolescents and young adults

(11-24 years); 1,000 mg/day for women between 25 and 50 years; 1,200-1,500 mg/day for pregnant or lactating women; and 1,000 mg/day for postmenopausal women on estrogen replacement therapy and 1,500 mg/day for postmenopausal women not on estrogen therapy. Recommended daily intake for men is 1,000 mg/day (25-65 years). For all women and men over 65, daily intake is recommended to be 1,500 mg/day, although further research is needed in this age group. These guidelines are based on calcium from the diet plus any calcium taken in supplemental form.

- Adequate vitamin D is essential for optimal calcium absorption. Dietary constituents, hormones, drugs, age, and genetic factors influence the amount of calcium required for optimal skeletal health.

- Calcium intake, up to a total intake of 2,000 mg/day, appears to be safe in most individuals.

- The preferred source of calcium is through calcium-rich foods such as dairy products. Calcium-fortified foods and calcium supplements are other means by which optimal calcium intake can be reached in those who cannot meet this need by ingesting conventional foods.

- A unified public health strategy is needed to ensure optimal calcium intake in the American population.

Introduction

It has been a decade since the 1984 Consensus Development Conference on Osteoporosis first suggested that increased intake of calcium might help prevent osteoporosis. Osteoporosis affects more than 25 million people in the United States and is the major underlying cause of bone fractures in postmenopausal women and the elderly. Previous surveys have revealed that the U.S. population experiences more than 1.5 million fractures annually at a cost in excess of $10 billion per year to the health care system. Two important factors that influence the occurrence of osteoporosis are optimal peak bone mass attained in the first two to three decades of life and the rate at which bone is lost in later years. Adequate calcium intake is critical to achieving optimal peak bone mass and modifies the rate of bone loss associated with aging. A number of publications have addressed the possible role of calcium intake in the prevention of disorders other than osteoporosis, including other bone diseases, oral bone loss, colon cancer, hypertension, and preeclampsia, a hypertensive disorder of pregnancy. The results of recent research investigating these issues indicate that the optimal amount of calcium intake may be greater than the amount consumed by most Americans. At the same time, the general public and scientists have been exposed to a body of information emphasizing the value of ensuring adequate calcium intake throughout life.

Calcium is an essential nutrient. Optimal calcium intake may vary according to a person's age, sex, and ethnicity. Other factors play a role in calcium intake, including vitamin D, which is needed for adequate calcium absorption. Many factors can negatively influence calcium availability, such as certain medications or food components. Optimal calcium intake may be achieved through diet, calcium-fortified foods, calcium supplements, or various combinations of these.

What Is the Optimal Amount of Calcium Intake?

Calcium is a major component of mineralized tissues and is required for normal growth and development of the skeleton and teeth. Optimal calcium intake refers to the levels of consumption that are necessary for an individual (a) to maximize peak adult bone mass, (b) to maintain adult bone mass, and (c) to minimize bone loss in the later years. Calcium requirements vary throughout an individual's lifetime, with greater needs during the periods of rapid growth in childhood and adolescence, during pregnancy and lactation, and in later adult life. Because 99 percent of total body calcium is found in bone, the need for calcium is largely determined by skeletal requirements. Most studies examining the efficacy of calcium intake on bone mass have used measures of external calcium balance and bone densitometry as primary outcomes. The results of balance studies suggest a threshold effect for calcium intake: Body retention of calcium increases with increasing calcium intake up to a threshold, beyond which further calcium intake causes no additional increment in calcium retention.

Infants (Birth-12 Months) and Young Children (1-10 Years)

Calcium intake of exclusively breast-fed infants during the first 6 months of life is in the range of 250-330 mg/day, with a fractional calcium absorption between 55 and 60 percent. A lower fractional absorption of 40 percent is found with cow milk-based formulas. These

Figure 17.2. Optimal Calcium Requirements

Group	Optimal Daily Intake (in mg of calcium)
Infant	
Birth-6 months	400
6 months-1 year	600
Children	
1-5 years	800
6-10 years	800-1,200
Adolescents/Young Adults	
11-24 years	1,200-1,500
Men	
25-65 years	1,000
Over 65 years	1,500
Women	
25-50 years	1,000
Over 50 years (postmenopausal)	
On estrogens	1,000
Not on estrogens	1,500
Over 65 years	1,500
Pregnant and nursing	1,200-1,500

formulas contain nearly twice the calcium content of human milk; this results in comparable calcium retentions of 150-200 mg/day from both formula and breast milk. Net calcium absorption from soy-based formulas is comparable to, or higher than, that of breast milk or cow milk formulas because of its considerably higher calcium content. For infants between the ages of 6 and 12 months, calcium intake ranges from 400 to 700 mg/day. On the basis of balance data, the current RDAs for calcium, 400 mg/day for infants from birth to 6 months and 600 mg/day for those from 6 to 12 months, seem sufficient to provide optimal calcium intake. However, special circumstances such as low birth weight may require higher calcium intake.

Available data suggest that optimal calcium intake in children 1-10 years of age is 800 mg/day. Limited data from one recent study suggest that in children 6-10 years old, intake above 800 mg/day may lead to increased rates of bone accumulation. Coupled with calcium balance data, this suggests that an intake of greater than 800 mg/day may be optimal for this age group. It should also be noted that poor calcium nutrition in childhood may be related to development of enamel hypoplasia and accelerated dental caries.

Children and Young Adults (11-24 Years)

Calcium accumulation in bone during preadolescence is between 140 and 165 mg/day and may be as high as 400-500 mg/day in the pubertal period. Fractional intestinal absorption is very efficient and estimated to be approximately 40 percent. Peak adult bone mass, depending on the skeletal site examined, is largely achieved by 20 years of age, although important additional bone mass may accumulate through the third decade of life. Furthermore, cross-sectional studies reveal a small but positive association between life-long calcium intake and adult bone mass. Therefore, optimal calcium intake in childhood and young adulthood is critical to achieving peak adult bone mass.

Recent evidence suggests that adding 500-1,000 mg/day to current calcium intake may, at least temporarily, increase bone accretion rates in preadolescent boys and girls. With this supplementation, total calcium intake in these studies exceeded the current RDA of 1,200 mg/day; however, it is unclear whether the effect on bone accretion rates persists beyond the reported 18-month to 3-year periods of treatment and whether these increased rates of bone formation translate into higher peak adult bone mass. Recent balance studies in adolescents indicate a calcium intake threshold in the range of 1,200-1,500 mg/day.

Collectively, these data suggest that calcium intake in the range of 1,200-1,500 mg/day might result in higher peak adult bone mass. Additional research is necessary, particularly longitudinal, long-term dose-ranging studies of the effects of varying calcium intake on bone mass, to more precisely define optimal calcium intake for this age group. Importantly, population surveys of girls and young women 12-19 years of age show their average calcium intake to be less than 900 mg/day, which is well below the calcium intake threshold. The consequences of low calcium intake during this crucial period of rapid skeletal accrual raise concerns that achievement of optimal peak adult peak bone mass may be seriously compromised. Special education and public measures aimed at improving dietary calcium intake in this age group are essential.

Calcium Intake in Adults (25-65 Years of Age)

Once peak adult bone mass is reached, bone turnover is stable in men and women such that bone formation and bone resorption are balanced. In women, resorption rates increase and bone mass declines beginning with the fall in estrogen production that is associated with the onset of menopause. The decline in circulating estradiol is the predominant factor in the accelerated bone loss that begins after the onset of menopause and continues for 6-8 years. Unlike hormone replacement therapy, supplemental calcium during this initial phase will not slow the decline in bone mass due to estrogen deficiency. Although the effects of calcium can be shown more clearly in postmenopausal women after the period when the effects of estrogen deficiency are no longer dominant (approximately 10 years after menopause), it is likely that the early postmenopausal years are also an important time to ensure optimal calcium intake. Between 25 and 50 years of age, women who are otherwise healthy should maintain a calcium intake of 1,000 mg/day. For postmenopausal women who are receiving estrogen replacement therapy, a calcium intake of 1,000 mg/day is recommended to maintain calcium balance and stabilize bone mass. For postmenopausal women who do not take estrogen, it is estimated that a calcium intake of 1,500 mg/day may limit loss of bone mass, but should not be considered a replacement for estrogen. Therefore, recommended calcium intake for postmenopausal women up to 65 years of age is 1,000 mg/day in conjunction with hormonal replacement and 1,500 mg/day in the absence of estrogen replacement.

Calcium Intake in Adults (Older Than 65 Years)

In men and women 65 years of age and older, calcium intake of less than 600 mg/day is common. Furthermore, intestinal calcium absorption is often reduced because of the effects of estrogen deficiency in women and the age-related reduction in renal 1,25-dihydroxyvitamin D production. Calcium insufficiency due to low calcium intake and reduced absorption can translate into an accelerated rate of age-related bone loss in older individuals. Among the homebound elderly and persons residing in long-term care facilities, vitamin insufficiency has been detected and may contribute to reduced calcium absorption. Calcium intake among women later in the menopause, in the range of 1,500 mg/day, may reduce the rates of bone loss in selected sites of the skeleton such as the femoral neck. (These findings also indicate that the calcium threshold for reducing bone loss may vary for different regions of the skeleton.)

The physiology of calcium homeostasis in aging men over 65 is similar to that of women with respect to the rate of bone loss, calcium absorption efficiency, declining vitamin D levels, and changes in markers of bone metabolism. It seems reasonable, therefore, to conclude that in aging men, as in aging women, prevailing calcium intakes are insufficient to prevent calcium-related erosion of bone mass. Thus, in women and in men over 65, calcium intake of 1,500 mg/day seems prudent.

Pregnant and Lactating Women

The current RDA for calcium intake during pregnancy and lactation is 1,200 mg/day. Pregnancy represents a significant physiological stress on maternal skeletal homeostasis. A full-term infant accumulates approximately 30 grams of calcium during gestation, most of which is assimilated into the fetal skeleton during the third trimester. Available data suggest that, with pregnancy, no permanent decline in body calcium occurs if recommended levels of dietary calcium intake are maintained. There is no association between parity and bone mass. Furthermore, there is no evidence to support changing the current recommendation of calcium intake for well-nourished pregnant women. There is, however, a large population of pregnant women who are not ingesting sufficient calcium, especially those who are undernourished. These women need to be identified, and appropriate adjustments in their calcium intake should be made. Data are not available regarding the calcium requirement for pregnant women at the extreme of reproductive years, for those who experience non-singleton births, and for those with closely spaced pregnancies.

During lactation, 160-300 mg/day of maternal calcium is lost through production of breast milk. Longitudinal studies in otherwise healthy women demonstrate acute bone loss during lactation that is followed by rapid restoration of bone mass with weaning and the resumption of menses. Women who are lactating should ingest at least 1,200 mg of calcium per day. Lactating adolescents and young adults should ingest up to 1,500 mg of calcium per day.

What Are the Important Cofactors for Achieving Optimal Calcium Intake?

Several cofactors modify calcium balance and influence bone mass. These include dietary constituents, hormones, drugs, and the level of physical activity. Unique host characteristics may also modify the effects of dietary calcium on bone health. These include the individual's age and ethnic and genetic background, the presence of gastrointestinal disorders such as malabsorption and the postgastrectomy syndrome, and the presence of liver and renal disease. Interactions among these diverse cofactors may affect calcium balance in either a positive or negative manner and thus alter the optimal levels of calcium intake.

Cofactors That Enhance Calcium Absorption

Vitamin D. Vitamin D metabolites enhance calcium absorption. 1,25-Dihydroxyvitamin D, the major metabolite, stimulates active transport of calcium in the small intestine and colon. Deficiency of 1,25-dihydroxyvitamin D, caused by inadequate dietary vitamin D, inadequate exposure to sunlight, impaired activation of vitamin D, or acquired resistance to vitamin D, results in reduced calcium absorption. In the absence of 1,25-dihydroxyvitamin D, less than 10 percent of dietary calcium may be absorbed. Vitamin D deficiency is associated with an increased risk of fractures. Elderly patients are at particular risk for vitamin D deficiency because of insufficient vitamin D intake from their diet, impaired renal synthesis of 1,25-dihydroxyvitamin D, and inadequate sunlight exposure, which is normally the major stimulus for endogenous vitamin D synthesis. This is especially evident in homebound or institutionalized individuals. Supplementation of vitamin D intake to provide 600-800 IU/day has been shown to improve calcium balance and reduce fracture risk in these individuals. Sufficient vitamin D should be ensured for all individuals, especially the elderly who are at greater risk for development of a deficiency. Sources of vitamin D, besides supplements, include sunlight, vitamin D fortified liquid dairy products, cod liver oil, and fatty fish. Calcium and vitamin D need not be taken together to be effective. Excessive doses of vitamin D may introduce risks such as hypercalciuria and hypercalcemia and should be avoided. Anticonvulsant medications may alter both vitamin D and bone mineral metabolism, particularly in certain disorders, in the institutionalized, and in the elderly. Although symptomatic skeletal disease is uncommon in noninstitutionalized settings, optimal calcium intake is advised for persons using anti-convulsants.

Sex Hormones. Sex hormone deficiency is associated with excessive bone resorption in women and men. Low calcium intake can exacerbate the deleterious consequences of sex hormone deficiency. One study suggested that calcium supplementation can decrease the minimum estrogen dosage required to maintain bone mass in postmenopausal women. However, oral calcium alone does not prevent the postmenopausal bone loss resulting from estrogen deficiency. In addition to estrogen, other endogenous cofactors that could enhance net calcium absorption include growth hormone, insulin-like growth factor-I, and parathyroid hormone.

Physical Activity. An interrelationship between physical activity and calcium balance has not been established conclusively. In a single study, increased physical activity enhanced the beneficial effect of oral calcium supplementation on bone mass in young adults. Thus far, studies of elderly individuals and peri-menopausal women have failed to establish a positive interaction between calcium intake and exercise to increase bone mass. Therefore, the positive effects of exercise on skeletal health are not likely to be related to calcium intake.

Immobilization. Immobilization has been shown to produce a rapid decrease in bone mass. This loss has been well documented in individuals placed on bed rest and in individuals with regional forms of immobilization such as that seen in para- and quadriplegia. Under these circumstances, the rate of bone loss may be rapid, which is in part related to an increase in bone resorption accompanied by a decrease in bone formation. There is concern that increased calcium intake may increase the risk of hypercalcemia, ectopic calcification, ectopic ossification, and nephrolithiasis in these individuals. Thus, any recommendations for increasing calcium intake are tempered in these individuals by the potential for undesirable consequences.

Factors That Decrease Calcium Availability

Calcium intake, intestinal absorption, urinary excretion, and endogenous fecal loss influence calcium balance. Intake and absorption account for only 25 percent of the variance in calcium balance, whereas urinary loss accounts for approximately 50 percent. The typical

American diet consists of high amounts of sodium and animal protein, both of which can significantly increase urinary calcium excretion. High oxalate and phytate in a limited number of foods can reduce the availability of calcium in these foods. With the exception of large amounts of wheat bran, fiber has not been found to affect calcium absorption significantly. Other dietary components, including fat, phosphate, magnesium, and caffeine, have not been found to affect calcium absorption or excretion significantly. Aluminum in the form of antacid medication, when taken in excess, may significantly increase urinary calcium loss. Glucocorticoids decrease calcium absorption. States of glucocorticoid excess are associated with negative calcium balance and a marked increase in fracture risk. In a recent study, oral calcium supplements plus 1,25-dihydroxyvitamin D decreased glucocorticoid-associated bone loss. On the basis of these observations and other studies, oral calcium supplements should be considered in all patients who are receiving exogenous glucocorticoids. The specific disease for which the glucocorticoid therapy is used (e.g., rheumatoid arthritis, inflammatory bowel disease, asthma) can be a determining factor in the occurrence and degree of bone loss.

Genetic and ethnic factors significantly influence many aspects of calcium and skeletal metabolism. Twin studies indicate a significant influence of genetic factors on peak bone mass. However, environmental factors appear to be more important in determining rates of bone loss in postmenopausal women. Racial and ethnic differences in bone mass and fracture incidence have been described, but these are not accounted for by differences in calcium intake. Whether there are genetic and ethnic differences in optimal calcium requirements needs to be determined.

What Are the Risks Associated with Increased Levels of Calcium Intake?

High levels of calcium intake have several potential adverse effects. The efficiency of calcium absorption decreases as intake increases, thereby providing a protective mechanism to lessen the chances of calcium intoxication. This adaptive mechanism can, however, be overcome by a calcium intake of greater than approximately 4 g/day. It is well known that calcium toxicity, with high blood calcium levels, severe renal damage, and ectopic calcium deposition (milk-alkali syndrome), can be produced by overuse of calcium carbonate, encountered clinically in the form of antacid abuse. Even at intake levels less than

4 g/day, certain otherwise healthy persons may be more susceptible to developing hypercalcemia or hypercalciuria. Likewise, subjects with mild or subclinical illnesses marked by dysregulation of 1,25-dihydroxyvitamin D synthesis (e.g., primary hyperparathyroidism, sarcoidosis) may be at increased risk from higher calcium intakes. Nevertheless, in intervention studies (albeit of relatively short duration—less than 4 years), no adverse renal effects of moderate supplementation up to 1,500 mg/day have been reported. Furthermore, one large study suggested that within the current ranges of calcium intake in the population, a higher calcium intake in men is associated with a decreased risk of stone formation. However, a dose-response relationship was not detected. Caution must be used, however, in supplementing individuals who have a history of kidney stones, because high calcium intakes can increase urinary calcium excretion and might increase the risk of stone formation in these patients.

The strategy of increasing calcium intake by increasing dairy products could tend to increase the intake of saturated fat. These potential problems can be averted by the use of low-fat dairy products. Reduced-fat or no-fat dairy products contain as much calcium per serving size as high-fat dairy products. The use of dairy products to increase calcium intake could increase side effects in people who are sensitive to milk products. Nondairy alternative sources are indicated in these individuals.

Concern has been raised that increased calcium intake might interfere with absorption of other nutrients. Iron absorption can be decreased by as much as 50 percent by many forms of calcium supplements or milk ingestion, but not by forms that contain citrate and ascorbic acid, which enhance iron absorption. Thus, increased intakes of specific sources of calcium might induce iron deficiency in individuals with marginal iron status. Population studies suggest that this is not a common or severe problem, but more study is needed. Whether calcium supplements interfere with absorption of other nutrients has not been thoroughly studied. Calcium may also interfere with absorption of certain medications, such as tetracycline.

Gastrointestinal side effects of calcium supplements have been observed, usually at relatively high dosages. A variable effect on the incidence of constipation has been reported in controlled studies of calcium supplements. The calcium ion stimulates gastrin secretion and gastric acid secretion, which can produce a "rebound hyperacidity" when calcium carbonate is used as an antacid. These side effects should not be major problems with a modest increase in calcium intake.

Certain preparations of calcium (e.g., bone meal and dolomite) can have significant contamination with lead and other heavy metals. However, most commercial calcium preparations are tested to ensure that they do not contain significant heavy metal contamination.

In conclusion, a modest increase in calcium intake should be safe for most people. Practices that might encourage total calcium intake to approach or exceed 2,000 mg/day seem more likely to produce adverse effects and should be monitored closely.

What Are the Best Ways to Attain Optimal Calcium Intake?

The preferred approach to attaining optimal calcium intake is through dietary sources. Additional strategies include the consumption of calcium-fortified foods and calcium supplements. For many Americans, dairy products are the major contributors of dietary calcium because of their high calcium content (e.g., approximately 250-300 mg/8 oz milk) and frequency of consumption. It may be necessary for individuals with lactose intolerance to limit or exclude liquid dairy foods, but adequate calcium intake can be achieved through the use of low-lactose-containing, dairy products (solid dairy food) or through milk rendered lactose deficient. Vegans who voluntarily limit their intake of dairy products can obtain dietary calcium through other sources. Other good food sources of calcium include some green vegetables (e.g., broccoli, kale, turnip greens, Chinese cabbage), calcium-set tofu, some legumes, canned fish, seeds, nuts, and certain fortified food products. Breads and cereals, while relatively low in calcium, contribute significantly to calcium intake because of their frequency of consumption.

Recommended calcium intake levels are based on the total calcium content of the food. To maximize calcium absorption, food selection decisions should include information on their bioavailability. Bioavailability (absorption) of calcium from food depends on the food's total calcium content and the presence of components that enhance or inhibit absorption. As mentioned previously, oxalic acid, which is present at high levels in some vegetables (e.g., spinach), has been found to depress absorption of the calcium present in the food but not of calcium in coingested dairy or other calcium-containing foods. Phytic acid also depresses calcium absorption but to a lesser extent. Dietary fiber, except for wheat bran, has little effect on calcium absorption. When present in high concentration, wheat bran has been found to depress calcium absorption from milk.

A number of calcium-fortified food products are currently available, including fortified juices, fruit drinks, breads, and cereals. Although some of these foods provide multiple nutrients and may be frequently consumed, their quantitative contribution and role in the total diet are not currently defined.

For some individuals, calcium supplements may be the preferred way to attain optimal calcium intake. Calcium supplements are available as various salts, and most preparations are well absorbed except when manufactured such that they do not disintegrate during oral ingestion. Absorption of calcium supplements is most efficient at individual doses of 500 mg or less and when taken between meals. Ingesting calcium supplements between meals supports calcium bioavailability, since food may contain certain compounds that reduce calcium absorption (e.g., oxalates). However, absorption of one form of calcium supplementation, calcium carbonate, is impaired in fasted individuals who have an absence of gastric acid. Absorption of calcium carbonate can be improved in these individuals when it is taken with certain food. The potential for calcium supplementation to interfere with iron absorption is an important consideration when it is ingested with meals. Alternatively, calcium supplementation in the form of calcium citrate does not require gastric acid for optimal absorption and thus could be considered in older individuals with reduced gastric acid production. In individuals with adequate gastric acid production, it is preferable to ingest calcium supplements between meals.

Maintenance of optimal bone health depends on an adequate supply of calcium and other essential nutrients. Current dietary intake data indicate that calcium intake is below recommended levels in most individuals. To attain the optimal calcium levels proposed, a change in dietary habits, including increased frequency of consumption of dairy products and/or calcium-rich vegetable sources, is needed. This approach of recommending the consumption of calcium-rich foods is consistent with current dietary guidelines (the U.S. Department of Agriculture (USDA) Food Guide Pyramid), which includes 2-3 servings per day of dairy products and 3-5 servings of vegetables. Recommendations for supplements should be made in the context of the total diet since recommendations are for calcium from all sources. The task for individuals to meet calcium requirements on a continuing daily basis is a formidable challenge.

What Public Health Strategies Are Available and Needed to Implement Optimal Calcium Intake Recommendations?

Optimizing the calcium intake of Americans is of critical importance. A large percentage of Americans still fail to meet currently recommended guidelines for calcium intake. The impact of suboptimal calcium intake on the health of Americans and the health care cost to the American public is a vital concern. It is thus appropriate that increasing calcium intake is a national health promotion and disease prevention objective in the Healthy People 2000 agenda (Department of Health and Human Services Publication Number 91.50212). Public health strategies to promote optimal calcium intake should have a broad outreach and should involve educators, health professionals, and the private and public sectors.

Public Education

A public education program is needed to do the following:

• Disseminate consensus recommendations to the public.

• Convene meetings of public leaders and representatives of national groups to disseminate information on optimal calcium intake for the general population and high-risk groups and to develop action plans for public education.

• Develop health education materials and programs to address the diverse linguistic and cultural needs of the multi-ethnic American population.

• Work with existing national organizations and the mass media to distribute information, decrease consumer confusion, and encourage consumers, including children, adolescent girls, postmenopausal women, and older Americans, to adopt health-promoting changes in their daily calcium intake.

Health Professionals

Primary care physicians, dentists, and other health professionals should play a strong role in educating their patients about bone health and calcium intake. An educational program to support this work of health professionals would:

- Disseminate consensus recommendations to health professionals.

- Develop and distribute educational materials, by serving as a clearinghouse for information on calcium-related research, and developing curricula for health professional training programs.

- Distribute educational materials through health professional organizations at their national and regional meetings.

- Initiate sessions at national meetings of health professionals focusing on promoting optimal calcium intake or initiating national meetings focusing specifically on calcium-related research.

Private Sector

The private sector can play an active part in promoting optimal calcium intake.

- Manufacturers and producers of food products should continue to develop and market a wide variety of calcium-rich foods to meet the needs and tastes of our multi-ethnic population.

- Restaurants, grocery stores, and other food outlets should increase the accessibility and visibility of calcium-rich products for the consumer.

- Biotechnology research groups should develop accessible cost-effective technologies to screen for populations who are at high risk of fracture and who would be candidates for increased calcium intake.

Public Sector

The Federal Government should take the following actions:

- The Government should ensure that guidelines for calcium intake across all agencies, departments, and institutions are consistent and that these guidelines reflect the current state of scientific knowledge.

- The National Center for Health Statistics and the USDA should widely disseminate their data on nutrient intakes and food consumption patterns, with respect to calcium, as well as their information on relevant trends in these nutrient intakes and food consumption patterns. To maximize educational programmatic, and policy efforts, these data should be specific to age, gender, ethnic group, region, and socioeconomic status where possible.

- Existing Federal food and food subsidy programs and federally regulated facilities for infants, children, low-income populations, and the elderly in the Department of Health and Human Services, the Veteran Administration, the Department of Defense and other agencies should ensure achievement of optimal calcium intake for program recipients. The USDA should direct school food services to promote calcium intake by serving calcium-rich foods and to urge that calcium be included in all nutrition education efforts within public schools.

- Government cafeterias should serve as models to promote optimal calcium intake by serving calcium-rich foods, labeling calcium content in single servings of those foods, and distributing brochures about the relationship between dietary calcium needs and good health to their customers.

- Address, within health care reform, the need for financial coverage of calcium supplements for those who cannot reach optimal calcium intake through foods alone and financial support for screening of target populations to identify individuals who are at high risk of fracture and who would be likely to benefit from increased calcium intake.

What Are the Recommendations for Future Research on Calcium Intake?

1. Prospective longitudinal studies to investigate long-term effects of calcium intake on regional (e.g., spine, hip, forearm) changes in bone mass and on fracture incidence in postmenopausal women and in older men.

2. Prospective longitudinal studies of adolescent girls and boys to investigate the long-term effects of different levels of calcium intake on the achievement of peak bone mass.

3. Studies to determine optimal calcium intake in the decade before the menopause and the potential role of declining estrogen levels during this time.

4. Evaluation of the long-term effects of calcium intake on bone remodeling.

5. Investigation of interactions between calcium supplementation and the absorption of other nutrients.

6. Evaluation of dose-response relationships between calcium intake and estrogen replacement therapy.

7. Determination of optimal calcium requirements in different ethnic populations.

8. Evaluation of the effect of long-term calcium supplementation on the development or prevention of kidney stones.

9. Studies on the effect of dietary calcium on bone mass and fracture incidence

10. Evaluation of the role of vitamin D metabolites in optimizing calcium balance.

11. Development of a cost-effective means by which calcium-deficient individuals can be identified at all ages.

12. Development of effective health-promoting programs to change population behavior with respect to calcium intakes that are tailored to specific age, sex, ethnic, socioeconomic status, and regional needs.

13. Improved methods to achieve and maintain optimal dietary intake of calcium by both nutritional and supplemental means.

Conclusions

- A large percentage of Americans fail to meet currently recommended guidelines for optimal calcium intake.

345

- On the basis of the most current information available, optimal calcium intake is estimated to be 400 mg/day (birth-6 months) to 600 mg/day (6-12 months) in infants, 800 mg/day in young children (1-5 years) and 800,200 mg/day for older children (6-10 years), 1,200,1500 mg/day for adolescents and young adults (11-24 years), 1,000 mg/day for women between 25 and 50 years, 1,200-1,500 mg/day for pregnant or lactating women, and 1,000 mg/day for postmenopausal women on estrogen replacement therapy and 1,500 mg/day for postmenopausal women not on estrogen therapy. Recommended daily intake for men is 1,000 mg/day (25-65 years). For all women and men over 65, daily intake is recommended to be 1,500 mg/day, although further research is needed in this age group. These guidelines are based upon calcium from the diet plus any calcium taken in supplemental form.

- Adequate vitamin D is essential for optimal calcium absorption. Dietary constituents, hormones, drugs, age, and genetic factors influence the amount of calcium required for optimal skeletal health.

- Calcium intake, up to a total intake of 2,000 mg/day, appears to be safe in most individuals.

- The preferred source of calcium is through calcium-rich foods such as dairy products. Calcium-fortified foods and calcium supplements are other means by which optimal calcium intake can be reached in those who cannot meet this need by ingesting conventional foods.

- A unified public health strategy is needed to ensure optimal calcium intake in the American population.

Section 17.5

Boning Up:
New Ways to Prevent Fractures
in Older Americans

NCRR Reporter, May/June 1994.

As we age, our bones age too. Because they are thinner and more brittle, they are far too easily broken in a fall. Often they heal slowly and painfully if they heal at all. The kind of fall that matters little to someone younger can bring independent living to an abrupt halt. In some cases, bones fracture spontaneously because they are unable to carry out their normal weight-supporting role.

Through studies that approach this problem from very different perspectives, two independent teams of NCRR-supported investigators have arrived at results that could help prevent bone fractures among older Americans.

Study 1

The first team of investigators, based at the General Clinical Research Center (GCRC) at the University of Texas Southwestern Medical Center at Dallas, has shown that an experimental treatment with sodium fluoride, the chemical that is added to drinking water, can stimulate mineral buildup and prevent new fractures in osteoporotic bones of the spinal column. Osteoporosis—the hollowing out of bones caused by reduced mineral content—affects more than 25 million Americans, including one of every three postmenopausal women.

At the beginning of the study, which included 110 postmenopausal osteoporotic patients, the average mineral content of the women's lower-back vertebrae was approximately 30 percent below that of a 30-year-old normal woman, and they all had spinal compression fractures. According to Dr. Charles Y. C. Pak, GCRC principal investigator and Distinguished Chair in Mineral Metabolism at the Southwestern Medical Center, painful spontaneous fractures often develop in the lower part of the spine in osteoporotic women. "The strength of the bone is not sufficient to sustain the weight-bearing function of the skeleton, so the spine becomes compressed and fractures develop," he explains. Fractures of the spine can cause back pain and deformity; damage to several vertebrae in the upper spine results in "dowager's hump."

Investigators conducting the ongoing trial randomized the 110 patients into two groups. One group (54 patients) receives slow release sodium fluoride tablets two times daily in repeated 14-month cycles (12 months treatment, 2 months withdrawal). The other group (56 patients) receives a placebo preparation on the same schedule. All patients receive calcium citrate tablets twice daily continuously as an optimally absorbable calcium supplement. Once a year the researchers determine how many spontaneous vertebral fractures the patients have developed and measure the mineral content of vertebrae and other bones. To date, 48 of the patients taking sodium fluoride have completed more than one cycle (mean of 2.5 cycles) of treatment. Eleven patients withdrew from the study prior to completing a full treatment cycle.

Interim analysis of the trial data in the remaining 99 patients shows that the treatment caused a continued 44 percent increase per cycle in vertebral bone mineral density in the fluoride-treated group, but did not result in any significant change in the placebo group. The fluoride-treated group developed substantially fewer spontaneous spinal fractures (10 new fractures) than did the placebo group (26 new fractures).

Researchers did not observe any significant side effects among treated patients, in contrast to earlier studies that have linked high levels of sodium fluoride intake with many side effects, including severe diarrhea, gastrointestinal bleeding, micro-fractures, and an increased rate of non-spinal fractures. Studies by other researchers have also previously reported that sodium fluoride administration promotes buildup of abnormal bone structure, but Dr. Pak and his colleagues use lower doses of a different type of sodium fluoride. "We use a slow-release preparation. Sodium fluoride leaks out of numerous tiny holes in the wax matrix tablets we use," he says. The slow release prevents high concentrations of fluoride in the stomach and blood.

If the concentration of sodium fluoride delivered to bone were high—as it was in other studies—and the amount of available calcium were low, the newly formed bone could be defective, Dr. Pak notes. "Sodium fluoride should not be given without adequate calcium. It could produce collagen, the bone matrix, but that would fail to mineralize, resulting in defective bone formation," he says. In addition, in contrast to the damaging effects on cortical bone seen by researchers in other studies, interim results in the current trial indicate "absolutely no change in cortical bone density and quality," says Dr. Pak. "Our findings show that this approach can greatly reduce new fractures, and they support the hypothesis we have had since the beginning of this work. That is, given in proper amounts with adequate calcium, fluoride is a means to form normal bone."

The Texas researchers plan to follow the patients through four cycles of treatment. The investigators have also initiated a similar study on a group of women who have lower than normal bone density but no compression fractures. They hope that the earlier treatment may prevent development of fractures.

Study 2

In the second investigation, a team of researchers has evaluated the mechanics of falls and suggested preventive methods to reduce the risk of hip fracture, the most devastating fall injury. Hip fracture, which affects more than 250,000 Americans each year, is the second leading cause of nursing home placement in the United States and exacts an estimated $8.7 billion annual cost to society.

Dr. Susan L. Greenspan and her colleagues at Beth Israel Hospital in Boston studied 149 ambulatory men and women who had fallen (126 women and 23 men aged 65 years or older). By falling, 72 patients broke their hips. These "case" patients were compared to 77 "control" patients who fell but did not break their hips.

By examining how people fell, the investigators found that a fall to the side carried a significant risk of hip fracture. In contrast, there was no increased risk of hip fracture associated with forward, backward, or straight-down falls, in which the individual collapses vertically to the floor.

It has been estimated that only about 5 percent of all falls by the elderly result in hip fracture. According to Dr. Greenspan, who is director of the Osteoporosis Prevention and Treatment Center at Beth Israel Hospital and assistant professor of medicine at Harvard Medical School, "The relatively low incidence of hip fracture in elderly fallers probably has a lot to do with factors other than osteoporosis. How people fall, where they land, and what they fall on—these factors all play a role. Many elderly persons may be able to break the fall or twist and turn the body to lessen the impact."

Not surprisingly, the mineral content, or bone mineral density (BMD), of hip bones was also an independent risk factor in predicting hip fracture and had a significance similar to that of fall mechanics in determining the risk of fracture among the study patients. The non-dominant role of BMD in predicting the risk of hip fracture may seem very surprising. But Dr. Greenspan emphasizes that, since the mean age of her study group was 83, the majority of women were likely to have had a BMD below the fracture threshold, the mineral density at which a bone easily breaks. Other factors, as a result, dominate in this statistical comparison between very similar people. "Osteoporosis is still very important, but our study shows that in addition to maintaining bone mass we need to focus on alternative methods to prevent hip fracture," she says.

People who broke their hips in a fall were generally taller and weighed slightly less than those who did not break their hips. From the weights and heights of the study participants, the investigators calculated the body mass index, BMI (kg/m2). Both women and men with hip fractures had significantly lower body mass indexes than those who did not break their hips.

The Boston investigators suggest that current approaches to prevent hip fracture should be modified. Today most efforts aim to retard bone loss rather than increase bone mass. In individuals older than 70 years the bone mineral density is already below a critical risk level for fracture, but the rate of bone loss has slowed. For these individuals preventive strategies could also focus on multi-disciplinary measures that are unrelated to bone mass. For example, education about environmental hazards such as throw rugs, loose electrical cords, poorly lit stairs, and high-heeled shoes might prevent many accidents.

Dr. Greenspan says that elderly people should also be encouraged to exercise their muscles to increase their strength in general and the strength of their thigh muscles in particular. In addition, their medication should be reviewed in order to eliminate drugs that affect balance or cause dizziness. Such medications can aggravate preexisting balance limitations that are common among the elderly and spring from many causes. "I think that many independent factors—such as cardiovascular, neuromuscular, and pharmacological problems—get compounded and lead to poor balance," says Dr. Greenspan.

Additional Reading

Pak, C.Y.C., Sakhaee, K., Piziak, V., et al. Randomized controlled trial of slow-release sodium fluoride in the management of postmenopausal osteoporosis. *Annals of Internal Medicine* 120:625-632, 1994.

Greenspan, S.L., Myers, E.R., Maitland, L.A., et al. Fall severity and bone mineral density as risk factors for hip fracture in ambulatory elderly. *JAMA* 271:128-133, 1994.

—by Ole Henriksen

Section 17.6

The Silent Epidemic of Hip Fractures

FDA Consumer, May 1988.

A silent epidemic may be hard to imagine. But that is how William G. Winter. M.D., describes the increasing number of hip fractures suffered by older people every year.

Winter, chief of orthopedics at the Denver Veterans Administration Hospital, feels other health problems that are frequently called epidemics get more attention because they affect younger people. "By the time people get around to breaking their hips, they are in the shadows of their lifetimes" he said. "Those people are no longer the focus of society."

But that doesn't mean the epidemic isn't there. Currently, over 200,000 hip fractures occur every year in the United States. Of those, almost 50 percent occur in persons who are 80 or older. Winter points out that "although [hip fractures] have always been a health problem, increasing numbers of older people will incur these injuries as our society steadily greys. We now have the ability to survive until our bones give out."

Most of those people will be women. According to Jennifer Kelsey, M.D., director of epidemiology at the Columbia University School of Public Health in New York, women account for 75 percent to 80 percent of all hip fractures, mainly because of the bone-weakening effects of osteoporosis, a disfiguring, often crippling condition that strikes women far more often than men. (This is due to hormone changes that occur in women after menopause.)

While medical technology offers an array of devices to help repair a broken hip, the best treatment is still prevention. Whether they occur in men or women, fractures of the hip are associated with more deaths, disability, and medical costs than all other fractures due to osteoporosis combined, according to Kelsey.

The National Center for Health Statistics reports that out of 112,000 people in nursing homes because of fractures in 1985, more than half—62,200—had suffered hip fractures.

One out of five of those who do not recover normal function after a hip fracture will die within a year. Of the people who survive hip fractures, 15 percent to 25 percent must remain in nursing homes for at least one year after the fracture. Even for those who are able to return home, about a third of them cannot get around on their own, but must depend on other people or special devices.

Repairing or Replacing the Fracture

There are medical devices—complete hips or parts of them—that can replace the damaged bones. These devices are especially important for older people whose bones can no longer grow back together or would take too long to do so.

But the decision to replace the real thing is not taken lightly. "The rule of thumb is whatever they can save, they save," says FDA's orthopedic devices branch director, Thomas Callahan, Ph.D. He says that in a young person whose otherwise healthy bone was broken in a fall, replacement might not be necessary at all—the fracture could be repaired by holding the bone together with a pin.

"That young person is one extreme," says Callahan. "The other extreme is the older patient who has advanced stages of a disease such as osteoarthritis, and all three elements [of the hip] are damaged. Then the physicians will probably go for a total hip replacement. Then there is a group of people in the middle where it is up to the physician to decide whether the bones that aren't replaced are good enough to last much longer."

Callahan says the trend is towards total hip replacements in the elderly. Winter, of the Denver VA Hospital, agrees. "For those people not strong enough to use crutches, a total replacement will allow them to walk a little without waiting for a fracture to heal," he said.

The three bones these devices replace are the shaft of the femur (thigh bone), the head of the femur, and the acetabular cup. The devices are made of metal, such as stainless steel, or alloys of cobalt, chrome and titanium.

Most of these prosthetic hips have smooth surfaces and must be anchored with a special bone cement. While they work well at first, the cement can loosen over time. "There is still a controversy in the field on whether it's the fault only of the bone cement itself or the fault of the bone cement in combination with the bone-cementing technique, but in either case the cement very often lets go after seven to 10 years," says Callahan.

However, a new hip replacement—the porous, coated prosthetic hip—is being used without cement. These hip replacement devices have rough surfaces that allow healthy bones to grow into them and hold them in place. "The idea is that if the bone can grow into it, it might make a more stable prosthesis [than the cemented hip] in the long run," says Callahan.

But that is only a theory. So far, the porous, coated hips are working as well as the cemented ones. However, "so far" is only five years, and problems with the cemented ones usually don't surface until the seventh year.

FDA is watching the performance of the porous, coated hips. The agency has approved only one such device, which has a rough bead-like surface. In addition, the Orthopedic and Rehabilitation Devices Panel, an FDA advisory committee, has recommended that the agency approve another hip that is covered in a metallic mesh.

The panel said it is not yet clear whether the bone actually holds the prosthesis in place or whether the device stays put because it is pressed very tightly in the femoral canal (a femur—thighbone—that has been surgically hollowed out). The panel also said any bone growth into the prosthesis may not be permanent. Blood vessels, necessary to nourish the bone, may not grow in with the bone or even if they do they might not be functional. This can cause the bone to be broken down by the body.

Determining the success of the bone growth into the porous, coated hip replacements is difficult. Any bone that might grow into the device is very difficult to see on an X-ray, so growth can only be measured if surgery is required for another reason or the patient dies.

The panel added that it hadn't seen any evidence that the porous hips were any better or worse than cemented ones.

In the meantime, research on all kinds of hip prostheses continues. According to the New York marketing research firm of Frost & Sullivan, Inc., new collagen-based materials, designed to induce bone regeneration, are the focus of a great deal of that research. FDA's Callahan says that the idea behind coating the prosthesis with collagen—a protein that is the chief constituent of skin, connective tissue, and bone—is to dupe the body into thinking the surface of the hip replacement is really bone. This allows the bone to grow into intimate contact with the prosthesis. Other research is looking into better cementing techniques and modular prostheses with interchangeable components to allow mixing and matching to fit individual patient needs.

"I think we'll see a wave of [new products] very soon," says Callahan.

But traditional devices are still very important and useful, according to Carl Larson, director of FDA's division of surgical and rehabilitation devices. Larson says that of all the people who might benefit from a hip replacement, 80 percent will get more traditional treatment.

Learning to Walk Again

Without the surgeon's work—repairing or replacing the damaged bone—a person with a hip fracture might never walk again. But even with surgery, a person who wants to walk must go through months of physical therapy after the operation.

How long does it take someone to get on their feet again? "It depends more on the patient than the device," says Fran Preidis of the National Hospital for Orthopaedics and Rehabilitation in Arlington, Va. Preidis, a clinical specialist in joint replacement, says that health and age can affect the length of recovery, as well as motivation.

Even in the highly motivated, it takes approximately three months for the patient to return to a normal level of activity—and that is with therapy that begins the very first day after surgery.

If there are no complications from the surgery, patients are encouraged to sit up on the side of the bed the day after the operation. By day two, they should try to stand. How much standing they should do and how much weight should be put on the leg depends on the type of prosthesis.

With cemented hip replacements, patients can put the amount of weight on the leg that feels comfortable to them whenever they want. This is because the cement fixes the prosthesis in place immediately.

With non-cemented hip replacements, however, bone growth is desired to hold the prosthesis in place, so patients must limit the amount of weight they put on their hips until the support is firm. Usually, therapy begins with six weeks on crutches or a walker, followed by one crutch for four weeks, and two weeks with a cane.

Patients with cemented hips may need to use crutches, too, but usually they're walking sooner than those with non-cemented prostheses.

How much weight should be placed on the hip at what time isn't based solely on the type of prosthesis. "It's up to the physician," says Preidis. "He knows what he has put in and what he wants the patient to accomplish."

Preidis says that some doctors have patients with porous-coated prostheses putting as much weight as possible on their legs as soon as possible after surgery to stimulate bone growth. At the same time, Preidis says that many physicians and therapists are changing the current practice for cemented hips and limiting the initial amount of weight allowed on the leg. This would allow the cement time to set, and any minor damage to the bone from the cement, which must be hot when applied to have the proper consistency, would have time to heal.

With both types of implants, exercise, such as riding a stationary bike and swimming, is added to the walking therapy after the first six weeks. These kinds of exercises are needed to increase the range of motion of the joint and strengthen the muscles.

Before the Fall

No matter what the advances in treatment, the best solution is to prevent hip fractures in the first place. The simplest form of prevention is to remove physical hazards from the home. The Office of Disease Prevention and Health Promotion, part of the U.S. Public Health Service, recommends that all staircases have handrails and that halls and staircases be well lit. Hazards caused by loose rugs, unstable furniture, and loose wires underfoot should be corrected. Medical conditions may also lead to falls. "Properly fitted eyeglasses and adequate podiatric [foot] care could reduce the risk of falls," the office said.

Recommendations for home safety measures to prevent falls in the elderly include:

- Provide handy light switches and good illumination
- Consider night light
- Eliminate extension cords by installing sufficient number of electrical outlets
- Provide toilet facility on same floor near bedroom
- Install high toilet seat
- Install handrails for toilet, bath, and stairways
- Remove castors from furniture; if castors are essential, put furniture against wall
- Make floors, bathtub, and carpets non-slip
- If possible, have home without steps inside or out, or have stairs with small gradient
- Make last step (up and down) a different color

Preventing the fragile bones that result from osteoporosis is a more difficult task. Proper calcium intake and exercise early in life can best prevent osteoporosis; however, there are steps that older people can take to slow bone loss.

"The most effective method of reducing postmenopausal bone loss is estrogen replacement," William E. Peck, M.D., professor of medicine at the Washington University School of Medicine in St. Louis, said at a February 1987 workshop on osteoporosis sponsored by the National Institutes of Health. Peck added that recent studies have shown that oral use of short-acting estrogen preparations (ones that are absorbed and have an effect within a day or two) reduces postmenopausal bone loss throughout the body, including the vertebrae, the hips, and the wrists.

A study reported in the Nov. 5, 1987, *New England Journal of Medicine* established that taking estrogens at any time after menopause cuts the risk of hip fracture by a third. The risk is cut to two-thirds after taking estrogens for two years. While the authors felt that the evidence of estrogen's protective effects was strong, they were unable "to determine the ideal duration and dose" of estrogen replacement.

However, estrogen use may be accompanied by side effects, the major one being an increased risk of endometrial cancer. Taking a second hormone, progestin, along with the estrogen reduces this risk, but Peck recommends even this combination therapy only for women at high risk of osteoporosis who have not had other medical problems such as breast or endometrial cancer, stroke, or unexplained vaginal bleeding. He adds that women who take estrogen must be conscientious about keeping appointments with their doctors to catch any side effects early.

Peck also promotes calcium and exercise. He says 1,500 milligrams of calcium daily and a program of frequent exercise may reduce the doses of oral estrogen needed to retard bone loss.

The best sources of calcium are dairy products. In addition to calcium, milk contains lactose and vitamin D, both of which help the body to absorb the calcium. Milk also contains magnesium and phosphorus, which are essential to bone growth.

"Drinking milk allows you to get more of these essential nutrients in the right proportions," says Mona Calvo, a staff fellow in experimental clinical nutrition at FDA's Center for Food Safety and Applied Nutrition. She adds that the same benefits that apply to milk apply to other dairy products.

In addition to dairy products, foods such as canned sardines (with bones), collards, broccoli, and canned salmon (with bones) are also good sources of calcium. The problem with getting enough calcium with foods is that a lot of calories come along for the ride. Those calories may be the reason that many people turn to calcium supplements. However, those supplements have their own set of problems.

Supplements made from bone meal and dolomite, which come from natural sources, can be contaminated with lead and other toxic trace elements. Also, some supplements don't dissolve quickly enough, and the calcium passes right through the body without ever being absorbed.

Even as research continues, however, Winter's silent epidemic of hip fractures should not be considered an unavoidable consequence of age. According to Winter, "Orthopedists need reminding that weakened osteoporotic bones might be preventable and that steady advances in osteoporosis investigations and management are occurring. But a fall is also an element responsible for most hip fractures; the consequences of this epidemic of falls in aged people should be examined, just as occupational safety and health experts might evaluate an industrial problem of similar magnitude."

—by Dori Stehlin

Section 17.7

Age Page: Osteoporosis, The Bone Thinner

National Institute on Aging Publication No. 1992-0-626-224.

One in four women over age 60 and nearly half of all people over 75 suffer from osteoporosis, the bone thinner. Osteoporosis is a major cause of fractures in the spine, hip, wrist, and other bones. To help prevent this condition, steps can be taken early in life and during the middle years. Also, treatment is available that may help older people who already have the disorder.

Osteoporosis develops over a period of many years. Gradually and without discomfort, the bones thin out until some of them break, causing pain and disability.

Bones maintain themselves through a process known as remodeling in which small amounts of old bone are removed and new bone is formed in its place. Beginning in the thirties, however, a little more bone is lost than is gained. This bone loss continues throughout life. In women, bone loss speeds-up around menopause—so that an early menopause, particularly when caused by the surgical removal of the ovaries, results in a greater risk of osteoporosis.

The cause of osteoporosis is not fully known. Falling hormone levels, too little calcium in the diet, and a lifetime of inactivity all play a role.

Who Gets It?

White and Asian women most often develop osteoporosis. Among this group, women who have had an early menopause or who have a family history of osteoporosis are at highest risk. Women with fair skin or small frames are also at greater risk than other people. Men are less likely than women to get osteoporosis for a variety of reasons such as their greater bone mass, and because they have no biological counterpart to menopause. However, men may face osteoporosis in their later years.

Diagnosis

An early sign of osteoporosis is loss of height. This happens when weakened bones of the spine (called vertebrae) collapse. Later, as these fractures mount up, a curving of the spine (often called "dowager's hump") may occur.

Osteoporosis may go unnoticed until there is a loss of height, the spine curves, or a fall results in a hip, wrist, or other fracture. Even a minor fall can result in a broken bone.

Tests are available to diagnose osteoporosis. The most common are single and dual-photon absorptiometry and dual-energy x-ray absorptiometry. Before an osteoporosis screening, consider factors such as insurance coverage and available equipment. Talk with your doctor if you are interested in a diagnostic test.

Prevention

Diet and exercise can help prevent osteoporosis. Foods that are high in calcium—such as low fat cheese, yogurt, and milk—should be a regular part of the diet.

Although the current recommended dietary allowance (RDA) for calcium is 800 mg daily, women who are nearing or have past menopause may need 1,000 to 1,500 mg. If the diet alone does not provide enough calcium, use a supplement. Keep in mind that some people—those who form kidney stones, for example—need to be careful about suddenly increasing their calcium intake.

It is also important to get enough vitamin D every day because it is needed by the body to absorb calcium. The RDA for vitamin D is 200 IU daily for people over 25. Vitamin fortified milk and cereals, egg yolk, saltwater fish, and liver are high in vitamin D. Fifteen minutes of mid-day sunshine may also meet the daily need for vitamin D.

Regular exercise is another important preventive measure. Walking, jogging, dancing, and bicycle riding are helpful because they place stress on the spine and the long bones of the body.

Women with osteoporosis risk factors (who have an early menopause or family members with this condition) should ask their doctor about tests to measure bone mass when nearing menopause. They should also discuss using an estrogen supplement.

Treatment

The goal in treating osteoporosis is to stop further bone loss and prevent falls, which are common in older people. Such falls often result in a fractured hip that causes hospitalization, both temporary and long-term disability, and dependence. Prevention and treatment for osteoporosis are based on similar goals. For example, exercise helps stimulate formation of new bone. If you already have had a fracture, a doctor should explain the type and amount of activity to be done.

Many doctors prescribe hormones, such as estrogen, which slow the rate of bone loss. Scientists are studying other drugs and combinations of calcium, vitamin D, and estrogen in the hope of finding a way to stop bone loss.

Research

Scientists are conducting studies on osteoporosis at universities, medical centers, and other research institutions around the country. In 1991 the National Institute on Aging (NIA) began a series of clinical trials, called STOP/IT (Sites Testing Osteoporosis Prevention/ Intervention Treatments), to test promising ways to lessen, prevent, or reverse osteoporosis in older people. This is one of the first osteoporosis studies to include large numbers of people over age 65.

Resources

More information on osteoporosis is available from NIA. Part of the National Institutes of Health (NIH), NIA supports research on osteoporosis and offers information on a range of health issues that concern older people, including Age Pages on estrogen therapy and preventing fractures. For a free list of publications, call 1-800-222-2225; or write to:

NIA Information Center
P.O. Box 8057
Gaithersburg, MD 20898-8057.

The National Institute of Arthritis and Musculoskeletal and Skin Diseases, part of NIH, also supports osteoporosis research. Contact:

NIAMS Clearinghouse at Box AMS
Bethesda, MD 20892
or call (301) 495-4484.

The National Institute of Diabetes and Digestive and Kidney Diseases is part of NIH. Contact:

National Digestive Diseases Information Clearinghouse,
Box NDDIC
Bethesda, MD 20892.

The National Osteoporosis Foundation offers nationwide programs to educate the public and health professionals about osteoporosis and related research. Contact:

National Osteoporosis Foundation
2100 M Street, NW., Suite 602
Washington, DC 20037
or call (202) 223-2226.

Section 17.8

Age Page: Preventing Falls and Fractures

National Institute on Aging, 1992.

An injury from falling can limit a person's ability to lead an active, independent life. This is especially true for older people. Each year thousands of older men and women are disabled, sometimes permanently, by falls that result in broken bones. Yet many of these injuries could be prevented by making simple changes in the home.

As people age, changes in their vision, hearing, muscle strength, coordination, and reflexes may make them more likely to fall. Older persons also are more likely to have treatable disorders that may affect their balance—such as diabetes or conditions of the heart, nervous system, and thyroid. In addition, compared with younger people, older persons often take more medications that may cause dizziness or lightheadedness.

Preventing falls is especially important for people who have osteoporosis, a condition in which bone mass decreases so that bones are more fragile and break easily. Osteoporosis is a major cause of bone fractures in women after menopause and older people in general. For people with severe osteoporosis, even a minor fall may cause one or more bones to break.

Steps to Take

Falls and accidents seldom "just happen," and many can be prevented. Each of us can take steps to make our homes safer and reduce the likelihood of falling. Here are some guidelines to help prevent falls and fractures.

- Have your vision and hearing tested regularly and properly corrected.

- Talk to your doctor or pharmacist about the side effects of the medicines you are taking and whether they affect your coordination or balance. Ask for suggestions to reduce the possibility of falling.

- Limit your intake of alcohol. Even a small amount of alcohol can disturb already impaired balance and reflexes.

- Use caution in getting up too quickly after eating, lying down, or resting. Low blood pressure may cause dizziness at these times.

- Make sure that the nighttime temperature in your home is at least 65°F. Prolonged exposure to cold temperatures may cause a drop in body temperature, which in turn may lead to dizziness and falling. Many older people cannot tolerate cold as well as younger people can.

- Use a cane, walking stick, or walker to help maintain balance on uneven or unfamiliar ground or if you sometimes feel dizzy. Use special caution in walking outdoors on wet and icy pavement.

- Wear supportive rubber-soled or low-heeled shoes. Avoid wearing smooth-soled slippers or only socks on stairs and waxed floors. They make it very easy to slip.

- Maintain a regular program of exercise to improve strength and muscle tone, and keep your joints, tendons, and ligaments more flexible. Many older people enjoy walking and swimming. Mild weight-bearing activities, such as walking or climbing stairs, may even reduce the loss of bone due to osteoporosis. Check with your doctor or physical therapist to plan a suitable exercise program.

Make Your Home Safe

Many older people fall because of hazardous conditions at home. Use this checklist to help you safeguard against some likely hazards.

Stairways, hallways, and pathways should have:

- good lighting and be free of clutter,

- a firmly attached carpet, rough texture, or abrasive strips to secure footing,

- tightly fastened handrails running the whole length and along both sides of all stairs, with light switches at the top and bottom.

Bathrooms should have:

- grab bars located in and out of tubs and showers and near toilets,

- nonskid mats, abrasive strips, or carpet on all surfaces that may get wet,

- nightlights.

Bedrooms should have:

- nightlights or light switches within reach of bed(s).

- telephones (easy to reach), near the bed(s).

Living areas should have:

- electrical cords and telephone wires placed away from walking paths,

- rugs well secured to the floor,

- furniture (especially low coffee tables) and other objects arranged so they are not in the way,

- couches and chairs at proper height to get into and out of easily.

Section 17.9

Gene Predicts Bone Density, Those at Risk for Osteoporosis

NIH Research News, Jan 19 1994.

Researchers have found a gene that may help to identify, early in life, individuals at high risk for osteoporosis. This gene strongly influences bone density, an important determinant of the risk of osteoporosis. Osteoporosis (porous, weak bone) affects more than 25 million people in the U.S.; it is the major underlying cause of bone fractures in postmenopausal women and the elderly. Osteoporosis usually results from two factors: the peak bone strength (density) attained in early life, and how rapidly a person loses bone in later life.

"The prospect of having a genetic marker of bone density that would permit early intervention to prevent osteoporosis is extremely exciting," says Dr. Lawrence E. Shulman, Director of the National Institute of Arthritis and Musculoskeletal and Skin Diseases at the National Institutes of Health, which funded the study.

Although heredity has long been suspected of playing a role in bone density, until now genes responsible for this trait have not been identified. As reported in the January 20th issue of the scientific journal *Nature*, Dr. John A. Eisman and colleagues at the Garvan Institute of Medical Research in Sydney, Australia, have now found that a single gene can account for up to 75 percent of the total genetic effect on bone density. This gene codes for the vitamin D receptor (VDR), a protein that enables vitamin D to exert its actions on bone and on calcium metabolism. Non-genetic factors such as hormones, calcium intake, and exercise also influence the density of bone.

Eisman and his colleagues measured bone densities in 70 pairs of identical twins and 55 non-identical twins. The researchers found that identical twins, who share 100 percent of their genes, had more similar bone densities than did non-identical twins, who do not share all genes. The researchers also found that there are two forms (alleles) of the VDR gene, one called "B" and the other called "b." Normal people have one copy of the VDR gene from each parent, and thus may have either the BB, Bb, or bb combination. The researchers then looked at the effect of the two forms of the VDR gene on bone density. They found a strong link between the "B" version of the VDR gene and low bone density in the spine and femur (thigh bone at the hip). Bone density was lowest in those with the BB combination, intermediate in those with Bb, and highest in those with bb. Non-identical twins that had the same alleles of the VDR gene were similar to identical twins in this regard, thus strengthening the importance of these receptor genes to bone density. It is not yet clear how the difference between the two forms of the VDR gene could affect bone density.

The researchers also examined 311 unrelated healthy women from the Sydney area. In this second population, the vitamin D receptor gene was also found to be a strong predictor of bone density, and again the "B" allele was associated with lower bone density. Eisman and colleagues predict that women with BB, having low bone density in early life, will, when they start to lose bone as they age, reach the "fracture threshold" of low bone density in the spine 11 years earlier, and in the hip 8 years earlier, than those with bb. The latter translates to a four-fold increase in the risk of hip fracture for BB individuals as compared to those with bb.

365

These findings need to be extended to other and larger populations in the United States and elsewhere. They may provide an important explanation for the wide variation in bone density, not only among individuals, but also among various ethnic groups. African-American women in the United States, for example, develop approximately 10 percent greater peak bone mass by age 35 than do Caucasian women.

Research is also needed to uncover the precise role of the vitamin D receptor in regulating bone density. These investigations open new frontiers in research on the underlying causes of osteoporosis, and in particular the critical role of vitamin D in bone formation and metabolism. They could also pave the way for developing new targeted approaches to the prevention and treatment of this common and debilitating disease, a major public health problem in the United States.

Chapter 18

What Women Should Know about Lupus

Do You or Someone You Know Have Signs of Lupus?

Lupus is a serious health problem that affects mainly young women. The disease often starts between the ages of 15 and 44.

People of all races may get lupus. However, lupus is three times more common in black women than in white women.

As many as one in 250 black women will get the disease.

What Is Lupus?

Lupus is a disease that can affect many parts of the body. It can affect the joints, the skin, the kidneys, the lungs, the heart, or the brain. Only a few of these parts of the body are affected in most people.

Something goes wrong with the body's immune system in lupus. We can think of the immune system as an army within the body with hundreds of defenders (known as antibodies). They defend the body from attack by germs and viruses. In lupus, however, the immune system becomes overactive and goes out of control. The antibodies attack healthy tissues in the body. This attack induces inflammation, causing redness, pain, and swelling in the affected parts of the body. This tendency for the immune system to become overactive may run in families.

What Does a Person with Lupus Look Like?

Many people with lupus look healthy.

NIH Pub No. 93-3219.

What Are the Signs of Lupus?

The signs of lupus differ from one person to another. Some people have just a few signs of the disease; others have more. Lupus may be hard to diagnose. It is often mistaken for other diseases. For this reason, lupus has often been called the "great imitator."

Common signs of lupus are:

- Red rash or color change on the face, often in the shape of a butterfly across the bridge of the nose and the cheeks.
- Painful or swollen joints.
- Unexplained fever.
- Chest pain with breathing.
- Unusual loss of hair.
- Pale or purple fingers or toes from cold or stress.
- Sensitivity to the sun.
- Low blood count.

These signs are more important when they occur together.

Other signs of lupus can include mouth sores, unexplained "fits" or convulsions, hallucinations or depression, repeated miscarriages, and unexplained kidney problems.

What Causes Lupus?

We don't know what causes the immune system to become overactive. In some people, lupus becomes active after exposure to sunlight, infections, or certain medications.

Can You Catch Lupus From Someone Else?

No, lupus is not catching. You can't give it to someone else. Also, it is not a form of cancer. It is not AIDS.

Does Lupus Run in Families?

Most relatives of lupus patients do not develop the disease, but in some families more than one member gets lupus. If a relative of a lupus patient develops signs of lupus, she or he should see a doctor.

How Serious Is Lupus?

Signs of lupus tend to come and go. There are times when the disease quiets down, or goes into remission. At other times, lupus flares up, or becomes active. Years ago, many people with lupus died. Now, with good medical care, most people with the disease can lead active, productive, and fulfilling lives.

Are There Different Kinds of Lupus?

There are three major types of lupus:

1. lupus that affects certain parts of the body (systemic lupus erythematosus),

2. lupus mainly of the skin (discoid or cutaneous lupus), and

3. lupus caused by medicine (drug-induced lupus).

Systemic lupus erythematosus, sometimes called SLE, is the most serious form of the disease. This type of lupus is the focus of this chapter. Systemic means that it may affect many parts of the body, such as the joints, skin, kidneys, lungs, heart, or the brain. This type of lupus can be mild or serious. If it is not treated, systemic lupus can cause damage to the organs inside your body.

Discoid and cutaneous lupus mainly affect the skin. The person may have a red rash or a color change of the skin on the face, scalp, or other parts of the body.

Drug-induced lupus is caused by a small number of prescription medications. The person with drug-induced lupus may have the same symptoms as the person with systemic lupus, but it is usually less serious. Usually when the medicine is stopped, the disease goes away. The most common drugs that can cause lupus are:

*   procainamide used for heart problems,
*   hydralazine used for high blood pressure, and
*   Dilantin used for seizures.

Drug-induced lupus is usually found in older men and women of all races.

Does Sunlight Cause Lupus?

In some people, no matter what shade of skin, an attack of lupus may be brought on by being in the sun, even for a short period of time.

Do Men Get Lupus?

Yes, men get all forms of lupus. However, nine out of ten people who have lupus are women.

Why Is Lupus More Common in Black Women Than White Women?

We do not know why the disease is more common in black women. However, research doctors supported by the National Institutes of Health are studying this problem. Researchers are studying why minorities are more inclined to get lupus, what causes it to start, and why is it mild in some and severe in others. Other researchers are studying why the signs of lupus differ between black women and white women.

What Should You Do if You Think You Have Lupus?

You should see a doctor or a nurse and be examined and tested for lupus. They will talk to you and take a history of your health problems. Many people have lupus for a long time before it is detected. It is important that you tell the doctor or nurse about your symptoms. (Photocopy the list of "Signs of Lupus" above and use it as a checklist which you can take to your doctor.)

How Is Lupus Treated?

The doctor may treat each lupus patient in a different way because the signs of lupus often differ from one person to another. The doctor may give aspirin or similar medicine to treat the painful, swollen joints and the fever. Creams may be prescribed for the rash, and stronger medicines prescribed for more serious problems.

Is There a Cure for Lupus?

At this point, lupus cannot be cured. However, in many cases, signs of the disease can be relieved. The good news is that with the correct medicine and by taking care of themselves, most lupus patients can hold a job, have children, and lead a full life.

Outlook

The outlook for lupus patients has greatly improved. Research doctors supported by the National Institutes of Health are studying many aspects of lupus, such as what goes wrong with the immune system, why the disease runs in families, how lupus causes damage in the body, and why it can lead to repeated miscarriages. Others are researching why lupus is so much more common in women, especially black women. Researchers have learned a great deal about lupus and are studying new ways to treat and, hopefully, prevent the disease. The future holds great promise for improving the health of all Americans who have lupus.

Awareness

Please share this information with your family and friends. Someone you know or care about may have lupus.

Other Resources

For further information on lupus, see your doctor or health clinic and contact your local chapter of the following organizations:

Lupus Foundation of America, Inc.
4 Research Place
Suite 800
Rockville, Maryland 20850-3226
(301) 670-9292
(800) 558-0121

The American Lupus Society
3914 Del Amo Blvd.
Suite 922
Torrance, California 90503
(310) 542-8891
(800) 331-1802

Both of these groups can provide more detailed information on lupus through free pamphlets and newsletters. They also have pamphlets in Spanish. The two groups also can refer people to doctors and clinics who see a lot of lupus patients.

Additional copies of this chapter are available free of charge as the booklet <u>What Black Women Should Know About Lupus</u>. The National Institute of Health encourages readers to duplicate and distribute this material as needed or to obtain as many booklets as needed from NIAMS Task Force on Lupus in High Risk Populations, National Institute of Arthritis and Muskoskeletal and Skin Diseases, Box AMS, 9000 Rockville Pike, Bethesda, Maryland 20892.

Chapter 19

Disorders of the Urinary Tract

Chapter Contents

Section 19.1

Urinary Tract Infections

NIH Publication No. 91-2097 (1991).

Urinary tract infections are a serious health problem affecting millions of people each year. They are also very common—only respiratory infections occur more often. Each year, urinary tract infections (UTI's) account for about 8 million doctor visits. Women are especially prone to UTI's for reasons that are poorly understood. One woman in five develops a UTI during her lifetime.

The urinary system consists of the kidneys, ureters, bladder, and urethra. The key players in the system are the kidneys, a pair of purplish-brown organs located below the ribs toward the middle of the back. The kidneys remove liquid waste from the blood in the form

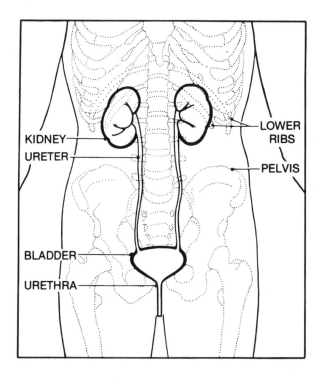

Figure 19.1. *The Urinary Tract.*

of urine, keep a stable balance of salts and other substances in the blood, and produce a hormone that aids the formation of red blood cells. Narrow tubes called ureters carry urine from the kidneys to the bladder, a triangle-shaped chamber in the lower abdomen. Urine is stored in the bladder and emptied through the urethra.

The average adult passes about a quart and a half of urine each day. The amount of urine varies, depending on the fluids and foods a person consumes. The volume formed at night is about half that formed in the daytime.

Causes of Urinary Tract Infection

Normal urine is sterile. It contains fluids, salts, and waste products, but it is free of bacteria, viruses, and fungi. An infection occurs when microorganisms, usually bacteria from the digestive tract, cling to the opening of the urethra and begin to multiply. Most infections arise from one type of bacteria, Escherichia coli (E. coli), which normally live in the colon.

In most cases, bacteria first begin growing in the urethra. An infection limited to the urethra is called urethritis. From there bacteria often move on to the bladder, causing a bladder infection (cystitis). If the infection is not treated promptly, bacteria may then go up the ureters to infect the kidneys (pyelonephritis).

Microorganisms called Chlamydia and Mycoplasma may also cause UTI's in both men and women, but these infections tend to remain limited to the urethra and reproductive system. Unlike E. coli, Chlamydia and Mycoplasma may be sexually transmitted, and infections require treatment of both partners.

The urinary system is structured in a way that helps ward off infection. The ureters and bladder normally prevent urine from backing up toward the kidneys, and the flow of urine from the bladder helps wash bacteria out of the body. In men, the prostate gland produces secretions that slow bacterial growth. In both sexes, immune defenses also prevent infection. Despite these safeguards, though, infections still occur.

Who Is at Risk?

Some people are more prone to getting a UTI than others. Any abnormality of the urinary tract that obstructs the flow of urine (a kidney stone, for example) sets the stage for an infection. An enlarged prostate gland also can slow the flow of urine, thus raising the risk of infection.

A common source of infection is catheters, or tubes, placed in the bladder. A person who cannot void, is unconscious or critically ill, often needs a catheter that stays in place for a long time. Some people, especially the elderly or those with nervous system disorders who lose bladder control, may need a catheter for life. Bacteria on the catheter can infect the bladder, so hospital staff take special care to keep the catheter sterile and remove it as soon as possible.

People with diabetes have a higher risk of a UTI because of changes of the immune system. Any disorder that suppresses the immune system raises the risk of a urinary infection.

UTI's may occur in infants who are born with abnormalities of the urinary tract, which sometimes need to be corrected with surgery. UTI's are rarely seen in boys and young men. In women, though, the rate of UTI's gradually increases with age. Scientists are not sure why women have more urinary infections than men. One factor may be that a woman's urethra is short, allowing bacteria quick access to the bladder. Also, a woman's urethral opening is near sources of bacteria from the anus and vagina. For many women, sexual intercourse seems to trigger an infection, although the reasons for this linkage are unclear.

According to several studies, women who use a diaphragm are more likely to develop a UTI than women who use other forms of birth control. Recently, researchers found that women whose partners use a condom with spermicidal foam also tend to have growth of E. coli bacteria in the vagina.

Recurrent Infections

Many women suffer from frequent UTI's. Nearly 20 percent of women who have a UTI will have another, and 30 percent of those will have yet another. Of the last group, 80 percent will have recurrences.

Usually, the latest infection stems from a strain or type of bacteria that is different from the infection before it, indicating a separate infection. (Even when several UTI's in a row are due to E. coli, slight differences in the bacteria indicate distinct infections.)

Research funded by the National Institutes of Health (NIH) suggests that one factor behind recurrent UTI's may be the ability of bacteria to attach to cells lining the urinary tract. A recent NIH funded study has also shown that women with recurrent UTI's tend to have certain blood types. Some scientists speculate that women with these blood types are more prone to UTI's because the cells lining the vagina and urethra may allow bacteria to attach more easily. Further research will show whether this association is sound and proves useful in identifying women at high risk for UTI's.

Infections in Pregnancy

Pregnant women seem no more prone to UTI's than other women. However, when a UTI does occur, it is more likely to travel to the kidneys. According to some reports, about 2 to 4 percent of pregnant women develop a urinary infection. Scientists think that hormonal changes and shifts in the position of the urinary tract during pregnancy make it easier for bacteria to travel up the ureters to the kidneys. For this reason, many doctors recommend periodic testing of urine.

Symptoms of Urinary Tract Infection

Not everyone with a UTI has symptoms, but most people get at least some. These may include a frequent urge to urinate and a painful, burning feeling in the area of the bladder or urethra during urination. It is not unusual to feel bad all over—tired, shaky, washed out—and to feel pain even when not urinating. Often, women feel an uncomfortable pressure above the pubic bone, and some men experience a fullness in the rectum. It is common for a person with a urinary infection to complain that, despite the urge to urinate, only a small amount of urine is passed. The urine itself may look milky or cloudy, even reddish if blood is present. A fever may mean that the infection has reached the kidneys. Other symptoms of a kidney infection include pain in the back or side below the ribs, nausea, or vomiting.

In children, symptoms of a urinary infection may be overlooked or attributed to another disorder. A UTI should be considered when a child or infant seems irritable, is not eating normally, has an unexplained fever that does not go away, has incontinence or loose bowels, or is not thriving. The child should be seen by a doctor if there are any questions about these symptoms, especially if there is a change in the child's urinary pattern.

Diagnosis

To find out whether you have a UTI, your doctor will test a sample of urine for pus and bacteria. You will be asked to give a "clean catch" urine sample by washing the genital area and collecting a "midstream" sample of urine in a sterile container. (This method of collecting urine helps prevent bacteria around the genital area from getting into the sample and confusing the test results.) Usually, the sample is sent to a laboratory, although some doctors' offices are equipped to do the testing.

In the urinalysis test, the urine is examined for white and red blood cells and bacteria. Then the bacteria are grown in a culture and tested against different antibiotics to see which drug best destroys the bacteria. This last step is called a sensitivity test.

Some microbes, like Chlamydia and Mycoplasma, can only be detected with special bacterial cultures. A doctor suspects one of these infections when a person has symptoms of a UTI and pus in the urine, but a standard culture fails to grow any bacteria.

When an infection does not clear up with treatment and is traced to the same strain of bacteria, the doctor will order a test that makes images of the urinary tract. One of these tests is an intravenous pyelogram (IVP), which gives x-ray images of the bladder, kidneys, and ureters. An opaque dye visible on x-ray film is injected into a vein, and a series of x-rays are taken. The film shows an outline of the urinary tract, revealing even small changes in the structure of the tract.

If you have recurrent infections, your doctor also may recommend an ultrasound exam, which gives pictures from the echo patterns of sound-waves bounced back from internal organs. Another useful test is cystoscopy. A cystoscope is an instrument made of a hollow tube with several lenses and a light source, which allows the doctor to see inside the bladder from the urethra.

Treatment of Urinary Tract Infection

UTI's are treated with antibacterial drugs. The choice of drug and length of treatment depends on the patient's history and the urine tests that identify the offending bacteria. The sensitivity test is especially useful in helping the doctor select the most effective drug. The drugs most often used to treat routine, uncomplicated UTI's are trimethoprim (Trimpex), trimethoprim/sufamethoxazole (Bactrim, Septra, Cotrim), amoxicillin (Amoxil, Trimox, Wymox), nitrofurantoin (Macrodantin, Furadantin), and ampicillin.

Often, a UTI can be cured with 1 or 2 days of treatment if the infection is not complicated by an obstruction or nervous system disorder. Still, many doctors ask their patients to take antibiotics for a week or two to assure that the infection has been cured. Single-dose treatment is not recommended for some groups of patients, for example, those who have delayed treatment or have signs of a kidney infection, patients with diabetes or structural abnormalities, or men who have prostate infections. Longer treatment is also needed by patients with infections caused by Mycoplasma or Chlamydia, which are usually treated with tetracycline, trimethoprim/sulfamethoxazole (TMP/SMZ), or doxycycline. A follow-up urinalysis helps to confirm that the urinary tract is infection-free. It is important to take the full course of treatment because symptoms may disappear before the infection is fully cleared.

Severely ill patients with kidney infections may be hospitalized until they can take fluids and needed drugs on their own. Kidney infections generally require several weeks of antibiotic treatment. Researchers at the University of Washington found that 2-week therapy with TMP/SMZ was as effective as 6 weeks of treatment with the same drug in women with kidney infections that did not involve an obstruction or nervous system disorder. In such cases, kidney infections rarely lead to kidney damage or kidney failure unless they go untreated.

Various drugs are available to relieve the pain of a UTI. A heating pad or a warm bath may also help. Most doctors suggest that drinking plenty of water helps cleanse the urinary tract of bacteria. For the time being, it is best to avoid coffee, alcohol, and spicy foods. (And one of the best things a smoker can do for his or her bladder is to quit smoking. Smoking is the major known cause of bladder cancer.)

Treatment of Recurrent Infections in Women

About 4 out of 5 women who have a UTI get another in 18 months. Many women have them even more often. A woman who has frequent recurrences (three or more a year) should ask her doctor about one of the following treatment options:

- Take low doses of an antibiotic such as TMP/SMZ or nitrofurantoin daily for 6 months or longer. (If taken at bedtime, the drug remains in the bladder longer and may be more effective.) NIH-supported research at the University of Washington has shown this therapy to be effective without causing serious side effects.

- Take a single dose of an antibiotic after sexual intercourse.

- Take a short course (1 or 2 days) of antibiotics when symptoms appear.

Dipsticks that change color when an infection is present are now available without prescription. The strips detect nitrite, which is formed when bacteria change nitrate in the urine to nitrite. The test can detect about 90 percent of UTI's and may be useful for women who have recurrent infections.

Doctors suggest some additional steps that a woman can take on her own to avoid an infection:

- Drink plenty of water every day. Some doctors suggest drinking cranberry juice, which in large amounts inhibits the growth of some bacteria by acidifying the urine. Vitamin C (Ascorbic Acid) supplements have the same effect.

- Urinate when you feel the need; don't resist the urge to urinate;

- Wipe from front to back to prevent bacteria around the anus from entering the vagina or urethra;

- Take showers instead of tub baths;

- Cleanse the genital area before sexual intercourse;

- Empty the bladder shortly before and after sexual intercourse; and

- Avoid using feminine hygiene sprays and scented douches, which may irritate the urethra.

Treatment of Infections in Pregnancy

A pregnant woman who develops a UTI should be treated promptly to avoid premature delivery of her baby and other risks such as high blood pressure. Some antibiotics are not safe to take during pregnancy. In selecting the best treatment, doctors consider various factors such as the drug's effectiveness, the stage of pregnancy, the mother's health, and potential effects on the fetus.

Treatment of Complicated Infections

Curing infections that stem from a urinary obstruction or nervous system disorder depends on finding and correcting the underlying problem, sometimes with surgery. If the root cause goes untreated, this group of patients is at risk of kidney damage. Also, such infections tend to arise from a wider range of bacteria, and sometimes from more than one type of bacteria at a time.

UTI's are unusual in men. They usually stem from an obstruction—for example, a urinary stone or enlarged prostate—or a medical procedure involving a catheter. The first step is to identify the infecting organism and the drugs to which it is sensitive. Usually, doctors recommend lengthier therapy in men than in women, in part to prevent infection of the prostate gland. Prostate infections (prostatitis) are harder to cure because antibiotics are unable to penetrate infected prostate tissue effectively. For this reason, men with prostatitis often need long-term treatment with a carefully selected antibiotic.

For Further Information

The NIDDK sponsors the National Kidney and Urologic Diseases Information Clearinghouse, which collects and produces information about kidney and urinary tract disorders for health professionals and the public. For information about kidney and urinary tract disorders, contact:

The National Kidney and Urologic Disease Information Clearinghouse
Box NKUDIC
9000 Rockville Pike
Bethesda, MD 20892
(301) 468-6345

Suggestions for Additional Reading

The following material can be found in medical libraries, many college and university libraries, and through interlibrary loan in most public libraries.

Corriere, J.N. Jr et al.(1988) Cystitis: Evolving Standard of Care. *Patient Care,* Feb. 29, 33-47.

Fowler, J.E. Jr. (1986) Urinary Tract Infections in Women. *Urologic Clinics of North America,* Nov. 673-683.

Gillenwater J.Y. et al. (1987) *Adult and Pediatric Urology,* vol. 1. Chicago: Yearbook Medical Publishers.

Goldman P.L. et al. (1991) Evaluating Dysuria in the Era of STDs. *Patient Care,* Jan. 15, 51-69.

Hooton T.M. et al. (1991) Escherichia coli Bacteriuria and Contraceptive Method. *Journal of the American Medical Association,* Jan. 2, 64-69.

Krieger, J.N. (1986) Complications and Treatment of Urinary Tract Infections During Pregnancy. *Urologic Clinics of North America,* Nov. 685-693.

Kunin, C.M. (1987) *Detection, Prevention and Management of Urinary Tract Infections.* 4th edition, Philadelphia: Lea and Febiger.

Prostate Enlargement: Benign Prostatic Hyperplasia. A patient education booklet prepared by the National Institute of Diabetes and Digestive and Kidney Diseases, NIH, 1991.

Sheinfeld J. et al. (1989) Association of the Lewis Blood-Group Phenotype with Recurrent Urinary Tract Infections in Women. *New England Journal of Medicine,* March 23, 773-776.

Spencer J.R. and Schaeffer A.J. (1986) Pediatric Urinary Tract Infections. *Urologic Clinics of North America,* Nov. 661-672.

Stamm W.E. et al. (1987) Acute Renal Infection in Women: Treatment with Trimethoprim-Sulfamethoxazole or Ampicillin for Two or Six Weeks: A Randomized Trial. *Annals of Internal Medicine,* March, 341-345.

Stapleton A. et al. (1990) Postcoital Antimicrobial Prophylaxis for Recurrent Urinary Tract Infection: a randomized, double-blind, placebo-controlled trial. *Journal of the American Medical Association,* August 8, 703-706.

Walsh P.C. et al. (1986) eds. *Campbell's Urology,* Vol 1, 5th edition. Philadelphia: W.B. Saunders.

Section 19.2

Interstitial Cystitis

NIH Pub. No. 94-3220, 1994.

The urinary system consists of the kidneys, ureters, bladder, and urethra. The kidneys, a pair of purplish-brown organs, are located below the ribs toward the middle of the back. The kidneys remove liquid waste from the blood in the form of urine, keep a stable balance of salts and other substances in the blood, and produce erythropoietin, a hormone that aids the formation of red blood cells. Narrow tubes called ureters carry urine from the kidneys to the bladder, a triangle-shaped chamber in the lower abdomen. Like a balloon, the bladder's elastic walls relax and expand to store urine and contract and flatten when urine is emptied through the urethra. The typical adult bladder can store about 1 1/2 cups of urine.

Adults pass about a quart and a half of urine each day. The amount of urine varies, depending on the fluids and foods a person consumes. The volume formed at night is about half that formed in the daytime.

Normal urine is sterile. It contains fluids, salts and waste products, but it is free of bacteria, viruses and fungi. The tissues of the bladder are isolated from urine and toxic substances by a coating that discourages bacteria from attaching and growing on the bladder wall.

People with interstitial cystitis (IC) have an inflamed, or irritated, bladder wall. This inflammation can lead to scarring and stiffening of the bladder, decreased bladder capacity, glomerulations (pinpoint bleeding) and, in rare cases, ulcers in the bladder lining.

IC, also known as painful bladder syndrome and frequency-urgency-dysuria syndrome, is a complex, chronic disorder that has baffled doctors for as long as it has been recognized.

Estimates of the number of people who have IC run as high as 500,000, but no one knows for sure how many people have it. About 90 percent of IC patients are women. While people of any age can be affected, about two-thirds of patients are in their twenties, thirties, or forties. IC is rare in children. In a few cases, IC has afflicted both mother and daughter, but there is no evidence that the disorder is hereditary, or genetically passed from parent to child.

Two Types of Interstitial Cystitis

Because IC varies so much in its symptoms and severity, most researchers believe that it is not one but several diseases. Two types of IC are usually described; they are mainly distinguished by whether ulcers have formed on the bladder wall. Most researchers believe that IC does not generally progress from the nonulcerative to the ulcerative form.

Nonulcerative IC

This disorder is the most common type of IC. It usually affects young to middle-age women who have a normal, near normal, or increased bladder capacity when measured under general anesthesia. Glomerulations can be seen in the bladder wall.

Ulcerative IC

This type of IC tends to be found in middle-age to older women. Bladder capacity is low (less than 1 1/2 cups) when measured under general anesthesia. The decrease is thought to result in part from fibrosis, the formation of threadlike tissue that makes the bladder stiff and small. Cracks, scars, and Hunner's ulcers (star-shaped sores) in the bladder wall may bleed when the bladder is filled to capacity during a cystoscopy.

Cause of Interstitial Cystitis

No one knows what causes IC, but doctors studying the disorder believe it is a real, physical problem—not a result, symptom, or sign of an emotional problem.

One area of research on the cause of IC has focused on the lining of the bladder called the glycocalyx, made up primarily of substances called mucins and glycosaminoglycans (GAGs). This layer normally protects the bladder wall from toxic effects of urine and its contents. Researchers at the University of California, San Diego, found that this protective layer of the bladder was "leaky" in about 70 percent of IC patients they examined and may allow substances in urine to pass into the bladder wall and trigger IC symptoms. The researchers also found that patients with Hunner's ulcers had "leakier" bladders than patients without the ulcers.

Some people are diagnosed with IC after taking antibiotics for a presumed urinary tract infection. Therefore, it has been suggested that antibiotics may damage the bladder wall and make it "leaky." This idea has been studied carefully, but antibiotics have never been found to harm the bladder wall. Thus, other ideas are more likely to explain why some IC patients are diagnosed after a urinary tract infection. It is possible that the infection started an autoimmune response against the bladder, the patient's original symptoms were from IC all along, or an infecting organism is in bladder cells but is not detectable through routine tests.

Symptoms of Interstitial Cystitis

The symptoms of IC vary greatly from one person to another but have some similarities to those of a urinary tract infection:

- decreased bladder capacity

- an urgent need to urinate frequently day and night

- feelings of pressure, pain, and tenderness around the bladder, pelvis, and perineum (the area between the anus and vagina or anus and scrotum), which may increase as the bladder fills and decrease as it empties

- painful sexual intercourse

- in men, discomfort or pain in the penis and scrotum.

In most women, symptoms usually worsen around the menstrual cycle. As with many other illnesses, stress may also intensify symptoms but does not cause them.

Diagnosis of Interstitial Cystitis

Because the symptoms of IC are similar to those of other disorders of the urinary system, and because there is no definitive test to identify IC, doctors must rule out other conditions before considering a

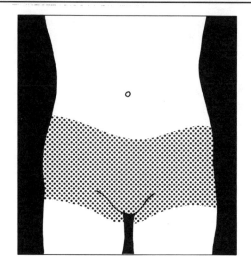

Figure 19.2. *Area of pain and pressure.*

diagnosis of IC. Among these disorders are urinary tract or vaginal infections, bladder cancer, bladder inflammation or infection caused by radiation to the abdomen, eosinophilic and tuberculous cystitis, kidney stones, endometriosis, neurological disorders, sexually transmitted diseases, low-count bacteriuria, and, in men, chronic bacterial and abacterial prostatitis.

The diagnosis of IC in the general population is based on

- presence of urgency, frequency or pelvic/bladder pain,
- cystoscopic evidence (under anesthesia) of bladder wall inflammation and glomerulations or Hunner's ulcers,
- absence of other diseases that may cause the symptoms.

Medical tests that help identify other conditions include a urinalysis, urine culture, cystoscopy, biopsy of the bladder wall and, in men, laboratory examination of prostate secretions.

Urinalysis and Urine Culture

These tests can detect and identify the most common organisms in the urine that may be causing symptoms. There are, however, organisms such as the bacteria chlamydia that can't be detected with these tests, so a negative culture does not rule out all types of infection. A urine sample is obtained either by catheterization or by the "clean catch" method. For a "clean catch," the patient washes the genital area before collecting urine "midstream" in a sterile container. White and red blood cells and bacteria in the urine may indicate an infection of the urinary tract, which can be treated with an antibiotic. If urine is sterile for weeks or months while symptoms persist, a doctor may consider a diagnosis of IC.

Culture of Prostate Secretions

In men, the doctor will obtain prostatic fluid from the patient. This fluid will be examined for signs of an infection, which can be treated with antibiotics.

Cystoscopy Under Anesthesia with Bladder Distension

During cystoscopy to diagnose IC, the doctor uses a cystoscope—an instrument made of a hollow tube about the diameter of a drinking straw with several lenses and a light—to see inside the bladder and urethra. The doctor will also distend or stretch the bladder to its capacity by filling it with a liquid or gas. Because bladder distension is painful in IC patients, before the doctor inserts the cystoscope through the urethra into the bladder, the patient must be given either regional or general anesthesia. These tests can detect inflammation; a thick, stiff bladder wall; Hunner's ulcers; and glomerulations (pinpoint bleeding) that may be seen only after the bladder is stretched.

The doctor may also test the patient's maximum bladder capacity, the amount of liquid or gas the bladder can hold under anesthesia. Without anesthesia, capacity is limited by either pain or a severe urge to urinate. Many people with IC have normal or large maximum bladder capacities under anesthesia. However, a small bladder capacity under anesthesia helps to support the diagnosis of IC.

Biopsy

A biopsy is a microscopic examination of tissue. Samples of the bladder and urethra may be removed during a cystoscopy and examined with a microscope later. A biopsy helps rule out bladder cancer and confirm bladder wall inflammation.

Treatment of Interstitial Cystitis

Scientists have not yet found a cure for IC, nor can they predict who will respond best to which treatment. Symptoms may disappear without explanation or coincide with an event such as a change in diet or treatment. Even when symptoms disappear, however, they may return after days, weeks, months, or years. Scientists do not know why.

Because doctors do not know what causes IC, treatments are aimed at relieving symptoms. Most people are helped for variable periods of time by one or a combination of treatments, many of which are described briefly here. However, as researchers learn more about IC, the list of potential treatments may change. Patients should discuss treatment options with a doctor.

Bladder Distension

Because some patients have noted an improvement in symptoms after a bladder distension done to diagnose IC, the procedure is often thought of as one of the first treatment attempts.

Researchers are not sure why distension helps, but some believe that the procedure may increase bladder capacity and interfere with pain signals transmitted by nerves in the bladder. Symptoms may temporarily worsen 24 to 48 hours after distension, but should then return to pre-distension levels or improve after 2 to 4 weeks.

Bladder Instillation

This procedure may also be called a bladder wash or bath. During a bladder instillation, the bladder is filled with a solution that is held for varying periods of time, from a few seconds to 15 minutes, before being drained through a narrow tube called a catheter.

The only drug approved by the U.S. Food and Drug Administration (FDA) for bladder instillation is dimethyl sulfoxide (DMSO, RIMSO®-50). With DMSO treatments a narrow tube (catheter) is guided up the urethra into the bladder. A measured amount of DMSO is passed through the catheter into the bladder, where it is retained for about 15 minutes before being expelled Treatments are given every week or two for 6 to 8 weeks, and repeated as needed. Most people with IC who respond to DMSO notice improvement of symptoms 3 or 4 weeks after the first 6- to 8-week cycle of treatments. Highly motivated patients who are willing to catheterize themselves may, after consultation with their doctor, be able to have DMSO treatments at home. Self-administration of DMSO is less expensive and more convenient than going to the doctor's office.

Doctors think DMSO works in several ways. Because it passes into the bladder wall, DMSO may more effectively reach tissue to reduce inflammation and block pain. It may also prevent muscle contractions that may cause pain, frequency, and urgency.

A bothersome but relatively insignificant side effect of DMSO treatments is a garlic-like taste and odor from the breath and skin. This may last up to 72 hours after a treatment. Long-term DMSO treatments have caused cataracts in animal studies, but this side effect has not appeared in humans. Blood tests, including a complete blood count and kidney and liver function tests, should be done about every 6 months.

A variety of other drugs have been used experimentally for bladder washes, including silver nitrate, sodium oxychlorosene (Clorpactin® WCS-90), heparin, and pentosanpolysulfate (Elmiron®).

Silver nitrate and oxychlorosene sodium are thought to work by first attacking the bladder lining. This triggers the body's immune system to step in and start the healing process. Some patients have been successfully treated with these drugs, but the frequent, painful treatments usually must be done under general anesthesia. Neither drug can be used in people who have urinary reflux, a condition in which urine flows backward up the ureters into the kidneys.

Heparin and pentosanpolysulfate are thought to work by replacing or repairing the "leaky" bladder lining.

Oral Drugs

There are no oral drugs approved by the FDA specifically for the treatment of IC, but a variety of drugs such as aspirin, ibuprofen, antihistamines, and the urinary tract pain reliever phenazopyridine (available by prescription as Pyridium® and over-the-counter as Azo-Standard™) may help lessen symptoms.

A blend of atropine, hyoseyamine, methenamine, methylene blue, phenyl salicylate and benzoic acid (Urised®) may inhibit the growth of organisms in the urine and reduce bladder spasms that cause frequency, urgency, and nighttime trips to the bathroom. Drugs such as oxybutynin chloride (Ditropan®) also may reduce bladder spasms. In separate studies of only a few patients each, hydroxyzine (Vistaril® and Atarax®), an antihistamine, and nifedipine (Procardia®), a heart disease and high blood pressure treatment, have been reported to reduce symptoms in some IC patients. But, as stated by the authors of these reports, further studies are needed to determine the drugs' true value in IC patients. All of these drugs must be prescribed by a physician.

Amitriptyline (Elavil®) is an FDA approved tricyclic antidepressant, but its ability to block pain and reduce bladder spasms makes it helpful in treating IC. Amitriptyline may cause drowsiness but can be taken at night to reduce this effect. Most people who respond to this drug show improvement 3 or 4 weeks after starting treatment. The dose may need adjustment for the best possible results

The experimental drug sodium pentosanpolysulfate (Elmiron®) is thought to repair the layer lining the bladder. In several studies, 19 percent to 65 percent of patients reported at least partial symptom relief. Most people who respond to pentosanpolysulfate see improvement within 6 to 8 weeks after starting treatment. There are few side effects, but the most common is skin rash. Clinical trials have been completed, and the drug's manufacturer has requested FDA approval to market pentosanpolysulfate as a treatment for IC. Until approved by FDA, doctors can prescribe the drug only by first obtaining approval for compassionate use in individual patients, or by having patients participate in an FDA-approved clinical trial.

Another experimental drug, nalmefene hydrochloride (Incystene™), blocks the body's receptors to pain, thus inhibiting the sensation of pain. Nalmefene is currently being evaluated in the treatment of IC in an FDA approved clinical study sponsored by the drug's manufacturer.

Because drugs have side effects, patients should always consult a doctor before using any drug for an extended time.

TENS (Transcutaneous Electrical Nerve Stimulation)

With TENS, mild electric pulses enter the body for minutes to hours two or more times a day either through wires placed on the lower back or the suprapubic region, between the navel and the pubic hair, or through special devices inserted into the vagina in women or into the rectum in men. Although scientists don't know exactly how it works, it has been suggested that the electric pulses may increase blood flow to the bladder, strengthen pelvic muscles that help control the bladder, and trigger the release of hormones that block pain.

TENS is relatively inexpensive and allows the patient to take an active part in treatment. Within some guidelines, the patient decides when, how long, and at what intensity TENS will be used. TENS has been most helpful in relieving pain and decreasing frequency in IC patients who have Hunner's ulcers. Smokers do not respond as well as nonsmokers. If TENS is going to help, change usually occurs in 3 to 4 months.

Diet

There is no scientific evidence linking diet to IC, but some doctors and patients believe that alcohol, tomatoes, spices, chocolate, caffeinated and citrus beverages, and high-acid foods may contribute to bladder irritation and inflammation. Some patients also notice a worsening of symptoms after eating or drinking products containing artificial sweeteners. Patients may try eliminating such products from their diet and reintroduce them one at a time to determine which, if any, affect symptoms. It is important, however, to maintain a well-balanced and varied diet.

Smoking

Many IC patients feel that smoking worsens their symptoms. (Because smoking is the major known cause of bladder cancer, one of the best things a smoker can do for the bladder is to quit smoking.)

Exercise

Many IC patients feel that regular exercise helps relieve symptoms and, in some cases, hastens remission.

Bladder Training

People who have found some relief from pain may be able to reduce frequency using bladder training techniques. Methods vary, but basically the patient decides to void at designated times and use relaxation techniques and distractions to help keep to the schedule. Gradually, the patient tries to lengthen the time between the scheduled voids. A diary of voids is usually helpful in keeping track of progress.

Surgery

This option is considered only if an IC patient has failed all available treatments and the pain is severe. Most doctors are reluctant to operate because the outcome is unpredictable in individual patients—some people have surgery and still have symptoms.

Anyone considering surgery should discuss the potential risks and benefits, side effects, and long and short-term complications with a surgeon and family, as well as with people who already have had the procedure. Surgery requires anesthesia, hospitalization, and weeks or months of recovery, and as the complexity of the procedure increases, so do the chances for complications and failure.

To locate a surgeon experienced in performing specific procedures, check with your doctor.

Transurethral fulguration and resection of ulcers. Fulguration involves burning Hunner's ulcers using electricity or a laser. When the area heals, the dead tissue and the ulcer fall off, leaving new, healthy tissue behind. Resection involves cutting around and removing the ulcers. Both treatments, done under anesthesia, use special instruments inserted into the bladder through a cystoscope. Laser surgery in the urinary tract should only be done by doctors who have the special training and expertise needed to perform the procedure.

Denervation. This is a complicated procedure done by surgeons who have special training and expertise. Rarely used in the treatment of IC, it involves cutting some of the nerves to the bladder, interfering with pain signals. Many approaches and techniques are used, each of which has its own advantages and complications that should be discussed with the surgeon.

Augmentation. This makes the bladder larger, most often by adding a section of the patient's small intestine, a tube-like structure that absorbs and transports nutrients from food for use by the body. With this treatment, scarred, ulcerated and inflamed sections of the patient's bladder are removed, leaving only healthy tissue and the base of the bladder. A piece of the patient's small intestine is removed, reshaped, and attached to what remains of the bladder. After the incisions heal, the patient may be able to void normally.

Even in carefully selected patients—those with small, contracted bladders—the pain, frequency, and urgency may remain or return after surgery and the patient may have additional problems with infections in the new bladder and difficulty absorbing nutrients from the shortened intestine. Some patients are incontinent while others cannot void at all and must insert a catheter into the urethra to empty urine from the bladder.

Bladder Removal (Cystectomy). Different methods can be used to reroute urine once the bladder has been removed. In most cases, the ureters are attached to a piece of bowel that opens onto the skin of the abdomen, called a stoma. Urine empties through the stoma into a bag outside the body. This procedure is called a urostomy. Some urologists are using a technique that also requires a stoma but allows urine to be stored in a pouch inside the abdomen. At intervals throughout the day, the patient puts a catheter into the stoma and empties the pouch. Patients with either type of urostomy must use very clean, or sterile, steps to prevent infections in and around the stoma.

With a third method, a new bladder is made from a piece of the patient's bowel (large intestine) and attached to the urethra in place of the removed bladder. After a time of healing, the patient may be able to empty the bladder by voiding at scheduled times or may insert a catheter into the urethra. Few surgeons have the special training and expertise needed to perform this procedure.

Even after total bladder removal, some patients still experience variable symptoms of IC. Therefore, the decision to undergo a cystectomy should only be undertaken after serious deliberation on the potential outcome.

Electrical Nerve Stimulation. This surgical treatment is a variation of TENS, described previously, but involves permanent implantation of electrodes and a unit that emits continuous electrical pulses. This relatively new procedure has variable short-term results, unknown long-term effects and, therefore, is not widely used.

Special Concerns

Cancer

There is no evidence that IC increases the risk of bladder cancer. However, the long-term effects of IC require further observation and research.

Pregnancy

Researchers have little information about pregnancy and IC, but believe that the disorder does not affect fertility or the health of the fetus. Some women have a remission from IC during pregnancy, while others have more pain and pressure during the third trimester, possibly due to the weight of the fetus on the bladder.

Working

Symptom flare-ups that result in frequent absences from work may make it difficult to get or keep a job. The Social Security Administration provides information on Social Security Disability benefits. The National Organization of Social Security Claimants' Representatives can refer you to a lawyer experienced with Social Security claims.

Coping

The emotional support of family, friends, and other people with IC is very important in helping patients cope with the disorder. Studies have found that IC patients who learn about the disorder and become involved in their own care do better than patients who do not. The Interstitial Cystitis Association can provide the address and phone number of the nearest support group.

Other Coping Tips:

- Find a health care team that is sympathetic, helpful, and receptive.
- Understand that your health care team does not know all the answers and may be as frustrated as you are.
- Don't become isolated from family and friends.
- Involve your family in treatment decisions.
- Do not allow IC to become the center of your life.
- Try to put IC in perspective—worse could happen.
- Talk to other people with IC about their experiences and ways of coping.
- Trust yourself.

Research

Although answers may seem slow in coming, researchers are working every day to solve the painful riddle of IC. Some scientists receive funds from the Federal Government to help support their research, and some receive support from other sources such as their employing institution, drug companies, and the Interstitial Cystitis Association Researchers and doctors around the country, regardless of who funds their work, may competently diagnose and treat IC.

The National Institute of Diabetes and Digestive and Kidney Diseases (NIDDK), a part of the National Institutes of Health (NIH), leads the Federal Government's research efforts on IC. Most studies funded by the NIDDK are a result of unsolicited grant applications sent to NIH by scientists at universities and medical centers throughout the United States. Other NIDDK-funded studies result from solicitations issued to encourage increased research on a certain topic.

By law, all applications sent to NIH are first reviewed by non-Government experts in the field of the proposed research for scientific merit and feasibility before being reviewed by the NIDDK's National Advisory Council. The council is made up of non-Government scientists, health professionals, and individuals who represent voluntary groups with an interest in the research of the institute. Approved applications are eligible for funding based on a scientific merit rating, or priority score, assigned by the initial reviewers. Applications are usually funded in priority score order, with the best applications funded first.

The NIDDK's investment in scientifically meritorious IC research has grown considerably since 1987, largely due to special solicitations. We now support research across the country that is looking at various aspects of IC, such as how urine contents may injure the bladder and what possible role organisms identified using nonstandard methods may have in causing IC. In addition to funding research, NIDDK sponsors scientific workshops where investigators share the results of their studies and discuss future areas for investigation.

Other Resources

American Foundation for Urologic Disease
The Bladder Health Council
300 West Pratt Street, Suite 401
Baltimore, MD 21201
410/727-2908 or 1-800-242-2383

American Pain Society
5700 Old Orchard Road
Skokie, IL 60077
708/966-5595

American Uro-Gynecologic Society
401 North Michigan Avenue
Chicago, IL 60611-4267
312/644-6610

International Pain Foundation
909 Northeast 43rd Street, Suite 306
Seattle, WA 98105-6020
206/547-2157

Interstitial Cystitis Association of America, Inc.
P.O. Box 1553
Madison Square Station
New York, NY 10159-1553
212/979-6057 or 1-800-ICA-1626

National Chronic Pain Outreach Association
7979 Old Georgetown Road, Suite 100
Bethesda, MD 20814
301/652-4948

National Kidney Foundation
30 East 33rd Street
New York, NY 10016
212/889-2210 or 1-800-622-9010

National Kidney and Urologic Diseases Information Clearinghouse
3 Information Way
Bethesda, MD 20892-3580
301/654-4415

Suggested Further Reading

The materials listed below may be found in medical libraries, many college and university libraries, through inter-library loan in most public libraries, and at book stores.

Articles and Book Chapters

Bavendam, TG. A Common Sense Approach To Lower Urinary Tract Hypersensitivity in Women. *Contemporary Urology,* 1992; 4(4):25-40.

Fleischmann, JD, et al. Clinical and Immunological Response to Nifedipine for the Treatment of Interstitial Cystitis. *The Journal of Urology,* 1991; 146:1235-1239.

Hanno, PM, et al. Diagnosis of Interstitial Cystitis. *The Journal of Urology,* 1990; 143(2):278-281.

Interstitial Cystitis Association. IC and Social Security Disability. *ICA Update,* 1988; 3(3):1

Messing, EM. Interstitial Cystitis and Related Syndromes. *Campbell's Urology.* Eds. Walsh, PC, et al. Philadelphia, WM Saunders Company, 1986. 1070-1083.

Mosedale, L. Embattled Bladders. *Health,* 1990; 22(5):40-78.

Parsons, CL. Managing Interstitial Cystitis. *Contemporary Urology,* March 1990; 2:45-49.

Perez-Marrero, R, Emerson, LE. Interstitial Cystitis. *The Canadian Journal of OB/GYN,* February 1990;4-10.

Ratner, V, et al. Interstitial Cystitis:A Bladder Disease Finds Legitimacy. *Journal of Women's Health,* 1992; 1(1):63-68.

Sant, GR. Interstitial Cystitis: Pathophysiology, Clinical Evaluation, and Treatment. *Urology Annual.* Ed. Rous, SN. Connecticut, Appleton & Lange, 1989. 171-196.

Schmidt, RA. Treatment of Unstable Bladder. *Urology,* 1991; 37(1): 28-32.

Schmidt, RA, Vapnek, JM. Pelvic Floor Behavior and Interstitial Cystitis. *Seminars in Urology,* 1991; 9(2):154-159.

Tanagho, EA. Interstitial Cystitis. *General Urology.* Eds Tanagho, EA, McAninch, JW. Connecticut, Appleton & Lange, 1988. 554-555.

Theoharides, TC. Hydroxyzine for Interstitial Cystitis. *Journal of Allergy and Clinical Immunology,* 1993; 91:686-687.

Books and Booklets

Budish, AD. *Avoiding the Medicaid Trap: How to Beat the Catastrophic Costs of Nursing Home Care.* New York, Holt, 1989.

Chalker, R, Whitmore, KE. *Overcoming Bladder Disorders.* New York, Harper & Row, 1990.

Gillespie, L., Blakeslee, D. *You Don't Have To Live With Cystitis!* New York, Avon Books, 1986.

Hanno, PM, et al., ed. *Interstitial Cystitis.* New York, Springer, Verlag, 1990.

National Institutes of Health, Office of Clinical Center Communications. *Relieving Pain.* Single copies are available from NIH/OCCC, Relieving Pain/IC, Building 10, Room 1C255, 9000 Rockville Pike, Bethesda, MD 20892.

Pitzele, SK. *We Are Not Alone—Learning To Live With Chronic Illness.* Minneapolis, Thompson, 1985.

Sant, GR, Guest ed. Interstitial Cystitis—1987. Supplement to *Urology.* 29(4). New Jersey, Hospital Publications, Inc., 1987.

Schrotenboer, K, Berkman, S. *The Woman Doctor's Guide To Overcoming Cystitis.* New York, Nal Penguin, Inc., 1987.

Section 19.3

Understanding Urinary Incontinence

Agency for Health Care Policy and Research Publication No. 96-0684, March 1996.

Many people lose urine when they don't want to. When this happens enough to be a problem, it is called urinary incontinence.

Urinary incontinence is very common. But some people are too embarrassed to get help. The good news is that millions of men and women are being successfully treated and cured.

How Your Body Makes, Stores, and Releases Urine

When you eat and drink, your body absorbs the liquid. The kidneys filter out waste products from the body fluids and make urine.

Urine travels down tubes called ureters into a muscular sac called the urinary bladder, which stores the urine.

When you are ready to go to the bathroom, your brain tells your system to relax.

Urine travels out of your bladder through a tube called the urethra. You release urine by relaxing the urethral sphincter and contracting the bladder muscles. The urethral sphincter is a group of muscles that tightens to hold urine in and loosens to let it out.

Causes of Urinary Incontinence

Urinary incontinence is not a natural part of aging. It can happen at any age, and can be caused by many physical conditions. Many causes of incontinence are temporary and can be managed with simple treatment. Some causes of temporary incontinence are:

- Urinary tract infection
- Vaginal infection or irritation

- Constipation
- Effects of medicine

Incontinence can be caused by other conditions that are not temporary. Other causes of incontinence are:

- Weakness of muscles that hold the bladder in place
- Weakness of the bladder itself
- Weakness of the urethral sphincter muscles
- Overactive bladder muscles
- Blocked urethra (can be from prostate enlargement)
- Hormone imbalance in women
- Neurologic disorders
- Immobility (not being able to move around)

In almost every case, these conditions can be treated. Your health care provider will help to find the exact cause of your incontinence.

Types of Incontinence

There are also many different types of incontinence. Some people have more than one type of incontinence. You should be able to identify the type of incontinence you have by comparing it to the list below.

Urge Incontinence

People with urge incontinence lose urine as soon as they feel a strong need to go to the bathroom. If you have urge incontinence you may leak urine:

- When you can't get to the bathroom quickly enough
- When you drink even a small amount of liquid, or when you hear or touch running water

You may also:

- Go to the bathroom very often; for example, every two hours during the day and night. You may even wet the bed.

Stress Incontinence

People with stress incontinence lose urine when they exercise or move in a certain way. If you have stress incontinence, you may leak urine:

- When you sneeze, cough, or laugh
- When you get up from a chair or get out of bed
- When you walk or do other exercise

You may also:

- Go to the bathroom often during the day to avoid accidents

Overflow Incontinence

People with overflow incontinence may feel that they never completely empty their bladder. If you have overflow incontinence, you may:

- Often lose small amounts of urine during the day and night
- Get up often during the night to go to the bathroom
- Often feel as if you have to empty your bladder but can't
- Pass only a small amount of urine but feel as if your bladder is still partly full
- Spend a long time at the toilet, but produce only a weak, dribbling stream of urine

Some people with overflow incontinence do not have the feeling of fullness, but they lose urine day and night.

Finding the Cause of Urinary Incontinence

Once you tell your health care provider about the problem, finding the cause of your urinary incontinence is the next step.

Your health care provider will talk with you about your medical history and urinary habits. You may be asked to keep a record of your usual habits in a bladder record. You probably will have a physical examination and urine tests. You may have other tests, as well. These tests will help find the exact cause of your incontinence and the best treatment for you. Below some of the tests you may be asked to take are listed.

Common Tests Used to Diagnose Urinary Incontinence

The following is a list of the different tests used to diagnose urinary incontinence.

1. **Blood tests.** These examine blood for levels of various chemicals.

2. **Cystoscopy.** This looks for abnormalities in bladder and lower urinary tract. It works by inserting a small tube into the bladder (because you may be uncomfortable during this part of the test, you may be given some medication to help relax you.) that has a telescope for the doctor to look through.

3. **Post-void residual (PVR) measurement.** This measures how much urine is left in the bladder after urinating by placing a small soft tube into the bladder or by using ultrasound (sound waves).

4. **Stress test.** This looks for urine loss when stress is put on bladder muscles usually by coughing, lifting, or exercise.

5. **Urinalysis.** This examines urine for signs of infection, blood, or other abnormality.

6. **Urodynamic** testing. This examines bladder and urethral sphincter function (may involve inserting a small tube into the bladder; x-rays also can be used to see the bladder).

Treating Urinary Incontinence

Once the type and cause of your urinary incontinence are known, treatment can begin. Urinary incontinence is treated in one or more of three ways: behavioral techniques, medication, and surgery.

Behavioral Techniques

Behavioral techniques teach you ways to control your own bladder and sphincter muscles. They are very simple and work well for certain types of urinary incontinence. Two types of behavioral techniques are commonly used:

1. Bladder training and
2. Pelvic muscle exercises.

You may also be asked to change the amount of liquid that you drink. You may be asked to drink more or less water depending on your bladder problem.

Bladder Training. Bladder training is used for urge incontinence, and may also be used for stress incontinence. Both men and women can benefit from bladder training. People learn different ways to control the urge to urinate. Distraction (thinking about other things) is just one example. A technique called prompted voiding—urinating on a schedule—is also used. This technique has been quite successful in controlling incontinence in nursing home patients.

Pelvic Muscle Exercises. Pelvic muscle exercises called Kegel exercises are used for stress incontinence. The Kegel exercises help to strengthen weak muscles around the bladder.

Medication

Some people need to take medicine to treat conditions that cause urinary incontinence. The most common types of medicine treat infection, replace hormones, stop abnormal bladder muscle contractions, or tighten sphincter muscles. Your health care provider may recommend medication for your condition. You will be taught how and when to take it.

Surgery

Surgery is sometimes needed to help treat the cause of incontinence. Surgery can be used to:

- Return the bladder neck to its proper position in women with stress incontinence
- Remove tissue that is causing a blockage
- Correct severely weakened pelvic muscles
- Enlarge a small bladder to hold more urine

There are many different surgical procedures that may be used to treat incontinence. The type of operation you may need depends on the type and cause of your incontinence. Your doctor will discuss the specific procedure you might need. *Be sure to ask questions so that you fully understand the procedure.*

Other Measures and Supportive Devices

Some other products can be used to help manage incontinence. These include pads and catheters. Catheters are used when a person cannot urinate. A catheter is a tube that is placed in the bladder to drain urine into a bag outside the body. The catheter usually is left inside the bladder, but some catheters are not left in. They are put in and taken out of the bladder as needed to empty it every few hours. Condom catheters (mostly used in men) attach to the outside of the body and are not placed directly in the bladder. Specially designed pads are available to help men and women with incontinence.

Catheters and pads are not the first and only treatment for incontinence. They should only be used to make other treatments more effective or when other treatments have failed.

What To Do Next

Your health care provider will tell you about the type of incontinence you have and will recommend a treatment. While you are being treated, be sure to:

- Ask questions
- Follow instructions
- Take all of your medicine
- Report side effects of your medicine, if any
- Report any changes, good and bad, to your health care provider

and remember, incontinence is not a natural part of aging. In most cases, it can be successfully treated and reversed.

Risks and Benefits of Treatment

Three types of treatment are recommended for urinary incontinence:

- Behavioral techniques
- Medicine
- Surgery

How well each of these treatments works depends on the cause of the incontinence and, in some cases, patient effort. The risks and benefits described below are based on current medical knowledge and expert opinion. How well a treatment works may also depend on the individual patient. A treatment that works for one patient may not be as effective for another patient. Therefore, it is important to talk with a health care provider about treatment choices.

Behavioral Techniques. There are no risks for this type of treatment.

Medicine. As with most drugs, there is a risk of having a side effect. If you are taking medicine for other conditions, the drugs could react with each other. Therefore, it is important to work with the health care provider and report all of your medicines and any side effects as soon as they happen.

Surgery. With any surgery there is a possibility of a risk or complication. It is important to discuss these risks with your surgeon.

Coping with Incontinence

Several national organizations help people with urinary incontinence. They may be able to put you in touch with local groups that can give you more information, ideas, and emotional support in coping with urinary incontinence.

Alliance for Aging Research (information on bladder training program)
2021 K Street, N.W.
Suite 305
Washington, DC 20006
202-293-2856

Bladder Health Council
c/o American Foundation for Urologic Disease
300 West Pratt Street, Suite 401
Baltimore, MD 21201
1-800-242-2383
410-727-2908

National Association for Continence
(formerly Help for Incontinent People)
P.O. Box 8310
Spartanburg, SC 29305
864-579-7900
1-800-BLADDER or 1-800-252-3337

International Continence Society
The Continence Foundation
2 Doughty Street
London WC1N 2PH
1144-1714-046875

Simon Foundation for Continence
Box 835
Wilmette, IL 60091
1-800-23-SIMON
708-864-3913

Section 19.4

Urinary Incontinence in Adults: Clinical Practice Guideline Update

Agency for Health Care Policy and Research Publication No. 96-R034,
March 1996.

In 1992, the Agency for Health Care Policy and Research (AHCPR) released its first guideline on urinary incontinence. Since then the guideline has become the standard of care for incontinence in many settings across the country.

This update of the guideline reflects new findings in the rapidly changing field of treatment for urinary incontinence. To develop the update, AHCPR convened a multi-disciplinary private-sector panel of physicians, nurses, allied health professionals, and health care consumers to study the effectiveness of diagnostic and treatment procedures for urinary incontinence, their costs, and how they affect patient outcomes.

The results of this research show that incontinence can be improved, and in some cases, even cured. Anecdotal evidence shows that long-term care facilities that have adopted the guideline have improved the quality of life of their patients and saved money at the same time.

What Is Urinary Incontinence?

Urinary incontinence (UI), or the unintentional loss of urine, is a problem for more than 13 million Americans—85 percent of them women. Although about half of the elderly have episodes of incontinence, bladder problems are not a natural consequence of aging, and they are not exclusively a problem of the elderly.

Incontinence has several causes. Women are most likely to develop incontinence either during pregnancy and childbirth, or after the hormonal changes of menopause, because of weakened pelvic muscles. Older men can become incontinent as the result of prostate surgery. Pelvic trauma, spinal cord damage, caffeine, or medications including cold or over-the-counter diet tablets also can cause episodes of incontinence.

But even though urinary incontinence can be improved in 8 out of 10 cases, fewer than half of those with bladder problems ever discuss the condition with their health care professional. The condition often goes untreated.

Facts about Incontinence

- 13 million Americans are incontinent; 11 million are women.
- 1 in 4 women ages 30-59 have experienced an episode of UI.
- 50% or more of the elderly persons living at home or in long-term care facilities are incontinent.
- $16.4 billion is spent every year on incontinence-related care: $11.2 billion for community-based programs and at home, and $5.2 billion in long-term care facilities.
- $1.1 billion is spent every year on disposable products for adults.

Types and Causes of UI

There are four common types of incontinence:

1. **Stress incontinence** happens when the bladder can't handle the increased compression during exercise, coughing, or sneezing. This kind of incontinence happens mostly to women under 60 and in men who have had prostate surgery.

2. **Urge incontinence** is caused by a sudden, involuntary bladder contraction. It is more common in older adults.

3. **Mixed incontinence** is a combination of both stress and urge incontinence, and is most common in older women.

4. **Overflow incontinence,** in which the bladder becomes too full because it can't be fully emptied, is rarer and is the result of bladder obstruction or injury. In men, it can be the result of an enlarged prostate.

5. Other factors can cause incontinence such as decreased mobility, cognitive impairment or medications.

Treatment Recommendations

Treatment for UI depends on the type of incontinence, its causes, and the capabilities of the patient. The guideline update recommends the following treatments:

Pelvic Muscle Rehabilitation

This is to improve pelvic muscle tone and prevent leakage. This includes:

- **Kegel exercises.** Regular, daily exercising of pelvic muscles can improve, and even prevent, urinary incontinence. This is particularly helpful for younger women. Should be performed 30-80 times daily for at least 8 weeks.

- **Biofeedback.** Used in conjunction with Kegel exercises, biofeedback helps people gain awareness and control of their pelvic muscles.

- **Vaginal weight training.** Small weights are held within the vagina by tightening the vaginal muscles. Should be performed for 15 minutes, twice daily, for 4 to 6 weeks.

- **Pelvic floor electrical stimulation.** Mild electrical pulses stimulate muscle contractions. Should be performed in conjunction with Kegel exercises.

Behavioral Therapies

These help people regain control of their bladder and include:

- Bladder training teaches people to resist the urge to void and gradually expand the intervals between voiding.
- Toileting assistance uses routine or scheduled toileting, habit training schedules, and prompted voiding to empty the bladder regularly to prevent leaking.

Pharmacologic Therapies

These improve incontinence medically and include:

- Oxybutynin (brand name Ditropan) prevents urge incontinence by relaxing sphincter muscles.
- Estrogen, either oral or vaginal, may be helpful in conjunction with other treatments for postmenopausal women with UI.

Surgical Therapies

These treat specific anatomical problems.

- Sling procedures, bulking injections (such as collagen) and other surgical procedures support or move the bladder to improve continence.

Treatment Recommendations for the Chronically Incontinent

Although many people will improve their continence through treatment, some will never become completely dry. They may need to take medications that cause incontinent episodes or have cognitive or physical impairments that keep them from being able to perform pelvic muscle exercises or retrain their bladders. Many will be cared for in long-term care facilities or at home. The guideline update makes the following recommendations to help caregivers keep the chronically incontinent drier and reduce their cost of care:

- **Scheduled toileting**—take people to the toilet every 2 to 4 hours or according to their toilet habits.

- **Prompted voiding**—check for dryness and encourage use of the toilet.

- **Improved access to toilets**—use equipment such as canes, walkers, wheelchairs, and devices that raise the seating level of toilets to make toileting easier.

- **Managing fluids and diet**—eliminate dietary caffeine (for those with urge incontinence) and encourage adequate fiber in the diet.

- **Disposable absorbent garments—use to keep people dry.**

Education

The guideline recommends that patients and professionals learn about the different treatment options for incontinence.

- Patients and their families should know that incontinence is not inevitable or shameful but is treatable or at least manageable. All management alternatives should be explained.

- Professional education about UI evaluation and treatment should be included in the basic curricula of undergraduate and graduate training programs of all health care providers, as well as continuing education program.

Part Five

Emotional and
Mental Health Concerns

Chapter 20

Eating Disorders

Chapter Contents

Section 20.1

Facts about Anorexia Nervosa

An NIH publication by Ms. Jody Dove, of the Office of Research Reporting.

Anorexia nervosa is a disorder of self-starvation which manifests itself in an extreme aversion to food and can cause psychological, endocrine and gynecological problems. It almost exclusively affects adolescent white girls, with symptoms involving a refusal to eat, large weight loss, a bizarre preoccupation with food, hyperactivity, a distorted body image and cessation of menstruation. Although the symptoms can be corrected if the patient is diagnosed and treated in time, about 10-15 percent of anorexia nervosa patients die, usually after losing at least half their normal body weight.

Anorexia nervosa patients typically come from white, middle to upper-middle class families that place heavy emphasis on high achievement, perfection, eating patterns and physical appearance. (There has never been a documented case of anorexia nervosa in a black male or female.) A newly diagnosed patient often is described by her parents as a "model child," usually because she is obedient, compliant, and a good student. Although most teenagers experience some feelings of youthful rebellion, persons with anorexia usually do not outwardly exhibit these feelings, tending instead to be childish in their thinking, in their need for parental approval, and in their lack of independence. Psychologists theorize that the patient's desire to control her own life manifests itself in the realm of eating—the only area, in the patient's mind, where she has the ability to direct her own life.

In striving for perfection and approval, a person with anorexia may begin to diet in order to lose just a few pounds. Dieting does not stop there, however, and an abnormal concern with dieting is established. Nobody knows what triggers the disease process, but suddenly, losing five or ten pounds is not enough. The anorectic patient becomes intent on losing weight. It is not uncommon for someone who develops this disorder to starve herself until she weighs just 60 or 70 pounds. Throughout the starvation process she either denies being hungry or claims to feel full after eating just a few bites.

Another related form of anorexia nervosa is an eating disorder known as "bulimia. " Patients with this illness indulge in "food binges," and then purge themselves through vomiting immediately after eating or through the use of laxatives or diuretics. While on the surface these patients may appear to be well adjusted socially, this serious disease is particularly hard to overcome because it usually has been a pattern of behavior for a long time.

Whom Does It Affect?

Most researchers agree that the number of patients with anorexia nervosa is increasing. Recent estimates suggest that out of every 200 American girls between the ages of 12 and 18, one will develop anorexia to some degree. Therapists find that persons with anorexia usually lack self-esteem and feel they can gain admiration by losing weight and becoming thin.

While most anorexia nervosa patients are female, about 6 percent are adolescent boys. Occasionally the disorder is found in older women and in children as young as eight years old.

Some researchers believe that certain characteristics are common to the families of persons who develop the disorder. Although this "typical" family model may not apply to all patients, it is common to many. Researchers describe these families as warm and loving on the surface. Evidently, this loving atmosphere masks a series of underlying problems in which family members are excessively involved in each other's lives, and overly dependent on one another. Apparently, they often are unable to deal with conflicts within the family. Either they deny that conflicts exist, or they become so overwhelmed by numerous petty conflicts that they are unable to recognize real problems.

What Are the Symptoms?

Psychological symptoms such as social withdrawal, obsessive-compulsiveness and depression often precede or accompany anorexia nervosa. The patient's distorted view of herself and the world around her are the cause of these psychological disturbances. Distortion of body image is another prevalent symptom. While most normal females can give an accurate estimate of their body weight, anorectic patients tend to perceive themselves as markedly larger than they really are. When questioned, most feel that their emaciated state (70-80 lbs.) is either "just right" or "too fat."

Profound physical symptoms also occur in cases of extreme starvation. These include loss of head hair, growth of fine body hair, constipation, intolerance of cold temperatures and low pulse rate.

Certain endocrine functions also become impaired. In females this results in a cessation of menstruation (amenorrhea) and the absence of ovulation. Menstruation usually will not resume until endocrine balance is restored. Ovulation is suppressed because production of certain necessary hormones decreases.

Anorexia in boys has effects similar to those in girls: severe weight loss, psycho-social problems and interruption of normal reproductive system processes.

Many differences in symptoms are apparent between anorectics and bulimics. Anorexia nervosa patients usually are not obese before onset of their illness. Typically, they are good students who become socially withdrawn before becoming ill and often come from families who fit the anorexia prototype described earlier. Bulimics, on the other hand, usually are extroverted before their illness, are inclined to be overweight, have voracious appetites and have episodes of binge eating. Anorexia patients often have a better chance of returning to normal weight because their eating patterns, unlike those of bulimics, have been altered for a relatively shorter time.

Causes of Anorexia

While the cause of anorexia is still unknown, a combination of psychological, environmental and physiological factors are associated with development of the disorder.

Researchers have discovered that a part of the brain called the hypothalamus begins to work improperly after the onset of anorexia. The hypothalamus controls such activities as maintenance of water balance, regulation of body temperature, secretion of the endocrine glands and sugar and fat metabolism. In anorexia patients, this improper functioning may result in lower blood pressure and body temperature, a lack of sexual interest and hormonal changes resulting in amenorrhea and reduced production of thyroid hormone.

Some scientists are studying the possibility that the abnormalities in certain endocrine functions may actually precede the onset of anorexia. Further studies are needed, however, to determine if anorexia patients have a biological predisposition to develop the illness.

Treatment of Anorexia

Treatment for anorexia nervosa is usually threefold, consisting of nutritional therapy, individual psychotherapy and family counseling. A team made up of pediatricians, psychiatrists, social workers and nurses often administers treatment. Some physicians hospitalize anorexia patients until they are nutritionally stable. Others prefer to work with patients in the family setting.

But no matter where therapy is started, the most urgent concern of the physician is getting the patient to eat and gain weight. This is accomplished by gradually adding calories to the patient's daily intake. If she is hospitalized, privileges are sometimes granted in return for weight gain. This is known as a behavioral contract, and privileges may include such desirable activities as leaving the hospital for an afternoon's outing.

Physicians and hospital staff make every effort to ensure that the patient does not feel overwhelmed and powerless. Instead, weight gain is encouraged in an atmosphere in which the patient feels in control of her situation, and in which she wants to gain weight.

Individual psychotherapy is necessary in the treatment of anorexia to help the patient understand the disease process and its effects. Therapy focuses on the patient's relationship with her family and friends, and the reasons she may have fallen into a pattern of self-starvation. As a patient begins to learn more about her condition she is often more willing to try to help herself recover. In cases of severe depression, drugs such as antidepressants are part of therapy. Behavior improvement generally occurs rapidly in these cases and the patient is able to respond more quickly to treatment.

The third aspect of treatment, family therapy, is supportive in nature. It examines how the patient and her parents relate to each other.

Persons with anorexia often become a source of family tension because refusals to eat cause frustration in the parents. The goal of family therapy is to help family members relate more effectively to one another, to encourage more mature thinking in the anorectic patient and to help all family members work together for the well-being of the patient and the family unit.

In treating anorexia, it is extremely important to remember that immediate success does not guarantee a permanent cure. Sometimes, even after successful hospital treatment and return to a normal weight, patients suffer relapses. Follow-up therapy lasting three to five years is recommended if the patient is to be completely cured.

Self-help groups for patients, parents, spouses and siblings can be a useful part of the overall treatment. Information on groups, treatment centers, hospitals, clinics and doctors specializing in anorexia can be obtained from any of the following voluntary organizations:

American Anorexia Nervosa Association, Inc.
133 Cedar Lane
Teaneck, N.J. 07666

National Anorexic Aid Society, Inc. (NAAS)
P.O. Box 29461
Columbus, Ohio 43229

Anorexia Nervosa and Associated Disorders (ANAS)
Suite 2020
550 Frontage Rd.
Northfield, Ill. 60093

Current Research

The National Institutes of Health is sponsoring research to determine the causes of anorexia, the best methods of treatment and ways to identify who might have a high risk of developing the disorder.

University scientists, sponsored by the National Institute of Child Health and Human Development, are examining the various factors in society, personality and families influencing persons who develop anorexia. Other projects are comparing weight gain in patients fed high-protein versus low-protein diets.

Researchers at the National Institute of Mental Health are studying the biological aspects and changes in brain chemistry which may control appetite. Although psychological or environmental factors may precipitate the onset of the illness, the study indicates that it may be prolonged by starvation-induced changes in body processes. Persons with anorexia are sometimes admitted for study and treatment at the Clinical Center, a research hospital located on the National Institutes of Health campus in Bethesda, MD.

The National Institutes of Health, through its Division of Research Resources, supports ten General Clinical Research Centers throughout the country in which anorexia research is underway. Topics currently under investigation include sexual maturation, endocrine evaluation, hypothalamic and pituitary aspects of anorexia nervosa and potassium levels in persons with anorexia.

The National Institute of Arthritis, Diabetes, and Digestive and Kidney Diseases sponsors studies in the endocrine disturbances of the hypothalamic, pituitary and ovarian function in the anorectic patient.

Section 20.2

Eating Disorders—When Thinness Becomes an Obsession

DHSS Publication No. 94-1181, January 1994.

Hula hoops, miniskirts, punk hair styles. Fads come and go, and most are harmless. But when it's a fad to self-induce symptoms of a severe illness, the current craze isn't harmless anymore.

That hazardous fad involves bulimia nervosa, a severe eating disorder of compulsive bingeing and purging. People with bulimia rapidly eat tremendous amounts of food and then get rid of the food by vomiting or other means. Bulimia symptoms are found in 40 to 50 percent of patients with another potentially life-threatening disorder called anorexia nervosa, or compulsive self-starvation.

"Bulimia almost has celebrity status, the 'in' thing to have," says Sue Bailey, M.D., medical director of Chevy Chase Associates, Washington, D.C., and clinical faculty member at Georgetown University School of Medicine in Washington, D.C. According to Bailey, victims think at first that they've found a great solution to weight control, that "they can eat whatever they want and get rid of it. Then, after a couple of years, it hits: 'I thought I could stop any time. But I can't.'"

Bailey was medical consultant to a Gallup Poll on eating disorders which projected that about 2 million American women 19 to 39 and 1 million teenagers are affected by some symptoms of bulimia or anorexia. In her own survey of several private schools in the Washington, D.C., area, Bailey found that 28 percent of one school's eighth graders said they would consider vomiting to lose weight. Many reported dieting since age 13, being dissatisfied with their bodies since age 10, and always trying to be perfect. "In other words," she says, "many girls were showing a real vulnerability to an eating disorder."

Some U.S. studies of female high school and college students suggest a bulimia prevalence ranging from 4.5 to 18 percent. But in the *Journal of the American Medical Association* (Sept. 4, 1987), David Schotte, Ph.D., and Albert Stunkard, M.D., reported that when they surveyed 1,965 students at the University of Pennsylvania, Philadelphia, they found only 1.3 percent of women met the American Psychiatric Association's diagnostic criteria for bulimia. "Thus," they wrote, "although bulimic behaviors may be quite common among college women, clinically significant bulimia is not. Also, research with college students has found that as many as 50 percent of college women who met diagnostic criteria for bulimia during the fall semester of their freshman year no longer met these criteria when reassessed nine months later."

Anorexia is estimated to affect as many as 1 out of every 100 females aged 12 to 18. Males are said to account for about 5 to 10 percent of bulimia and anorexia cases. (Because male victims are so few, we'll refer to all patients as females.) More research is needed to determine the exact incidence of bulimia and anorexia.

People of all races can develop bulimia and anorexia, but the vast majority of patients diagnosed with the disorders are white, which may reflect socioeconomic, rather than racial, factors. Yet the illnesses are not restricted to females with certain occupational or educational backgrounds. What causes the illnesses and why they occur primarily in females are unknown.

The disorders are obsessive—that is, most victims can't stop their self-destructive behavior without professional medical help. Left untreated, the disorders can become chronic and lead to severe health damage. The National Center for Health Statistics reported 70 deaths from anorexia nervosa in 1990, the latest year for which statistics are available. No deaths from bulimia were reported.

According to the American Psychiatric Association, all of the following criteria must be met for a diagnosis of bulimia or anorexia.

For the syndrome of bulimia nervosa:

- recurrent episodes of binge eating (rapid consumption of a large amount of food in a discrete period of time)

- a feeling of lack of control over eating behavior during the eating binges

420

- regularly engaging in either self-induced vomiting, use of laxatives or diuretics, strict dieting or fasting, or vigorous exercise in order to prevent weight gain

- a minimum average of two binge-eating episodes a week for at least three months

- persistent overconcern with body shape and weight.

For the syndrome of anorexia nervosa:

- refusal to maintain body weight over a minimal normal weight for age and height—for example, weight loss leading to maintenance of body weight 15 percent below that expected; or failure to make expected weight gain during period of growth, leading to body weight 15 percent below that expected

- intense fear of gaining weight or becoming fat, even though underweight

- disturbance in the way in which one's body weight, size or shape is experienced—for example, the person claims to "feel fat" even when emaciated, believes that one area of the body is "too fat" even when obviously underweight

- in females, absence of at least three consecutive menstrual cycles when otherwise expected to occur (primary or secondary amenorrhea). (A woman is considered to have amenorrhea if her periods occur only following administration of estrogen or other hormones.)

Ordinarily, bulimia begins in adolescence or the early 20s. However, because many bulimics successfully hide their bingeing and purging, an actual diagnosis may not be made until a patient is well into her 30s or 40s. In *Cosmopolitan* (January 1985), for example, actress Jane Fonda revealed that she had been a secret bulimic from age 12 until her recovery at age 35-bingeing and purging as much as 20 times a day, she said.

Bulimia usually begins in conjunction with a diet. But once a binge-purge cycle becomes established, it can get out of control.

Some bulimic patients may be somewhat underweight and few may be obese, but many maintain a nearly normal weight. In many, the menstrual cycle becomes irregular. Sexual interest may diminish.

Although bulimics appear healthy and successful—"perfectionists" at whatever they do—in reality, they have low self-esteem and are often depressed. They may exhibit other compulsive behaviors. One physician reports, for example, that a third of his bulimia patients regularly engage in shoplifting, and that a quarter of the patients have suffered from alcohol abuse or addiction at some point in their lives.

Binges can last as long as eight hours and result in an intake of 20,000 calories (that's roughly 210 brownies, or 5 1/2 layer cakes, or 18 dozen macaroons). One study, however, showed the *average* binge to be slightly less than 1 1/4 hours and slightly more than 3,400 calories (an entire pecan pie, for instance). Most binges are carried out in secret. Some bulimics spend $50 or more a day on food and even steal (food or money) to support the obsession.

To lose the gained weight, the bulimic begins purging, which may include using laxatives—from 50 to 100 or more tablets at one time— or diuretics (drugs to increase urination) or self-induced vomiting caused by gagging, using an emetic (a chemical substance that causes vomiting), or simply mentally willing the action. Between binges, the person may fast or exercise excessively.

Bulimia's binge-purge cycle can be devastating to health in a number of ways. It can upset the body's balance of electrolytes—such as sodium, magnesium, potassium, and calcium—which can cause fatigue, seizures, muscle cramps, irregular heartbeat, and decreased bone density, which can lead to osteoporosis. Repeated vomiting can damage the esophagus and stomach, cause the salivary glands to swell, make the gums recede, and erode tooth enamel. In some cases, all of the teeth must be pulled prematurely because of the constant wash by gastric acid. Other effects may be rashes, broken blood vessels in the cheeks, and swelling around the eyes, ankles and feet. For diabetics, bingeing on high-carbohydrate foods and sweets is particularly hazardous, since their bodies cannot properly metabolize the starches and sugars.

Bulimia's severe health risks and potential for becoming obsessive do not bode well for a decision to "try it out." Dr. Bailey points out, "Very rarely do I hear someone say, 'Oh yes, I had bulimia for three years and I just stopped one day and now I'm fine.' It's very hard to give up the behavior. Once somebody tells me they've done this several times—in my mind, they're probably hooked."

While anorexia nervosa most commonly begins in adolescence, onset also is reported (albeit far less frequently) in people ranging in age from about 8 to 60. The incidence in 8- to 11-year-olds is said to be increasing.

Anorexia may be a single, limited episode—that is, the person may lose a drastic amount of weight within a few months and then recover. Or the illness may gradually work itself into the victim's life and go on for years. A person may diet normally for several weeks, for instance, and then increasingly restrict her food intake until the diet gets out of control. Anorexia may fluctuate between spells of improvement and worsening, or it may become steadily more severe.

Anorectics are described as having low self-esteem and feeling that others are controlling their lives. Some may be very overactive—exercising excessively. The preoccupation with food usually prompts strange food-related patterns, or rituals: crumbling food, moving it about on the plate, cutting it into very tiny pieces to prolong eating, and not eating with the rest of the family. The anorectic sometimes becomes a gourmet cook, preparing elaborate meals for others while eating low-calorie food herself.

The anorectic becomes obsessed with a fear of fat and with losing weight. In her mind's eye, she sees normal folds of flesh as fat that must be eliminated. She may have trouble sleeping. Because there's no longer a fat tissue padding, sitting or lying down brings discomfort, not rest. As her obsession increasingly controls her life, she may become isolated from friends and family.

Many of the anorectic's peculiar behaviors and bodily changes are typical of any starvation victim. Thus, some functions are often restored to normal when sufficient weight is regained. Meanwhile, the starving body tries to protect itself—especially its two main organs, the brain and the heart—by slowing down or stopping less vital body processes. Thus, menstruation ceases (often before weight loss becomes noticeable), blood pressure and respiratory rate slow down, and thyroid activity diminishes—resulting in brittle hair and nails, dry skin, slowed pulse rate, cold intolerance, and constipation. With depletion of fat, the body temperature is lowered. Soft hair called lanugo forms over the skin. Electrolyte imbalance can become so severe that irregular heart rhythm, heart failure, and decreased bone density occur. Other physical signs and symptoms can include mild anemia, swelling of joints, reduced muscle mass, and light-headedness.

When anorectics adopt the bulimic bingeing and purging, they impair their health even further. Some use the emetic syrup of ipecac to induce vomiting after a binge. The late recording artist Karen Carpenter was an anorectic who died of syrup of ipecac abuse. Building up over time, the alkaloid emetine in the ipecac irreversibly damaged her heart muscle, which eventually led to her death by cardiac arrest.

Suggested Causes of Anorexia and Bulimia

As to the causes of anorexia and bulimia, there are many theories. One is that many young women feel abnormal pressure to be as thin as the "ideal" portrayed by magazines, movies and television.

David Jimerson, M.D., director of research, Department of Psychiatry at Beth Israel Hospital in Boston and associate professor of psychiatry at Harvard Medical School, suggests that a certain biological factor that is linked to clinical depression may contribute to the development or persistence of symptoms in anorexia and bulimia. Jimerson explains that a biological change in some people may predispose them to depression. "We're looking at whether that same biological predisposition, or some related alteration, might also predispose to the onset of an eating disorder." In fact, says Jimerson, 7 of 10 anorectics and bulimics are depression-prone, as are many of their relatives.

Jimerson points out that the neurotransmitter (a chemical involved in sending nerve "messages" to and from the brain) serotonin is linked to both mood and eating functions and that decreased serotonin activity has been linked to impulsive behavior. Bulimics are often impulsive.

Several other theories suggest biological factors. For instance, malfunctioning of the hypothalamus occurs in anorexia and may precede onset of the illness. The hypothalamus is a part of the brain that controls such bodily functions as hormonal secretions, temperature and water balance regulation, and sugar and fat metabolism. Also, endorphin hormones, which are released during purging and excessive exercise (causing the famous jogger's "high"), are believed to be addictive.

Anorexia and bulimia may be triggered by an inability to cope with a situation in life: puberty, the first sexual contact, ridicule over weight, death of a loved one, or separation from family because of college. It's been suggested that choices afforded by the women's movement may be misinterpreted as obligations, thus creating another stress with which anorectics-to-be cannot cope.

In her book *Eating Disorders*, the late Hilde Bruch, M.D., offered this explanation: "The urgent need to lose weight is a cover-up symptom, expressing an underlying fear of being despised or disregarded, or of not getting or even deserving respect. Desperate about their inability to solve their problems, the patients begin to worry about their weight and get a sense of accomplishment from manipulating their body."

Bruch also maintained that patients with anorexia learned to eat, not to satisfy hunger, but to satisfy the expectations of others; thus, their eating or not eating involved their self-esteem. She described anorectics as struggling against over-controlling parents to gain a sense of "leading a life of their own."

Some studies have found these characteristics in families of anorectics: poor communicating skills, conflict avoidance, overconcern with appearances, overemphasis on high achievement, and over-involvement with one another. But there are differences of opinion as to the significance of many of these observations.

And while opinions differ also about treatments for anorexia and bulimia, they agree on one point—that early treatment is vital. As either disorder becomes more entrenched, its damage becomes less reversible.

How Then to Treat These Disorders?

According to Bruch, "A realistic body-image concept is a pre-condition for recovery in anorexia nervosa." Considering the anorectic's tenacious denial of being too thin or eating too little, convincing her that she needs to gain weight is no small task. A prime example of resistance is this defense by one of Bruch's patients, "Of course I had breakfast; I ate my Cheerio." In contrast, bulimics usually cooperate with the medical staff; they may even seek treatment voluntarily.

Several approaches are usually used to treat both disorders, including motivating the patient, enlisting family support, and providing nutrition counseling and psychotherapy. Behavior modification therapy may be used as well.

No drugs are approved specifically for bulimia nervosa or anorexia nervosa, but several, including some antidepressants, are being investigated for this use.

Hospitalization may be required for patients who have life-threatening complications or extreme psychological problems. If the patient's life is not in danger, treatment for either disorder is usually on an outpatient basis. Treatment may take a year or more. However, in their book, *New Hope for Binge Eaters*, Harrison Pope, Jr., M.D., and James Hudson, M.D., reported that more than 80 percent of their patients with bulimia responded to antidepressant drug therapy within three to four weeks. For anorectics, however, they write that the benefits of antidepressants "must be regarded as tentative" and that precautions should be taken to determine whether the patient's undernourished body can handle the drugs.

Psychotherapy may be in many forms. In individual sessions, the patient explores attitudes about weight, food, and body image. Then, as she becomes aware of her problems in relating to others and dealing with stress, her attention is centered on feelings she may have about self-esteem, guilt, anxiety, depression, or helplessness. Constructive, non-judgmental feedback is given to encourage growth and independence. In behavior modification therapy, the focus is on eliminating self-defeating behaviors. Patients may improve their stress management by learning skills in relaxation and assertiveness. Family therapy is designed to improve overall family functioning. Group psychotherapy may help reduce a sense of isolation and secrecy and is especially effective for bulimics.

The National Association of Anorexia Nervosa and Associated Disorders (ANAD), a support group, says it's important for the patient to have confidence in the type of therapy used as well as rapport with the therapist. If some improvement isn't apparent after a reasonable time, says ANAD, the patient (or patient advocate, such as a parent) shouldn't hesitate to discuss this with the therapist and, if need be, change therapists. Local places to ask for help in finding a therapist are: the psychiatry department of a nearby medical school; local hospitals; family physician; priest, rabbi or minister; county or state mental health or health and social services departments; and private welfare agencies.

Self-help, or support, groups are an adjunct to primary treatment. Through sharing of experiences, members give mutual emotional support, exchange information, and diminish feelings of isolation. Services may include: information on symptoms and treatment, lists of therapists, newsletters, book reviews, and bibliographies.

Tips for Parents

Whether their child is 10 or 20, parents of a patient with bulimia or anorexia may find it difficult to deal with such a constant, long-term problem. From the American Anorexia/Bulimia Association, Inc., here are some tips that may help:

- Do not urge your child to eat, or watch her eat, or discuss food intake or weight with her. Your involvement with her eating is her tool for manipulating parents.

- Do not allow yourself to feel guilty. Once you have checked out her physical condition with a physician and made it possible for her to begin counseling, getting well is her responsibility.

- Do not neglect your spouse or other children. Focusing on the sick child can perpetuate her illness and destroy the family.

- Do not be afraid to have the child separated from you, either at school or in separate housing, if it becomes obvious that her continued presence is undermining the emotional health of the family. Don't allow her to intimidate the family with threats of suicide. (But don't ignore the threats, either.)

- Do not put the child down by comparing her to her more "successful" siblings or friends. Do not ask questions such as "How are you feeling?" or "How is your social life?"

- Love your child as you should love yourself.

- Trust your child to find her own values, ideals and standards, rather than insisting on yours.

- Do everything to encourage her initiative, independence and autonomy.

- Be aware of the long-term nature of the illness. Families must face months and sometimes years of treatment and anxiety.

Requests for information from the following nonprofit associations should be accompanied by a stamped, self-addressed. business-size envelope.

American Anorexia/Bulimia Association, Inc.
418 E. 76th St.
New York NY 10021
(212) 734-1114

Anorexia Nervosa and Related Eating Disorders, Inc.
P.O. Box 5102
Eugene, OR 97405
(503) 344-1144

National Anorexic Aid Society
1925 E. Dublin-Granville Road
Columbus, OH 43229
(614) 436-1112

National Association of Anorexia Nervosa and Associated Disorders
(ANAD)
P.O. Box 7
Highland Park, IL 60035
(1-708) 831-3438

Bulimia, Anorexia Self-Help
6125 Clayton Ave., Suite 215
St. Louis, MO 63139
1-800-227-4785

—by Dixie Farley

Section 20.3

On the Teen Scene—Eating Disorders Require Medical Attention

FDA Consumer, March 1992.

For reasons that are unclear, some people—mainly young women—develop potentially life-threatening eating disorders called bulimia nervosa and anorexia nervosa. People with bulimia, known as bulimics, indulge in bingeing (episodes of eating large amounts of food) and purging (getting rid of the food by vomiting or using laxatives). People with anorexia whom doctors sometimes call anorectics, severely limit their food intake. About half of them also have bulimia symptoms.

The National Center for Health Statistics (NCHS) estimates that 10,000 bulimia cases and 11,000 anorexia cases were diagnosed in 1989, the latest year for which statistics are available. Studies indicate that by their first year of college, 4.5 to 18 percent of women and 0.4 percent of men have a history of bulimia and that as many as 1 in 100 females between the ages of 12 and 18 have anorexia.

Males account for only 5 to 10 percent of bulimia and anorexia cases. While people of all races develop the disorders, the vast majority of those diagnosed are white.

Most people find it difficult to stop their bulimic or anorectic behavior without professional help. If untreated, the disorders may become chronic and lead to severe health problems, even death. NCHS reports 67 deaths from anorexia in 1988, the latest year for which it has figures, but does not have similar information on bulimia.

As to the causes of bulimia and anorexia, there are many theories. One is that some young women feel abnormally pressured to be as thin as the "ideal" portrayed by magazines, movies and television. Another is that defects in key chemical messengers in the brain may contribute to the disorders' development or persistence.

The Bulimia Secret

Once people begin bingeing and purging, usually in conjunction with a diet, the cycle easily gets out of control. While cases tend to develop during the teens or early 20s, many bulimics successfully hide their symptoms, thereby delaying help until they reach their 30s or 40s. Several years ago, actress Jane Fonda revealed she had been a secret bulimic from age 12 until her recovery at 35. She told of bingeing and purging up to 20 times a day.

Many people with bulimia maintain a nearly normal weight. Though they appear healthy and successful—"perfectionists" at whatever they do—in reality, they have low self-esteem and are often depressed. They may exhibit other compulsive behaviors. For example, one physician reports that a third of his bulimia patients regularly engage in shoplifting and that a quarter of the patients have suffered from alcohol abuse or addiction at some point in their lives.

While normal food intake for a teenager is 2,000 to 3,000 calories in a day, bulimic binges average about 3,400 calories in 1 1/4 hours, according to one study. Some bulimics consume up to 20,000 calories in binges lasting as long as eight hours. Some spend $50 or more a day on food and may resort to stealing food or money to support their obsession.

To lose the weight gained during a binge, bulimics begin purging by vomiting (by self-induced gagging or with an emetic, a substance that causes vomiting) or by using laxatives (50 to 100 tablets at a time), diuretics (drugs that increase urination), or enemas. Between binges, they may fast or exercise excessively.

Extreme purging rapidly upsets the body's balance of sodium, potassium, and other chemicals. This can cause fatigue, seizures, irregular heartbeat, and thinner bones. Repeated vomiting can damage the stomach and esophagus (the tube that carries food to the stomach), make the gums recede, and erode tooth enamel. (Some patients need all their teeth pulled prematurely). Other effects include various skin rashes, broken blood vessels in the face, and irregular menstrual cycles.

Complexities of Anorexia

While anorexia most commonly begins in the teens, it can start at any age and has been reported from age 5 to 60. Incidence among 8- to 11-year-olds is said to be increasing.

Anorexia may be a single, limited episode with large weight loss within a few months followed by recovery. Or it may develop gradually and persist for years. The illness may go back and forth between getting better and getting worse. Or it may steadily get more severe.

Anorectics may exercise excessively. Their pre-occupation with food usually prompts habits such as moving food about on the plate and cutting it into tiny pieces to prolong eating, and not eating with the family.

Obsessed with weight loss and fear of becoming fat, anorectics see normal folds of flesh as "fat" that must be eliminated. When the normal fat padding is lost, sitting or lying down brings discomfort not rest, making sleep difficult. As the disorder continues, victims may become isolated and withdraw from friends and family.

The body responds to starvation by slowing or stopping certain bodily processes. Blood pressure falls, breathing rate slows, menstruation ceases (or, in girls in their early teens, never begins), and activity of the thyroid gland (which regulates growth) diminishes. Skin becomes dry, and hair and nails become brittle. Light-headedness, cold intolerance, constipation, and joint swelling are other symptoms. Reduced fat causes the body temperature to fall. Soft hair called lanugo forms on the skin for warmth. Body chemicals may get so imbalanced that heart failure occurs.

Anorectics who additionally binge and purge impair their health even further. The late recording artist Karen Carpenter, an anorectic who used syrup of ipecac to induce vomiting, died after buildup of the drug irreversibly damaged her heart.

Getting Help

Early treatment is vital. As either disorder becomes more entrenched, its damage becomes less reversible.

Usually, the family is asked to help in the treatment, which may include psychotherapy, nutrition counseling, behavior modification, and self-help groups. Therapy often lasts a year or more—on an outpatient basis unless life-threatening physical symptoms or severe psychological problems require hospitalization. If there is deterioration or no response to therapy, the patient (or parent or other advocate) may want to talk to the health professional about the plan of treatment.

There are no drugs approved specifically for bulimia or anorexia, but several, including some antidepressants, are being investigated for this use.

If you think a friend or family member has bulimia or anorexia, point out in a caring, non-judgmental way the behavior you have observed and encourage the person to get medical help. If you think you have bulimia or anorexia, remember that you are not alone and that this is a health problem that requires professional help. As a first step, talk to your parents, family doctor, religious counselor, or school counselor or nurse.

—by Dixie Farley

Section 20.4

Binge Eating Disorder

NIH Publication No. 94-3589, November 1993.

Binge eating disorder ia a newly recognized condition that affects millions of Americans. People with binge eating disorder frequently eat large amounts of food while feeling a loss of control over their eating. This disorder is different from binge-purge syndrome (bulimia nervosa) because people with binge eating disorder usually do not purge afterward by vomiting or using laxatives.

How Does Someone Know If He or She Has Binge Eating Disorder?

Most of us overeat from time to time, and many people feel they frequently eat more than they should. Eating large amounts of food, however, does not mean that a person has binge eating disorder. Doctors are still debating the best ways to determine if someone has binge eating disorder. But most people with serious binge eating problems have:

1. Frequent episodes of eating what others would consider an abnormally large amount of food.

2. Frequent feelings of being unable to control what or how much is being eaten.

3. Several of these behaviors or feelings:
    - Eating much more rapidly than usual.
    - Eating until uncomfortably full.
    - Eating large amounts of food, even when not physically hungry.
    - Eating alone out of embarrassment at the quantity of food being eaten.
    - Feelings of disgust, depression, or guilt after overeating.

Episodes of binge eating also occur in the eating disorder bulimia nervosa. Persons with bulimia, however, regularly purge, fast, or engage in strenuous exercise after an episode of binge eating. *Purging* means vomiting or using diuretics (water pills) or laxatives in greater-than-recommended doses to avoid gaining weight. *Fasting* is not eating for at least 24 hours. *Strenuous exercise*, in this case, is termed as exercising for more than an hour solely to avoid gaining weight after binge eating. Purging, fasting, and strenuous exercise are dangerous ways to attempt weight control.

How Common Is Binge Eating Disorder, and Who Is at Risk?

Although it has only recently been recognized as a distinct condition, binge eating disorder is probably the most common eating disorder. Most people with binge eating disorder are obese (more than 20 percent above a healthy body weight), but normal weight people also can be affected. Binge eating disorder probably affects 2 percent of all adults, or about 1 million to 2 million Americans. Among mildly obese people in self-help or commercial weight loss programs, 10 to 15 percent have binge eating disorder. The disorder is even more common in those with severe obesity.

Binge eating disorder is slightly more common in women, with three women affected for every two men. The disorder affects blacks as often as whites; its frequency in other ethnic groups is not yet known. Obese people with binge eating disorder often became overweight at a younger age than those without the disorder. They also may have more frequent episodes of losing and regaining weight (yo-yo dieting).

What Causes Binge Eating Disorder?

The causes of binge eating disorder are still unknown. Up to half of all people with binge eating disorder have a history of depression. Whether depression is a cause or effect of binge eating disorder is unclear. It may be unrelated. Many people report that anger, sadness, boredom, anxiety or other negative emotions can trigger a binge episode. Impulsive behavior and certain other psychological problems may be more common in people with binge eating disorder.

Dieting's effect on binge eating disorder is also unclear. While findings vary, early research suggests that about half of all people with

433

binge eating disorder had binge episodes before they started to diet. Still, strict dieting may worsen binge eating in some people.

Researchers also are looking into how brain chemicals and metabolism (the way the body burns calories) affect binge eating disorder. These areas of research are still in the early stages.

What Are the Complications of Binge Eating Disorder?

The major complications of binge eating disorder, are the diseases that accompany obesity. These include diabetes, high blood pressure, high cholesterol levels, gallbladder disease, heart disease, and certain types of cancer.

People with binge eating disorder are extremely distressed by their binge eating. Most have tried to control it on their own but have not succeeded for very long. Some people miss work, school, or social activities to binge eat. Obese people with binge eating disorder often feel bad about themselves, are preoccupied with their appearance, and may avoid social gatherings. Most feel ashamed and try to hide their problem. Often they are so successful that close family members and friends don't know they binge eat.

Should People with Binge Eating Disorder Try to Diet?

People who are not overweight or only mildly obese should probably avoid dieting, since strict dieting may worsen binge eating. However, many people with binge eating disorder are severely obese and have medical problems related to their weight. For these people, losing weight and keeping it off are important treatment goals. Most people with binge eating disorder, whether or not they want to lose weight, may benefit from treatment that addresses their eating behavior.

What Treatment Is Available for People with Binge Eating Disorder?

Several studies have found that people with binge eating disorder may find it harder than other people to stay in weight loss treatment. Binge eaters also may be more likely to regain weight quickly. For these reasons, people with the disorder may require treatment that focuses on their binge eating before they try to lose weight. Even those who are not overweight are frequently distressed by their binge eating and may benefit from treatment.

Several methods are being used to treat binge eating disorder. **Cognitive-behavioral** therapy teaches patients techniques to monitor and change their eating habits as well as to change the way they respond to difficult situations. **Interpersonal psychotherapy** helps people examine their relationships with friends and family and to make changes in problem areas. **Treatment with medications** such as anti-depressants may be helpful for some individuals. **Self-help** groups also may be a source of support. Researchers are still trying to determine which method or combination of methods is the most effective in controlling binge eating disorder. The type of treatment that is best for an individual is a matter for discussion between the patient and his or her health care provider.

If you believe you have binge eating disorder, it's important you realize that you are not alone. Most people who have the disorder have tried unsuccessfully to control it on their own. You may want to seek professional treatment. [See Figure 20.1. Treatment Centers for Eating Disorders on the next page.]

Additional Reading

Marcus MD. *Binge Eating in Obesity*. In: Fairburn CG, Wilson GT (eds). Binge eating: nature, assessment, and treatment. New York: Guilford Press, 1993.

de Zwann MD, Mitchell JE. Binge Eating in the Obese. Annals of Medicine. Vol. 24:303-308, 1992.

Stunkard AJ. Eating Patterns and Obesity. Psychiatric Quarterly, 1958, Vol. 33:284-295. This classic paper provides one of the first descriptions of binge eating in obese individuals.

	Program Type						Treatment Used			Patients Treated					
	Inpatient	Day Hospital	Outpatient	Individual Therapy	Group Therapy	Family/Couple Therapy	Cognitive Behavior Therapy	Interpersonal Therapy	Drug Therapy	Males	Females	Children (under 12)	Adolescents (12-17)	Adults (18 and up)	Conducting Clinical Studies
Behavioral Medicine Stanford University School of Medicine Department of Psychiatry TD209 Stanford, CA 94305 Tel: 415-723-5868	●	●	●	●	●	●	●	●	●	●	●		●	●	●
Binge Eating Program Western Psychiatric Institute and Clinic 3811 O'Hara Street Pittsburgh, PA 15213 Tel: 412-624-2823			●	●			●	●			●			●	●
Eating Disorders Clinic New York State Psychiatric Institute Columbia Presbyterian Medical Center 722 W. 168th St., Unit #98 New York, NY 10032 Tel: 212-960-5739/5746			●	●			●		●	●	●			●	●
Eating Disorder Research Program University of Minnesota 2701 University Ave., S.E., Suite 102 Minneapolis, MN 55414 Tel: 612-627-4494				●		●	●			●	●			●	●
Nutrition Research Clinic Baylor College of Medicine 6535 Fannin St., MS F700 Houston, TX 77030 Tel: 713-798-5757			●	●	●		●	●	●	●	●			●	●
Rutgers Eating Disorders Clinic GSAPP, Rutgers University Box 819 Piscataway, NJ 08854 Tel: 908-932-2292			●	●	●		●			●	●		●	●	●
Women's Recovery Center 110 N. Essex Ave. Narberth, PA 19072 Tel: 215-664-5858		●	●	●	●	●	●	●	●[1]		●		●[2]	●	
Yale Center For Eating and Weight Disorders P.O. Box 11A, Yale Station New Haven, CT 06520 Tel: 203-432-4610			●	●	●	●	●	●	●	●	●			●	●

Footnotes:
1. Only through referrals to psychiatrists and physicians in their own practices
2. Adolescents age 16-17 only.

Figure 20.1. Treatment Centers for Eating Disorders

Chapter 21

Depression: What Every Woman Should Know

More Than the Blues

Life is full of emotional ups and downs and everyone experiences the "blues" from time to time. But when the "down" times are long lasting or interfere with an individual's ability to function at home and at work, that person may be suffering from a common, serious illness—depression.

Clinical depression affects mood, mind, body, and behavior. Research has shown that in the United States more than 17 million people—one in ten adults—experience depression each year, and nearly two thirds do not get the help they need. Treatment can alleviate the symptoms in over 80 percent of cases. Yet, because it often goes unrecognized, depression continues to cause unnecessary suffering.

Women are disproportionately affected by depression, experiencing it at roughly twice the rate of men. Research continues to explore how the illness affects women and to identify new areas that hold promise of deepening our understanding. At the same time, it is important to increase women's awareness of what is already known about depression, so that they seek early and appropriate treatment.

To grasp the specifics of depression in women, it is essential to have a broad understanding of the illness itself. To this end, this chapter presents an overview of depression as a pervasive and impairing illness that affects women and men in similar fashion. It then focuses

NIH publication No. 95-3871 (1995).

on special issues—biological, life cycle, and psychosocial—that are unique to women and may be associated with depression.

A Picture of Depression

Jane slowly walked into the house, as though her body ached in every muscle. Jeff had already tucked the kids in bed. When he asked why she was late, Jane told him she was trying to catch up at work. She was too tired to say more, and too scared to admit that she could hardly concentrate or remember what she was supposed to be doing. Jeff had cooked dinner—again—but Jane had no appetite. She felt guilty as she pushed away her plate, apologized, and went to bed.

Sitting in silence was familiar to Jeff. He was reluctant to speak because Jane often flew off the handle these days, so unlike the good humored woman she used to be. Jeff and her coworkers had noticed the change in Jane—the way she kept to herself, her forced smile, her pessimism and loss of interest in things. As she struggled through her days, neither Jane nor Jeff understood what was happening to her. She felt alone and empty, often plagued by negative thoughts and bad feelings about herself. One day she said she couldn't see the point in living anymore. That was when Jeff became alarmed and encouraged Jane to seek professional help. They found out that she had clinical depression.

What Is Depression?

Jane, our fictional patient, experienced many of the symptoms that characterize depressive illness. Her story depicts how depression alters not just mood but one's entire existence, and how it impacts not just the affected individual but family and coworkers. Most importantly, it illustrates the importance of awareness of the illness, so that early recognition and appropriate treatment can keep depressive symptoms and their impact to a minimum.

No two people become depressed in exactly the same way. Many have only some of the symptoms, varying in severity and duration. For some, symptoms occur in time-limited episodes; for others, symptoms can be present for long periods if no treatment is sought. The age at which depression first appears also varies. There is evidence that in individuals born after 1945, it occurs at a younger age than in previous generations. Common to all age groups, affecting rich and poor alike, depressive illness occurs most frequently in adults between the ages of 25 and 44.

The Symptoms of Depression and Mania

Depression

- Persistent sad, anxious, or "empty" mood
- Loss of interest or pleasure in activities, including sex
- Feelings of hopelessness, pessimism
- Feelings of guilt, worthlessness, helplessness
- Sleeping too much or too little, early-morning awakening
- Appetite and/or weight loss or overeating and weight gain
- Decreased energy, fatigue, feeling "slowed down"
- Thoughts of death or suicide, or suicide attempts
- Restlessness, irritability
- Difficulty concentrating, remembering, or making decisions
- Persistent physical symptoms that do not respond to treatment, such as headaches, digestive disorders, and chronic pain

Mania

- Abnormally elevated mood
- Irritability
- Severe insomnia
- Grandiose notions
- Increased talking
- Racing thoughts
- Increased activity, including sexual activity
- Markedly increased energy
- Poor judgement that leads to risk-taking behavior
- Inappropriate social behavior

A thorough diagnostic evaluation is needed if five or more of these symptoms persist for more than two weeks, or if they interfere with work or family life. An evaluation involves a complete physical checkup and information gathering on family health history.

Having some depressive symptoms does not mean a person is clinically depressed. For example, it is not unusual for those who have lost a loved one to feel sad, helpless, and disinterested in regular activities. Only when these symptoms persist for an unusually long time is there reason to suspect that grief has become depressive illness. Similarly, living with the stress of potential layoffs, heavy workloads, or financial or family problems may cause irritability and "the blues." Up to a point, such feelings are simply a part of human experience.

But when the symptoms increase in number, duration and intensity, so that an individual is unable to function as usual, a temporary mood has very likely become a clinical illness.

Types of Depressive Illness

Major Depression, Jane's illness, emerges in episodes. Some people have one episode in a lifetime; others have recurrent episodes. While initial symptoms may not always seem significant, eventually the individual will experience emotional pain and misery, and impairment in productivity at work and home and in relationships with family and friends.

Sometimes the episodes appear seasonally—typically with depression occurring in fall and winter and diminishing in the spring. Women seem to be especially prone to this kind of depression, known as Seasonal Affective Disorder (SAD).

Manic-Depressive Illness, also called bipolar disorder, involves cycles similar to major depression alternating with inappropriate "highs." Unlike other depressions, women and men are equally vulnerable. During manic episodes, people become overly active, euphoric, irritable, talkative and may spend money irresponsibly and get involved in sexual misadventures.

Dysthymia involves symptoms similar to those of major depression. They are milder but longer lasting, with a minimum duration of two years. People with dysthymia are frequently lacking in zest and enthusiasm for life, living joyless and fatigued existences that seem almost natural outgrowths of their personalities. If, in addition, they have a major depressive episode, as often happens, they are sometimes referred to as having "double depression."

Causes of Depression

Genetic Factors

There is a risk for developing depression when there is a family history of the illness, indicating that a biological vulnerability may be inherited. The risk is somewhat higher for those with bipolar disorder. However, not everybody with a family history develops the illness. In addition, major depression can occur in people who have had no family members with the illness. This suggests that additional factors, possibly biochemistry, environmental stressors, and other psychosocial factors, are involved in the onset of depression.

Biochemical Factors

Evidence indicates that brain biochemistry is a significant factor in depressive disorders. It is known, for example, that individuals with major depressive illness typically have too little or too much of certain brain chemicals, called neurotransmitters. Additionally, sleep patterns, which are biochemically influenced, are typically different in people with mood disorders. Depression can be induced or alleviated with certain medications, and some hormones have mood-altering properties. What is not yet known is whether the "biochemical disturbances" of depression are of genetic origin, or are secondary to stress, trauma, physical illness, or some other environmental condition.

Environmental and Other Stressors

Significant loss, a difficult relationship, financial problems, or a major change in life pattern have all been cited as contributors to depressive illness. Sometimes the onset of depression is associated with acute or chronic physical illness. In addition, some form of substance abuse disorder occurs in about one third of people with any type of depressive disorder.

Other Psychosocial Factors

Persons with certain characteristics—pessimistic thinking, low self-esteem, a sense of having little control over life events, and proneness to excessive worrying—are more likely to develop depression. These attributes may heighten the effect of stressful events or interfere with taking action to cope with them or with getting well. Upbringing or sex role expectations may contribute to the development of these traits. It appears that negative thinking patterns typically develop in childhood or adolescence.

The Many Dimensions of Depression in Women

Women at Risk

Many factors that appear to contribute to depression are common to both women and men, while the specific causes of depression in women remain unclear. However, varied factors unique to women's lives are suspected to contribute to depression—developmental, reproductive, hormonal, genetic, and other biological factors; abuse and oppression; interpersonal factors; and certain psychological and personality characteristics.

Regardless of contributing factors, depression is a highly treatable illness and the types of treatment discussed later in this chapter are effective for a majority of women.

Developmental Roles

The Issues of Adolescence. The higher incidence of depression in females begins in adolescence, when there are dramatic changes in roles and expectations along with other physical, intellectual and hormonal changes. The added stresses of adolescence include forming an identity, confronting sexuality, separating from parents, and making decisions for the first time. These significant issues are generally different for boys and girls. Studies show that female high school students have significantly higher rates of depression, anxiety disorders, eating disorders, and adjustment disorders than male students, who have higher rates of disruptive behavior disorders.

Adulthood: Relationships and Work Roles. Stress in general can contribute to depression in persons biologically vulnerable to the illness. Some have theorized that the higher incidence of depression in women is not due to greater vulnerability, but to the multidimensional stresses that many women face, such as major responsibilities at home and work, single parenthood, and caring for children and aging parents. How these factors uniquely affect women is not yet fully understood.

For both women and men, rates of major depression are highest among the separated and divorced, and lowest among the married, while remaining always higher for women than for men. The quality of a marriage, however, may contribute significantly to depression. Lack of an intimate, confiding relationship, as well as marital disputes, have been shown to be related to depression in women. In fact, rates of depression were shown to be highest among unhappily married women.

Reproductive Life Cycle

Significant events in women's reproductive life cycle include menstruation, pregnancy, the post-pregnancy period, and menopause.

These events bring fluctuations in mood that for some women include depression. Further, infertility and the decision not to have children can also bring about changes in mood. Researchers have confirmed that hormones have an effect on the brain chemistry that controls emotions and mood; a specific biological mechanism explaining hormonal involvement is not known, however.

Menstruation and Premenstrual Syndrome. Many women experience certain normal behavioral and physical changes associated with phases of their menstrual cycles. Some women, however, regularly experience a significant number of extreme changes, including depressed feelings, irritability, and other emotional and physical manifestations. Though not considered a disorder in the most recent diagnostic manual for psychiatry, these extreme changes are generally called premenstrual syndrome (PMS) or premenstrual dysphoric disorder (PMDD). The changes typically begin after ovulation and become gradually worse until menstruation starts. Scientists are exploring how the cyclical rise and fall of estrogen and other hormones may affect the brain chemistry that is associated with depressive illness.

Pregnancy. Pregnancy (if it is desired) seldom contributes to depression, and having an abortion does not appear to lead to a higher incidence of depression. Women with infertility problems may be subject to extreme anxiety or sadness, though it is unclear if this contributes to a higher rate of depressive illness.

Postpartum Depression. Following childbirth, women may experience sadness that ranges from transient "blues" to an episode of major depression to severe, incapacitating, psychotic depression. Studies suggest that women who experience depressive illness after childbirth very often have had prior depressive episodes, though they may not have been diagnosed and treated. For most women, postpartum depressions are transient with no adverse consequences.

Maternal Depression. Because women typically carry the primary responsibility for child care, the impact of their depressive illness on their parenting ability is of particular concern. Evidence suggests that maternal depression may have a negative effect on a child's behavior, and psychological and social development. These findings give additional emphasis to the importance of women recognizing the need for and seeking treatment for depression.

Menopause. A definitive study has shown that, in general, menopause is not associated with an increased risk of depression. In fact, while once considered a unique disorder, research has shown that depressive illness at menopause is no different than at other ages. The women more vulnerable to change-of-life depression are those with a history of past depressive episodes.

Specific Cultural Considerations

As in depression in general, the prevalence rate of depression in African American and Hispanic women remains about twice that of men. There is some indication, however, that major depression and dysthymia may be diagnosed less frequently in African American and slightly more frequently in Hispanic than in Caucasian women. Prevalence information for other racial and ethnic groups is not definitive.

Possible differences in symptom presentation may effect the way depression is recognized and diagnosed among minorities. For example, African Americans are more likely to report somatic symptoms, such as appetite change. In addition, people from various cultural backgrounds may view depressive symptoms in different ways. Such factors should be considered when working with women from special populations.

Personality and Psychology

As mentioned earlier, persons with certain characteristics appear to be more likely to develop or have difficulty overcoming depression. Some experts have suggested that the traditional upbringing of girls might foster these traits and that may be a factor in the higher rate of depression.

Others have suggested that women are not more vulnerable to depression than men, but simply express or label their symptoms differently. Women may be more likely to admit feelings of depression, brood about their feelings, or seek professional assistance. Men, on the other hand, may be socially conditioned to deny such feelings or to bury them in alcohol, as reflected in the higher rates of alcoholism in men. There is currently insufficient scientific data to verify this theory.

Victimization

It is known that far more women than men are sexually abused as children. Studies show that women molested as children are more likely to have clinical depression at some time in their lives than those with no such history. In addition, there appears to be a higher incidence of depression among women who were raped as adults. Women who experience other, commonly occurring forms of abuse, such as physical abuse and sexual harassment on the job, also may experience higher rates of depression. It has been suggested that abuse may lead to depression by fostering low self-esteem, a sense of helplessness, self-blame, and social isolation. Research is needed to understand the connection between victimization and depression.

Poverty

Low economic status brings with it many stresses, including isolation, uncertainty, frequent negative events, and poor access to helpful resources. It is known that depressive feelings and demoralization are common among the poor, the deprived, and those lacking social supports, and yet it is not clear whether depressive illnesses are more prevalent among victims of such environmental stressors. In fact, one very large study has shown that these illnesses tend to equally effect the poor and the rich.

Depression in Later Adulthood

Close examination of the facts casts doubt on "the empty nest syndrome" as an explanation for depression in older women. The lack of increased rates of depression among women at this stage of life suggests that most women do not get depressed when children leave home.

As with younger age groups, more elderly women than men suffer from depressive illness. Similarly, for all age groups, being unmarried (which includes widowhood) is also a risk factor for depression. Despite this, depression should not be dismissed as a normal consequence of the physical, social and economic problems of later life. In fact, studies show that the rate of clinical depression in older people is lower than that of the general population, and that most older people feel satisfied with their lives.

About 800,000 persons are widowed each year, most of them are older, female, and experience varying degrees of depressive symptomatology. Most do not need formal treatment, but many who are moderately or severely sad appear to benefit from self-help groups or various psychosocial treatments. Remarkably, a third of widows/widowers meet criteria for major depressive episode in the first month after the death of a spouse, but only half of these remain clinically depressed one year later. These depressions respond to standard anti-depressant medications, although the optimal timing of the intervention is a matter of clinical judgement.

Depression Is a Treatable Illness

Even severe depression can be highly responsive to treatment. Indeed, believing one's condition is "incurable" is often part of the hopelessness that accompanies serious depression. Such patients should be provided with the information about the effectiveness of treatments for depression. As with many illnesses, the earlier treatment begins, the more effective it is and the greater the likelihood of preventing serious recurrences. Of course, treatment will not eliminate life's inevitable stresses and ups and downs; but it can greatly enhance the ability to manage such challenges and lead to greater enjoyment of life.

As a first step, a thorough physical examination may be recommended to rule out any physical illnesses that may cause depressive symptoms.

Types of Treatment for Depression

The most commonly used treatments for depression are antidepressant medication, psychotherapy, or a combination of the two. Which of these is the right treatment for an individual case depends on the nature and severity of the depression and, to some extent, on individual preference. In mild or moderate depression, one or both of these treatments may be useful, while in severe or incapacitating depression, medication is generally recommended as a first step in treatment. In combined treatment, medication can relieve physical symptoms quickly, while psychotherapy allows the opportunity to learn more effective ways of handling problems.

Medications

The medications used to treat depression include tricyclic antidepressants, monoamine oxidase inhibitors (MAOIs), serotonin re-uptake inhibitors (SRIs), and bupropion. Each acts on different chemical pathways of the brain related to moods. Anti-depressant medications are not habit-forming. To be effective, medications must be taken for at least 4-6 months (in a first episode), carefully following the doctor's instructions. Medications must be monitored to ensure the most effective dosage and to minimize side effects.

The prescribing doctor will provide information about possible side-effects and dietary restrictions. In addition, other medications being used should be reviewed because some can interact negatively with anti-depressant medication. There may be restrictions during pregnancy.

Psychotherapy

In mild to moderate cases, psychotherapy is also a treatment option. Some short-term (10-20 week) therapies have been very effective in several types of depression. "Talking" therapies help patients gain insight and resolve problems through verbal give-and-take with the therapist. "Behavioral" therapies help patients learn new behaviors that lead to more satisfaction in life and "unlearn" counterproductive behaviors.

Research has shown that two short-term psychotherapies, Interpersonal and Cognitive/Behavioral, are helpful for some forms of depression. Interpersonal therapy works to change interpersonal relationships that cause or exacerbate depression. Cognitive/Behavioral therapy helps change negative styles of thinking and behaving that may contribute to the depression.

Other Treatments

Despite the unfavorable publicity electroconvulsive therapy (ECT) has received, research has shown that there are circumstances in which its use is medically justified and can even save lives. This is particularly true for those at high risk for suicide or with psychotic agitation, severe weight loss or physical debilitation due to other physical illness. ECT may also be recommended for persons who cannot take or do not respond to medication.

People who experience Seasonal Affective Disorder (SAD) can also be helped by a new form of therapy using lights, called phototherapy.

Treating Recurrent Depression

Even when treatment is successful, depression may recur. Studies indicate that certain treatment strategies are very useful in this instance. Continuation of anti-depressant medication at the same dosage that successfully treated the acute episode can often prevent recurrence. Monthly interpersonal psychotherapy can lengthen the time between episodes in patients not taking medication.

The Path to Healing

Reaping the benefits of treatment begins by recognizing the signs of depression. The list of symptoms earlier in this chapter can be used for this purpose.

The next step is to be evaluated by a qualified professional. Depression can be diagnosed and treated by psychiatrists, psychologists, clinical social workers, and other mental health professionals, as well as by primary care physicians.

Treatment is a partnership between the patient and the health care provider. An informed consumer knows her treatment options and discusses concerns with her provider as they arise.

If you don't feel some improvement after several weeks of treatment, or if symptoms worsen, discuss this with your treatment provider. Trying another treatment approach, or getting a second opinion from another health or mental health professional, may be in order.

Helping Resources

General

- Physicians
- Mental health specialists
- Health maintenance organizations
- Community mental health centers
- Hospital departments of psychiatry or outpatient psychiatric clinics
- University or medical school-affiliated programs
- State hospital outpatient clinics
- Family service/social agencies
- Private clinics and facilities
- Employee assistance programs
- Clergy

Professional Organizations

- American Psychiatric Association
- American Psychological Association
- National Association for Social Workers
- American Nurses Association
- American Mental Health Counselors Association
- American Orthopsychiatric Association

Advocacy Groups

- National Mental Health Association
- National Alliance for the Mentally Ill
- National Foundation for Depressive Illness
- National Depressive and Manic Depressive Association

Helping Yourself

Depressive illnesses make you feel exhausted, worthless, helpless and hopeless. Such feelings make some people want to give up. It is important to realize that these negative views are part of the depression and will fade as treatment begins to take effect.

Along with professional treatment, there are other things you can do to help yourself get better. Some people find participating in support groups very helpful. It may also help to spend some time with other people and to participate in activities that make you feel better, such as mild exercise. Just don't overdo it or expect too much from yourself right away. Feeling better takes time. Your treating professional can also suggest other self-help strategies.

Helping the Depressed Person

The most important thing anyone can do for the depressed person is to help him or her get appropriate diagnosis and treatment. This may involve encouraging the person to seek professional help or to stay in treatment once it is instituted.

The second most important thing is to offer emotional support. This involves understanding, patience, affection, and encouragement. Engage the depressed person in conversation or activities and be gently insistent if you meet with resistance. Remind that person that with time and help, he or she will feel better.

Remember...

Here, again, are the steps to healing:

- Check your symptoms against the list.
- Talk to a health or mental health professional.
- Consider yourself a partner in treatment and be an informed consumer.
- If you do not start to feel better after several weeks of treatment, discuss this with your provider. Different or additional treatment may be recommended.
- If you experience a recurrence, remember what you know about coping with depression, and don't shy away from seeking help again.

For Further Information on Depression

National Institute of Mental Health
5600 Fishers Lane
Room 10-85
Rockville, MD 20857
(301)443-4140

References

Blehar, M.D. and Lozovsky, D.B. Guest Eds. (1993). Special edition: toward a new psychobiology of depression in women. *Journal of Affective Disorders,* 29:75-211.

Frank, E., Karp, J.F., and Rush, A.J. (1993). Efficacy of treatments for major depression. *Psychopharmacology Bulletin,* 29:457-475.

Lewinsohn, P.M., Hyman, H.,Roberts, R.E., Seeley, J.R., and Andrews, J.A. (1993). Adolescent psychopathology: Prevalence and incidence of depression and other DSM-III-R disorders in high school students. *Journal of Abnormal Psychology,* 102:133-144.

NIH Consensus Development Panel on Depression in Late Life (1992). Diagnosis and treatment of depression in late life. *JAMA,* 268:1018-1024.

Regier, D.A., Narrow, W.E., Rae, D.S. Manderscheid, R.W., Locke, B.Z., and Goodwin, F.K. (1993). The de facto U.S. mental and addictive disorders service system: Epidemiological Catchment Area prospective 1-year prevalence rates of disorders and services. *Archives of General Psychiatry,* 50:85-94.

Rosenthal, N.E. (1993). Diagnosis and treatment of Seasonal Affective Disorder. *JAMA,* 270:2717-2720.

Weissman. M. Epidemiology of depression: frequency, risk groups and risk factors. *Perspectives on Depressive Disorders,* U.S. Department of Health and Human Services, National Institute of Mental Health, 1-21.

Chapter 22

Plain Talk about Handling Stress

You *need* stress in your life! Does that surprise you? Perhaps so, but it is quite true. Without stress, life would be dull and unexciting. Stress adds flavor, challenge, and opportunity to life. Too much stress, however, can seriously affect your physical and mental well-being. A major challenge in this stress-filled world of today is to make the stress in your life work *for* you instead of against you.

Stress is with us all the time. It comes from mental or emotional activity and physical activity. It is unique and personal to each of us. So personal, in fact, that what may be relaxing to one person may be stressful to another. For example, if you are an executive who likes to keep busy all the time, "taking it easy" at the beach on a beautiful day may feel extremely frustrating, nonproductive, and upsetting. You may be emotionally distressed from "doing nothing." Too much emotional stress can cause physical illness such as high blood pressure, ulcers, or even heart disease; physical stress from work or exercise is not likely to cause such ailments. The truth is that physical exercise can help you to relax and to handle your mental or emotional stress.

Hans Selye, M.D., a recognized expert in the field, has defined stress as a "non-specific response of the body to a demand." The important issue is learning how our bodies respond to these demands. When stress becomes prolonged or particularly frustrating, it can become harmful—causing *distress* or "bad stress." Recognizing the early signs of distress and then doing something about them can make

DHHS Pub. No. (ADM) 91-502

453

an important difference in the quality of your life, and may actually influence your survival.

Reacting to Stress

To use stress in a positive way and prevent it from becoming distress, you should become aware of your own reactions to stressful events. The body responds to stress by going through three stages: (1) alarm, (2) resistance, and (3) exhaustion.

Let's take the example of a typical commuter in rush-hour traffic. If a car suddenly pulls out in front of him, his initial alarm reaction may include fear of an accident, anger at the driver who committed the action, and general frustration. His body may respond in the alarm stage by releasing hormones into the bloodstream which cause his face to flush, perspiration to form, his stomach to have a sinking feeling, and his arms and legs to tighten. The next stage is resistance, in which the body repairs damage caused by the stress. If the stress of driving continues with repeated close calls or traffic jams, however, his body will not have time to make repairs. He may become so conditioned to expect potential problems when he drives that he tightens up at the beginning of each commuting day. Eventually, he may even develop a physical problem that is related to stress, such as migraine headaches, high blood pressure, backaches, or insomnia. While it is impossible to live completely free of stress and distress, it is possible to prevent some distress as well as to minimize its impact when it can't be avoided.

Helping Yourself

When stress does occur, it is important to recognize and deal with it. Here are some suggestions for ways to handle stress. As you begin to understand more about how stress affects you as an individual, you will come up with your own ideas of helping to ease the tensions.

Try physical activity. When you are nervous, angry, or upset, release the pressure through exercise or physical activity. Running, walking, playing tennis, or working in your garden are just some of the activities you might try. Physical exercise will relieve that "up tight" feeling, relax you, and turn the frowns into smiles. Remember, your body and your mind work together.

Share your stress. It helps to talk to someone about your concerns and worries. Perhaps a friend, family member, teacher, or counselor can help you see your problem in a different light. If you feel your problem is serious, you might seek professional help from a psychologist, psychiatrist, social worker, or mental health counselor. Knowing when to ask for help may avoid more serious problems later.

Know your limits. If a problem is beyond your control and cannot be changed at the moment, don't fight the situation. Learn to accept what is—for now—until such time when you can change it.

Take care of yourself. You are special. Get enough rest and eat well. If you are irritable and tense from lack of sleep or if you are not eating correctly, you will have less ability to deal with stressful situations. If stress repeatedly keeps you from sleeping, you should ask your doctor for help.

Make time for fun. Schedule time for both work and recreation. Play can be just as important to your well-being as work; you need a break from your daily routine to just relax and have fun.

Be a participant. One way to keep from getting bored, sad, and lonely is to go where it's all happening. Sitting alone can make you feel frustrated. Instead of feeling sorry for yourself, get involved and become a participant. Offer your services in neighborhood or volunteer organizations. Help yourself by helping other people. Get involved in the world and the people around you, and you'll find they will be attracted to you. You will be on your way to making new friends and enjoying new activities.

Check off your tasks. Trying to take care of everything at once can seem overwhelming, and, as a result, you may not accomplish anything. Instead, make a list of what tasks you have to do, then do one at a time, checking them off as they're completed. Give priority to the most important ones and do those first.

Must you always be right? Do other people upset you—particularly when they don't do things your way? Try cooperation instead of confrontation; it's better than fighting and always being "right." A little give and take on both sides will reduce the strain and make you both feel more comfortable.

It's OK to cry. A good cry can be a healthy way to bring relief to your anxiety, and it might even prevent a headache or other physical consequence. Take some deep breaths; they also release tension.

Create a quiet scene. You can't always run away, but you can "dream the impossible dream." A quiet country scene painted mentally, or on canvas, can take you out of the turmoil of a stressful situation. Change the scene by reading a good book or playing beautiful music to create a sense of peace and tranquility.

Avoid self-medication. Although you can use prescription or over-the-counter medications to relieve stress temporarily, they do not remove the conditions that caused the stress in the first place. Medications, in fact, may be habit-forming and also may reduce your efficiency, thus creating more stress than they take away. They should be taken only on the advice of your doctor.

The Art of Relaxation

The best strategy for avoiding stress is to learn how to relax. Unfortunately, many people try to relax at the same pace that they lead the rest of their lives. For a while, tune out your worries about time, productivity, and "doing right." You will find satisfaction in just *being*, without striving. Find activities that give you pleasure and that are good for your mental and physical well-being. Forget about always winning. Focus on relaxation, enjoyment, and health. If the stress in your life seems insurmountable, you may find it beneficial to see a mental health counselor. *Be good to yourself.*

—by Louis E. Kopolow, M.D.

Part Six

Tips for Maintaining a Healthy Lifestyle

Chapter 23

The Healthy Heart Handbook for Women

The Healthy Heart

You owe it to yourself to take this handbook to heart. For coronary heart disease is a woman's concern. Every woman's concern. It is not something that only affects your husband, your father, your brother, your son. This handbook tells you why you should be concerned about your own heart health, and what you can do to prevent coronary disease. A little prevention can have a big payoff—a longer, healthier, more active life.

Each year, 245,000 women die of coronary heart disease, making it the number one killer of American women. Another 90,000 women die each year of stroke. Although death rates from coronary heart disease and stroke have declined in recent years, these conditions still rank first and third, respectively, as causes of death for women.

Overall, about 10 million American women of all ages suffer from heart disease. One in ten women 45 to 64 years of age has some form of heart disease, and this increases to one in four women over 65. Each year, one-half million women suffer heart attacks. Cardiovascular diseases and their prevention, therefore, are pressing personal concerns for every woman.

What Are Cardiovascular Diseases?

Cardiovascular diseases are diseases of the heart and blood vessel system, such as coronary heart disease, heart attack, high blood

Taken from NIH Pub. No. 92-2720.

pressure, stroke, angina (chest pain), and rheumatic heart disease. Coronary heart disease—the primary subject of this handbook—is a disease of the blood vessels of the heart that causes heart attacks. A heart attack happens when an artery becomes blocked, preventing oxygen and nutrients from getting to the heart. A stroke results from a lack of blood to the brain, or in some cases, bleeding in the brain.

Who Gets Cardiovascular Diseases?

Some women have more "risk factors" for cardiovascular diseases than others. Risk factors are traits or habits that make a person more likely to develop a disease. Some risk factors for heart-related problems cannot be changed, but others can be. The three major risk factors for cardiovascular disease that you can do something about are cigarette smoking, high blood pressure, and high blood cholesterol. Other risk factors, such as overweight, diabetes, and physical inactivity, also are conditions you have some control over. Although growing older is a risk factor that cannot be changed, it is important to realize that other risks can be reduced at any age. This handbook identifies some key risk factors that you can control, and suggests changes in living habits to lessen your chances of developing cardiovascular diseases.

Some groups of women are more likely to develop cardiovascular diseases than other groups. Black women are 24 percent more likely to die of coronary heart disease than white women, and their death rate for stroke is 83 percent higher. Older women have a greater chance of developing cardiovascular diseases than younger women, partly because the tendency to have heart-related problems increases with age. Older women, for example, are more likely to develop high blood pressure and high blood cholesterol levels, to be diabetic, to be overweight, and to exercise less than younger women. Also, after menopause, women are more apt to get cardiovascular diseases, in part because their bodies produce less estrogen. Women who have had early menopause, either naturally or by means of a hysterectomy, are twice as likely to develop coronary heart disease as women of the same age who have not begun menopause.

While any one risk factor will raise your chances of developing heart-related problems, the more risk factors you have, the more concerned you should be about prevention. If you smoke cigarettes and have high blood pressure, for example, your chance of developing coronary heart disease goes up dramatically. Having all three major changeable risk factors—smoking, high blood pressure, and high blood cholesterol—can boost your risk to eight times that of women who have no risk factors.

We're Making Progress

Changing habits isn't easy—but experience shows that it works. As Americans have learned to control blood pressure and make healthful changes in their eating, smoking, and exercise habits, death rates for heart attack and stroke have dropped dramatically. Between 1970 and 1988 the death rate for women from coronary heart disease was cut in half. During the same period, the death rate for stroke went down 55 percent.

Cardiovascular diseases remain the leading cause of death for American women. But the message is clear: by taking an active role in your own heart health, you can make a difference. Beginning with the section titled "Self-Help Strategies for a Healthy Heart," this handbook supplies a number of practical tips to help you get started. Also, for information about other organizations and materials available to help you, see the section titled "Resources for a Healthy Heart."

Major Risk Factors

Smoking

Cigarette smoking has been described as "the most important individual health risk in this country." Approximately 26 million American women smoke. Although the smoking rate for women dropped 8 percent between 1965 and 1988, women who smoke today are apt to smoke more heavily than they did in the past.

Surprising as it may seem, smoking by women in the United States causes almost as many deaths from heart disease as from lung cancer. Women who smoke are two to six times as likely to suffer a heart attack as nonsmoking women, and the risk increases with the number of cigarettes smoked per day. Smoking also boosts the risk of stroke.

Cardiovascular diseases are not the only health risks for women who smoke. Cigarette smoking greatly increases the chances that a woman will develop lung cancer. In fact, the lung cancer death rate for women is now higher than the death rate for breast cancer, the chief cause of cancer deaths in women for many years. Cigarette smoking is also linked with cancers of the mouth, larynx, esophagus, urinary tract, kidney, pancreas, and cervix. Smoking also causes 80 percent of cases of chronic obstructive lung disease, which includes bronchitis and emphysema.

Smoking is also linked to a number of reproductive problems. Women who smoke are more apt to have problems getting pregnant and to begin menopause at a slightly younger age. Further, cigarette use during pregnancy poses serious risks for the unborn. Babies of women who smoked during pregnancy tend to weigh less at birth than babies of nonsmokers. Smoking while pregnant also increases risks of bleeding, miscarriage, premature delivery, stillbirth, and sudden infant death syndrome, or "crib death." Moreover, young children who are exposed to a parent's cigarette smoke have more lung and ear infections.

There is simply no "safe way" to smoke. Although low-tar and low-nicotine cigarettes may reduce the lung cancer risk to some extent, they do not lessen the risks of heart diseases or other smoking-related diseases. The only safe and healthful course is not to smoke at all.

High Blood Pressure

High blood pressure, also known as hypertension, is another major risk factor for coronary heart diseases and the most important risk factor for stroke. Even slightly high levels double the risk. High blood pressure also boosts the chances of developing kidney disease.

Nearly 58 million Americans have high blood pressure, and about half of them are women. Older women have a higher risk, with more than half of all women over the age of 55 suffering from this condition. High blood pressure is more common and more severe in black women than it is in white women. Use of birth control pills can contribute to high blood pressure in some women.

Blood pressure is the amount of force exerted by the blood against the walls of the arteries. Everyone has to have some blood pressure, so that blood can get to the body's organs and muscles. Usually, blood pressure is expressed as two numbers, such as 120/80, and is measured in millimeters of mercury (mmHg). The first number is the systolic blood pressure, the force used when the heart beats. The second number, or diastolic blood pressure, is the pressure that exists in the arteries between heartbeats. Depending on your activities, blood pressure may move up or down in the course of a day. Blood pressure is considered high when it stays above normal levels over a period of time.

High blood pressure is sometimes called the "silent killer" because most people have it without feeling sick. Therefore, it is important to have it checked each time you see your doctor or other health professional. Blood pressure can be easily measured by means of the familiar stethoscope and inflatable cuff placed around one arm. However, since blood pressure changes so often and is affected by many factors, your health professional should check it on several different days before deciding if your blood pressure is too high. If your blood pressure stays at 140/90 mmHg or above, you have high blood pressure.

Although high blood pressure can rarely be cured, it can be controlled with proper treatment. If your blood pressure is not too high, you may be able to control it entirely through weight loss if you are overweight, regular exercise, and cutting down on alcohol, table salt, and sodium. (Sodium is an ingredient in salt that is found in many packaged foods, baking soda, and some antacids.)

However, if your blood pressure remains high, your doctor will probably prescribe medicine in addition to the above changes. The amount you take may be gradually reduced, especially if you are successful with the changes you make in your lifestyle. While few people like the idea of taking any medicine for a long time, the treatment benefits are real and will reduce the risk of stroke, heart attack, and kidney disease. If you are prescribed a drug to control high blood pressure and find you have any uncomfortable side effects, ask your doctor about changing the dosage or possibly switching to another type of medicine.

During pregnancy, some women develop high blood pressure for the first time. Between 10 and 20 percent of first-time mothers develop a high blood pressure problem during pregnancy called preeclampsia. Other women who already have high blood pressure may find that it worsens during pregnancy. If untreated, these conditions can be life-threatening to both mother and baby. Since a woman can feel perfectly normal and still have one of these conditions, it is important to get regular prenatal checkups so that your doctor can discover and treat a possible high blood pressure problem.

Small Dose, Big Benefit

If you are one of the 3 million older Americans with a tyr~
blood pressure called isolated systolic hypertensior ~
good news. A recent study shows that treatin~ ~
a common blood pressure-lowering ~
thalidone, cut the risk of strok~ ~

the risk of coronary heart disease by 27 percent. The dose of the diuretic used in the study was only half of the smallest dose usually given to patients. One in five patients also took a low dose of a second drug, a beta-blocker, to help lower their blood pressure.

If you have ISH and are already doing well on another type of blood pressure-lowering drug, you should not necessarily switch medicines. But you may want to discuss with your doctor whether the treatment used successfully in this study might work for you.

High Blood Cholesterol

High blood cholesterol is a third important risk factor for coronary heart diseases that you can do something about. Although young women tend to have lower cholesterol levels than young men, between the ages of 45 and 55, women's cholesterol levels begin to rise higher than men's. After age 55, the gap between women and men becomes still wider. Today, about one-third of American women have blood cholesterol levels high enough to pose a serious risk for coronary heart diseases. The higher your blood cholesterol level, the higher your heart disease risk. For all adults, a desirable blood cholesterol level is less than 200 mg/dL. A level of 240 mg/dL or above is considered "high" blood cholesterol. But even levels in the "borderline-high" category (200-239 mg/dL) boost the risk of heart disease.

The body needs cholesterol to function normally. It is found in all foods that come from animals—that is all meats and dairy products. However, the body can make all of the cholesterol that it needs. Over a period of years, extra cholesterol and fat circulating in the blood settle on the inner walls of the arteries that supply blood to the heart. These deposits make the arteries narrower and narrower. As a result, less blood gets to the heart and the risk of coronary heart disease increases.

Ask your health professional to check your blood cholesterol level once every 5 years. This simple test involves taking a small blood sample and measuring the amount of cholesterol. The cholesterol level is expressed as, for example, "215 mg/dL" or 215 milligrams of cholesterol per deciliter of blood. Be sure to ask what your cholesterol number is and whether you should take steps to lower it. Before age 45, the total blood cholesterol level of women averages below 220 mg/dL. But between the ages of 45 and 55, women's average cholesterol levels soar to between 240 and 260 mg/dL. Women between 45 and 74 years of age who have a cholesterol level over 240 mg/dL are more than twice as likely to develop coronary heart disease as women with levels below 200 mg/dL.

Total blood cholesterol is the first measurement used to identify persons with high blood cholesterol. As you read above, a blood cholesterol level of 240 or more means you have "high" blood cholesterol. But even "borderline-high" levels (200-239) boost your risk of coronary heart disease. If your total blood cholesterol is in the high or borderline-high category and you have other risk factors for coronary heart disease, your doctor will want a more complete "cholesterol profile" before making a decision about treatment. Specifically, your doctor will measure your LDL and HDL levels after an overnight fast.

Cholesterol travels in the blood in packages called lipoproteins. Cholesterol packaged in low density lipoprotein (LDL) is often called "bad cholesterol" because LDL carries most of the cholesterol in the blood and if not removed, cholesterol and fat can build up in the arteries. Another type of cholesterol, which is packaged in high density lipoprotein (HDL), is known as "good cholesterol." That is because HDL helps remove cholesterol from the blood, preventing it from piling up in the arteries.

A "cholesterol profile" includes measurements of both HDL and LDL levels. An LDL level below 130 mg/dL is desirable. LDL levels of 130-159 mg/dL are "borderline-high." Levels of 160 mg/dL or above mean you have a high risk of developing coronary heart disease. As with total cholesterol, the higher the LDL number, the higher the risk. On the other hand, the lower your HDL number is, the greater your risk for coronary heart disease. Any HDL level below 35 mg/dL is considered too low. After studying your LDL- and HDL-cholesterol levels and other risk factors for coronary heart disease, your doctor may recommend a specific treatment program for you.

For many people, a change in eating habits is the only step needed to lower blood cholesterol levels. Cutting back on foods rich in fat, especially saturated fat, and in cholesterol, can lower both total and LDL-cholesterol. Weight loss for overweight persons also will lower blood cholesterol levels. Losing extra weight, as well as quitting smoking and becoming more active, also may help boost your HDL-cholesterol levels. Although we don't know for sure that raising HDL levels in this way will reduce the risk of coronary heart disease, these measures are likely to be good for your heart in any case.

While changing the way you eat is the first and most important action you can take to improve your blood cholesterol levels, your doctor may also suggest that you take cholesterol-lowering medications. This recommendation will depend on how much your new diet lowers your blood cholesterol and whether you have any other risk factors for coronary heart disease. If your doctor does prescribe medicines, you must also continue your cholesterol-lowering diet because the combination may allow you to take less medicine. Also, because diet is still the safest treatment, you should always try to lower your cholesterol levels with diet changes before adding medication.

Triglycerides are another type of fat found in the blood and in food. Triglycerides in food are made up of saturated, polyunsaturated, and monounsaturated fats. The liver also produces triglycerides. When alcohol is consumed or when excess calories are taken in, the liver produces more triglycerides. A number of studies have found that some people with coronary heart disease have high triglyceride levels. However, more research is needed to determine whether high triglycerides cause narrowing of the arteries or are just associated with other risk factors like low levels of HDL-cholesterol and being overweight.

Extremely high levels of triglycerides can cause a dangerous inflammation of the pancreas called pancreatitis.

To reduce blood triglyceride levels, doctors recommend a low-fat, low-calorie diet, weight control, increased exercise, and no alcohol. Occasionally drugs are needed.

Other Risk Factors

Overweight (obesity) is a proven risk factor for cardiovascular diseases. People who are obese—more than 30 percent overweight—are more likely to develop heart-related problems even if they have no other risk factors. According to an important study of cardiovascular diseases called the Framingham Heart Study, overweight in women is linked with coronary heart disease, stroke, congestive heart failure, and death from heart-related causes.

The Framingham Heart Study found that the more overweight a woman was, the higher her risk for heart disease. This was true for women of all ages, but especially for women under age 50. Among women younger than 50, the heaviest group was two and a half times more likely to develop coronary heart disease than the group with desirable weight. Overweight women under age 50 had more than four times the stroke rate of the group with desirable weight.

Overweight contributes not only to cardiovascular diseases, but to other risk factors as well. For example, overweight women under age 50 are three times as likely to develop high blood pressure as women of desirable weight. Overweight women also are more apt to have high blood cholesterol levels and diabetes. Fortunately, these conditions often can be controlled with weight loss and regular exercise.

What is a healthy weight for you? Currently, there is no exact answer. Researchers are trying to develop better ways to measure healthy weight. In the meantime, [if you have questions about you the proper weight for you, check published tables or consult with your doctor].

Research also suggests that body shape as well as weight affects heart health. "Apple-shaped" individuals with extra fat at the waistline may have a higher risk than "pear-shaped" people with heavy hips and thighs. If your waist is larger than the size of your hips, you may have a higher risk for coronary heart disease.

Diabetes

Diabetes, or high blood sugar, is a serious disorder that raises the risk of coronary heart disease. More than 80 percent of people who have diabetes die of some type of cardiovascular disease, usually heart attack. The risk of death from coronary heart disease is doubled in women with diabetes. Compared with nondiabetic women, diabetic women are also more apt to suffer from high blood pressure and high blood cholesterol. Besides helping to cause coronary heart disease, untreated diabetes can contribute to the development of kidney disease, blindness, problems in pregnancy and childbirth, nerve and blood vessel damage, and difficulties in fighting infection.

Diabetes is often called a "woman's disease" because after age 45, about twice as many women as men develop diabetes. The type of diabetes that develops in adulthood is usually "noninsulin-dependent diabetes mellitus," or NIDDM. This type of diabetes, in which the pancreas makes insulin but the body is unable to use it well, is the most common form of the disease. For unknown reasons, the risks of heart disease and heart-related death are higher for diabetic women than for diabetic men.

While there is no cure for diabetes, there are steps one can take to control it. Eighty-five percent of all NIDDM diabetics are at least 20 percent overweight. It appears that overweight and growing older promote the development of diabetes in certain people. Losing excess weight and boosting physical activity may help postpone or prevent the disease. For lasting weight loss, get regular, brisk exercise and eat a diet that is limited in calories and fat, especially saturated fat.

Stress

In recent years, we have read and heard much about the connection between stress and coronary heart disease. In particular, we have heard that "type A" behavior—aggressiveness, a need to compete, a constant concern about time—is linked to the development of heart disease. Some studies have shown such a relationship in men. But recent research on type A behavior in women shows no link between this kind of behavior and coronary heart disease.

Another factor that has often been connected to women's heart disease is employment outside the home. The "price of liberation" for working women, according to many media reports, is a high level of stress leading to soaring rates of coronary heart disease. But research from the Framingham Heart Study shows no difference in rates of coronary heart disease between housewives and employed women.

But it is too early to rule out stress as a risk factor for women. Certainly, some common ways of coping with stress, such as overeating and heavy drinking, are bad for your heart. On the other hand, stress-relieving activities such as exercise can lower your risk of heart disease. Researchers will need to study larger groups of women over time to find out whether certain behaviors, personality types, or stressful situations are linked to the development of coronary heart disease in women.

Birth Control Pills

Studies show that women who use high-dose birth control pills (oral contraceptives) are more likely to have a heart attack or a stroke because blood clots are more likely to form in the blood vessels. These risks are lessened once the birth control pill is stopped: Using birth control pills also may worsen the effects of other risk factors, such as smoking, high blood pressure, diabetes, high blood cholesterol, and overweight.

Much of this information comes from studies of birth control pills containing higher doses of hormones than those commonly used today. Still, the risks of using low-dose birth control pills are not fully known. Therefore, if you are now taking any kind of birth control pill or are considering using one, keep these guidelines in mind:

Smoking and "the pill" don't mix. If you smoke cigarettes, stop smoking or choose a different form of birth control. Cigarette smoking boosts the risks of serious cardiovascular problems from birth control pill use, especially the risk of blood clots. This risk increases with age and with the amount smoked. For women over 35, the risk is particularly high. Women who use oral contraceptives should not smoke.

Pay attention to diabetes. Glucose metabolism, or blood sugar, sometimes changes dramatically in women who take birth control pills. Any woman who is diabetic, or has a close relative who is, should have regular blood sugar tests if she takes birth control pills.

Talk with your doctor. If you have a heart defect, if you have suffered a stroke, or if you have any other kind of cardiovascular disease, oral contraceptives may not be a safe choice. Be sure your doctor knows about your condition before prescribing birth control pills for you.

Alcohol

Over the last several years, a number of studies have reported that moderate drinkers—those who have one or two drinks per day-are less likely to develop heart disease than people who don't drink any alcohol. Alcohol may help protect against heart disease by raising levels of "good" HDL cholesterol. On the other hand, it may also raise blood pressure which could lead to stroke.

If you are a nondrinker, this is not a recommendation to start using alcohol. And certainly, if you are pregnant or have another health condition that could make alcohol use harmful, you should not drink. But if you're already a moderate drinker, evidence suggests that you may be at a lower risk for heart attack.

But remember, moderation is the key. Heavy drinking can definitely cause heart-related problems. More than two drinks per day can raise blood pressure, and recent research shows that binge drinking can lead to stroke. It is well-known that people who drink heavily on a regular basis have higher rates of heart disease than either moderate drinkers or nondrinkers.

Keep in mind, too, that alcohol provides no nutrients—only extra calories. Most drinks contain 100-200 calories each. Women who are trying to control their weight may want to cut down on alcohol and substitute calorie-free iced tea, mineral water, or seltzer with a squeeze of lemon or lime.

What is moderate drinking? For women, "moderate drinking" is no more than one drink per day according to the U.S. Dietary Guidelines for Americans.

Count as one drink:

- 12 ounces of beer
- 5 ounces of wine
- 1 1/2 ounces of hard liquor (80 proof)

Source: *Dietary Guidelines for Americans*, U.S. Department of Agriculture/U.S. Department of Health and Human Services, 1990.

Prevention: A Personal Project

Preventing heart disease, by and large, means making changes in the way we live. For each individual a healthy heart requires a personal action plan. But where does one begin? A complete medical checkup is a sensible first step. With the help of your doctor or other health professional, you can find out if you have any cardiovascular disease risk factors, and if so, work out a practical treatment plan. Even if you don't have any risk factors now, you can discuss ways to lessen your chances of developing them. Good communication with your health professional is very important. Choose someone you trust who will listen to your questions, answer them fully, and take your concerns seriously.

But while advice from a health professional is important, the final responsibility for heart health lies with each woman. Only you can make the kinds of lifestyle changes—changes in eating, drinking, smoking, and exercise habits—that will help protect against cardiovascular diseases. To learn about the many organizations and reading materials available to help you, see [the section titled] "Resources for a Healthy Heart." In the meantime, keep reading. The self-help suggestions that follow can help you get started on a personal program for a healthy heart.

To Do!

The *Healthy Heart Action Plan:*

- Quit smoking
- Cut back on foods high in fat, saturated fat, and cholesterol
- Check blood pressure and blood cholesterol levels
- Get more exercise
- Lose weight if you are overweight

Self Help Strategies for a Healthy Heart

Kicking the Smoking Habit

There is nothing easy about giving up cigarettes. But as hard as quitting may be, the results are well worth it. In the first year after stopping smoking, the risk of coronary heart disease drops sharply. It then gradually returns to "normal"—that is, the same risk as someone who never smoked. This means that no matter what your age, quitting will lessen your chances of developing heart disease.

Quitting will also save you money. Over 10 years, a two-pack-a-day smoker can spend more than $7,500 on cigarettes. And that price tag doesn't take into account the extra costs of smoking-related illness, such as doctors' bills, medicines, and lost wages.

Take some time to think about other benefits of being an ex-smoker. Check the reasons that apply to you in the [list] that follows. Add any others you think are important. This is an important first step in kicking the smoking habit—figuring out for yourself what you have to gain.

- I will greatly lessen my chances of having a heart attack or stroke.
- I will greatly lessen my chances of getting lung cancer, emphysema, and other lung diseases.
- I will have fewer colds or flu each year.
- I will have better smelling clothes, hair, breath, home, and car.
- I will climb stairs and walk without getting out of breath.
- I will have fewer wrinkles.
- I will be free of my morning cough.
- I will reduce the number of coughs, colds, and earaches my children will have.
- I will have more energy to pursue physical activities I enjoy.
- I will have more control over my life.

Many women fear that if they stop smoking they will gain unwanted weight. But you do not have to gain a lot of weight. Here are the facts:

- The average weight gain for ex-smokers is only about 5 pounds.
- Only about 3 percent of women gain a lot of weight (more than 20 pounds) after quitting.

Weight gain may be partly due to changes in the way the body uses calories after smoking stops. Also, some people eat more when quitting because they substitute high-calorie food for cigarettes. Choosing more foods lower in calories and boosting your exercise level will help guard against weight gain. And if you do gain some weight, you can work on losing it after you have become comfortable as a non-smoker. When you think about the enormous health risks of smoking, the possibility of putting on a few pounds is not a reason to continue.

Getting Ready to Quit

Once you decide to stop smoking, a few preparations are in order. Set a target date for quitting—perhaps the first day of a month. Don't choose a time when you know you will be under a lot of stress. To help you stick to your quit date, write [and date a contract like the one] that follows and have someone sign it with you. And don't forget to list how you'll reward yourself for becoming an ex-smoker.

Consider asking your contract cosigner—or another friend or family member—to give you special support in your efforts to quit. Plan to get in touch with your supporter regularly to share your progress and to ask for encouragement. Give your "cheerleader" a copy of your list of "Why I Want to Quit" so that he or she can remind you of your goals. If possible, quit with a spouse or a friend.

Ex-Smoker's Contract

I WILL QUIT SMOKING ON: (date)

I WILL REWARD MYSELF FOR NOT SMOKING AS FOLLOWS:

First 3 days of not smoking:

Each week of not smoking:

Each month of not smoking:

Signed by:

Cosigned by:

Breaking the Habit

Surviving "Day One." On the evening before your quit day, "clean house." Throw away all cigarettes, matches, and lighters and give away your ashtrays. Plan some special activities for the next day to keep you busy, such as a long walk, a bike ride, a movie, or an outing with a good friend. Ask family members and friends not to offer you cigarettes or to smoke in front of you. Your goal is to get through that first important day smoke-free. If you succeed on the first day, it will help give you the confidence to succeed on the second-and on each day after that.

Know yourself. To quit successfully, you need to know your personal smoking "triggers." These are the situations and feelings that typically bring on the urge to light up. Some common triggers include drinking coffee, finishing a good meal, watching television, having an alcoholic drink, talking on the phone, or watching someone else smoke. Stress can also be a trigger. Make a list of the situations and feelings that particularly tempt you to smoke. Especially during the first weeks after quitting, try to avoid as many triggers as you can.

Find new habits. Replace "triggers" with new activities that you don't associate with smoking. For example, if you always had a cigarette with a cup of coffee, switch to tea for awhile. If you always smoked at the table after dinner, get up as soon as the meal is over and go out for a walk. If you're feeling tense or angry, try a relaxation exercise such as deep breathing to calm yourself. (Take a slow, deep breath, count to five, and release it. Repeat 10 times.)

Keep busy. Get involved in projects that require you to use your hands: needlework, gardening, jigsaw puzzles. Try out new physical activities that make smoking impossible, such as swimming, jogging, tennis, or aerobic dancing. When you feel the need to put something in your mouth, have low-calorie substitutes on hand, such as vegetable sticks, apple slices, or sugarless gum. Some people find it helpful to inhale on a straw or chew on a toothpick until the urge passes.

Know what to expect. During the first few weeks after quitting, you may experience some temporary withdrawal symptoms, such as headaches, irritability, tiredness, constipation, and trouble concentrating. These symptoms may come and go, and be stronger or weaker on different days. While these feelings are not pleasant, it is important to know that they are signs that your body is recovering from smoking. Most symptoms end within 2 to 4 weeks.

Two things to help you. Nicotine chewing gum and a nicotine patch are both available by prescription. [For information on over-the-counter products, see you doctor or pharmacist.] The gum and the patch can help you stay off cigarettes by lessening your withdrawal symptoms. They give you nicotine at a lower, more even dose than your cigarettes did. Gradually, you should chew fewer pieces of the gum each day until you stop using it altogether. Similarly, you gradually use patches with a lower dose of nicotine. Nicotine gum and the nicotine patch are not for everyone—talk to your health professional about using them. Pregnant women, nursing mothers, and people with serious heart problems cannot use them safely. But for those who can, both the gum and the patch can help one "over the hump" and on the road to smoke-free living.

More help is available. There are a number of free or low-cost programs available to help you stop smoking. They include programs offered by local chapters of the American Lung Association and the American Cancer Society (see "Resources for a Healthy Heart"). Other low-cost programs can be found through hospitals, health maintenance organizations (HMOs), workplaces, and community groups. Some programs offer special support groups for women.

Be good to yourself. Get plenty of rest, drink lots of fluids, and eat three balanced, healthful meals per day. If you are not as productive or cheerful as usual during the first several weeks after quitting, don't feel guilty. Give yourself a chance to adjust to your new nonsmoking lifestyle. Ask your friends and family to give you lots of praise for kicking the habit—and don't forget to pat yourself on the back. You are making a major change in your life, and you deserve a lot of credit.

If You "Slip"

A "slip" means that you have had a small setback and smoked a cigarette after your quit date. Don't worry. It doesn't mean that you've become a smoker again. Most smokers "slip" three to five times before they quit for good. But to get right back on the nonsmoker track, here are some tips:

Don't get discouraged. Having a cigarette or two doesn't mean you have failed. It doesn't mean you can't quit smoking. A slip happens to many, many people who successfully quit. Keep thinking of yourself as a nonsmoker. You are one.

Learn from experience. What was the trigger that made you light up? Were you driving home from work, having a glass of wine at a party, feeling angry at your boss? Think back on the day's events until you remember what the specific trigger was.

Take charge. Make a list of things you will do the next time you are in that particular situation—and other tempting situations as well. Sign a new contract with your support person to show yourself how determined you are to kick the habit. Reread your list of all the reasons you want to quit. You're on your way.

Getting Physical

Regular exercise can help you reduce your risk of coronary heart disease. Exercise helps women take off extra pounds, helps to control blood pressure, lessens a diabetic's need for insulin, and boosts the level of "good" HDL-cholesterol.

Some studies also show that being inactive boosts the risk of heart attack.

Exercise has many other benefits. It strengthens the lungs, tones the muscles, keeps the joints in good condition, and helps many people cope better with stress.

While many physical activities are fun, only regular, brisk exercise will improve heart health. This is called "aerobic" exercise and includes jogging, swimming, jumping rope, and cross-country skiing. Walking, biking, and dancing can also strengthen your heart, if you do them fast enough and long enough. Choose an activity that you think you will enjoy and that will fit most easily into your schedule.

Most people do not need to see a doctor before they start a gradual, sensible exercise program. Some people, however, should get medical advice. For example, if you have heart trouble or have had a heart attack, if you are over 50 years old and are not used to energetic activity, or if you have a family history of developing heart disease at a young age, check with your doctor before you start.

Eating for Health

The health of your heart has a lot to do with the food you eat. Changing your eating habits according to the Dietary Guidelines for Americans lessens your risk of heart disease in three ways:

- It helps reduce high blood cholesterol levels.
- It helps control high blood pressure.
- It helps take off extra pounds.

As a bonus, the kinds of eating habits that are good for your heart may also help prevent certain types of cancer and a number of other health problems.

Dietary Guidelines for Americans

- Eat a variety of foods
- Maintain a healthy weight
- Choose a diet low in fat, saturated fat, and cholesterol
- Choose a diet with plenty of vegetables, fruits, and grain products
- Use sugars only in moderation
- Use salt and sodium only in moderation
- If you drink alcoholic beverages, do so in moderation

Use these seven guidelines together as you choose a healthful and enjoyable diet.

Controlling Blood Pressure

More than half of American women will develop high blood pressure at some point in their lives. Women who have the highest risk include those who are black, have a family history of high blood pressure, are overweight, or have "high-normal" blood pressure. To help keep blood pressure under control, take these steps:

- Lose weight, if you are overweight.

- If you drink alcohol, have no more than one drink per day—that means no more than 12 ounces of beer, 5 ounces of wine, or 1 1/2 ounces of hard liquor.

- Exercise regularly. A regular aerobic exercise program—for example, brisk walking, bicycling, jogging, or swimming—helps weight control and is good for your entire cardiovascular system.

- Use salt in small amounts, if at all, in cooking and at the table. Try seasoning foods instead with pepper, garlic, ginger, minced onion or green pepper, and lemon juice. Keep in mind that sodium, an ingredient in salt, is "hidden" in many foods such as cured meats, cheese, canned vegetables and soups, frozen dinners, prepared snacks, and condiments such as catsup, soy sauce, pickles, and olives. Check product labels for the amount of sodium in each serving, or buy products labeled "no sodium," or "reduced in sodium."

- While salt substitutes containing potassium chloride may be useful for some individuals, they can be harmful to people with certain medical conditions. Ask your doctor before trying salt substitutes.

- If your doctor prescribes medication, take it regularly as directed.

Losing Weight: Four Ways to Win

If you are overweight, taking off pounds can lower the chances of developing cardiovascular disease in several ways. First, since being overweight raises the risk of heart disease, losing weight will directly lower your risk. Secondly, weight loss will also help reduce the risk of developing diabetes and help control it. Third and fourth, shedding pounds can lower both high blood pressure and cholesterol. In fact, if your blood pressure or blood cholesterol count is not too high, weight loss along with other changes in your diet may be the only treatment you will need. But even if medication is required, the more healthful your weight, the less medication you may need.

In a society so concerned about thinness, it may be hard to listen to yet more advice about the need to take off pounds. But too often, women are pressured to lose too much weight and for the wrong reasons: to look better in trendy clothes, to attract male attention, to have today's super-slim athletic look. The aim here is not to promote the false and discouraging idea that "thin is beautiful," but to show the link between reasonable weight and good health—especially the health of your heart.

Weight loss is advised only to reach a healthy weight, not to drop to an extreme level.

Taking off pounds—and especially keeping them off—can be quite a challenge. Here are some suggestions for making weight loss an easier, safer, and more successful process:

Eat for health. Choose a wide variety of low-calorie, nutritious foods in moderate amounts from each food group. Make sure that these foods are low in fat, since fat is the richest source of calories. To make every calorie count cut out snack foods that are high in calories but provide few other nutrients. If you have a lot of weight to lose, ask your doctor, a nutritionist, or registered dietitian to help you develop a sensible, well-balanced plan for gradual weight loss. To lose weight you will need to take in fewer calories than you burn. That means that you must either choose food with fewer calories or boost your physical activity—and preferably, do both.

Keep milk on the menu. Don't cut out dairy products in trying to reduce calories and fat. Dairy products are rich in calcium, a nutrient that is particularly important for women. Instead, choose low-fat, lower calorie dairy products. For instance, if you are used to drinking whole milk, gradually cut back to 2 percent milk, move to 1 percent, and then perhaps to skim milk. This way the calories are reduced while the amount of calcium remains the same.

Beyond dieting. To keep the pounds off, change your basic eating habits rather than simply "go on a diet." Keep a food diary of what, how much, when, and why you eat to help you understand your eating patterns and what affects them. Learn to recognize social and emotional situations that trigger overeating and figure out ways to cope with them. Set short-term goals at first.

Forget the fads. Tempting as their promises are, fad diets are not the answer. Most provide poor nutrition and cause a number of side effects, especially those with less than 800 calories. Although fad diets can give quick and dramatic results, much of the weight loss is due to water loss. The weight returns quickly once you stop dieting.

Steer clear of diet pills. Studies show that most diet medicines have troublesome side effects and don't work for long-term weight loss.

Get a move on. Although physical activity alone won't take off many pounds, exercise can help burn calories, tone muscles, and control appetite. (It will also give you something to do when you feel that familiar urge for a slice of chocolate fudge cake.) Even moderate activity, such as brisk walking, will burn up calories and help control weight.

Ask for support. Tell your family and friends about your weight-loss plans and let them know how they can be most helpful to you. You might also want to join a self-help group devoted to weight control. These groups provide companionship, support, and practical suggestions on changing eating habits and long-term weight loss.

Other Prevention Issues

Hormones and Menopause

Should menopausal women use "hormone replacement therapy"? There is no simple answer to this question.

Menopause is caused by a decrease in estrogen and other hormones produced by a woman's ovaries. It happens naturally in most women between the ages of 45 and 55, and it also occurs in any woman whose ovaries are removed by an operation. As estrogen levels begin to drop, some women develop uncomfortable symptoms such as "hot flashes" and mood changes. Hormone replacement therapy—a term for prescription hormone pills that are taken daily—can be used to relieve these symptoms. Some women are prescribed pills that contain only estrogen. Others take estrogen combined with a second hormone called progestin.

Estrogen pills have several important benefits. They can help you feel more comfortable as your body adjusts to lower estrogen levels. They also help to prevent osteoporosis, a thinning of the bones that makes them more likely to break in later life. Many studies also have found that estrogen pills help protect women from developing coronary heart disease, but more research is needed before we will know this for sure.

Estrogen therapy also has risks. It may increase the chances of developing gallbladder disease, and it may worsen migraine headaches. It may also increase the risk of breast cancer. But by far, the biggest risk of taking estrogen pills is cancer of the uterus. Women on estrogen therapy after menopause are up to six times more likely to develop uterine cancer than women not on this treatment. It is important to point out that women are much more likely to die of coronary heart disease than from uterine cancer. Still, the cancer risk exists and must be taken seriously and discussed with your doctor.

Because of the risk of uterine cancer, some doctors now prescribe estrogen in combination with the hormone progestin. When progestin is taken along with estrogen, the risk of cancer of the uterus is reduced. While this is good news, we don't yet know how this newer "combo" treatment affects other aspects of women's health. We don't know, for example, whether the progestin-estrogen combination is a safe and effective way to prevent heart disease. We don't know whether the combined hormones are as successful as estrogen alone in protecting women from osteoporosis. Finally, we don't yet know whether this combination will boost the risk of breast cancer. Studies are now under way to find answers to these important questions.

In the meantime, a woman and her doctor must decide whether the benefits of hormone therapy are worth the risks. If you are considering this treatment, you will need to consider your overall health and your personal and family history of heart disease, uterine and breast cancer, and osteoporosis.

If you are now on hormone therapy, check with your doctor to be sure you are taking the lowest possible effective dose. At least every 6 months, you and your doctor should discuss whether you need to continue treatment. Be alert for signs of trouble—abnormal bleeding, breast lumps, shortness of breath, dizziness, severe headaches, pain in your calves or chest-and report them immediately. See your doctor at least once a year for a physical examination.

The Aspirin Question

You may have heard that taking aspirin regularly can help prevent heart attacks. Is this a good idea for you? Maybe.

A recent study of more than 87,000 women found that those who took a low dose of aspirin regularly were less likely to suffer a first heart attack than women who took no aspirin. Older women appeared to benefit most: those over age 50 had a 32 percent lower risk of heart attack, while women overall had a 25 percent lower risk. While earlier research has shown that aspirin can help prevent heart attacks in men, this was the first study to suggest a similar benefit for women. Other recent research suggests that only a tiny daily dose of aspirin may be needed to protect against heart attacks. One study found that for both women and men, taking only 30 mg of aspirin daily—one-tenth the strength of a regular aspirin—helped prevent heart attacks as effectively as the usual 300 mg dose. The smaller dose also caused less stomach irritation.

While these recent reports are encouraging, more study is needed before we can be sure that aspirin is safe and effective in preventing heart attacks in women. What is known for sure is that you should not take aspirin to prevent a heart attack without first discussing it with your doctor. Aspirin is a powerful drug with many side effects. It can increase your chances of getting ulcers and stroke from a hemorrhage. Only a doctor who knows your complete medical history and current health can judge whether the benefit you may gain from aspirin outweighs the risks.

Research: New Focus on Women

As you have read through this handbook, you may have noticed the recurring words: "more research is needed." This is true. Until very recently, men were the main subjects of heart disease research. We now know, however, that coronary heart disease is indeed a woman's concern. We know that we need to understand more about women's heart problems if we are to prevent and treat these problems successfully. As a result, several major research projects are now under way. They include studies on:

- The effects of hormone replacement therapy on cardiovascular diseases, uterine cancer, breast cancer, and osteoporosis. Both estrogen pills and estrogen-progestin combinations are being studied.

- Whether low doses of aspirin can safely and successfully protect women from heart attacks.

- The effect of a low-saturated-fat diet on preventing coronary heart disease in women.

- Whether commonly used programs to encourage exercise, weight control, and quitting smoking are successful for women.

- Possible links between stress, hormonal changes, and risk for coronary heart disease in women.

These and other important research projects will give us new information and tools to better protect ourselves from coronary heart disease. They will also help doctors identify and treat women's heart

481

problems more successfully. Where women's hearts are concerned, knowledge is power—the power to improve our health and enrich our lives.

The Heart of the Matter

Getting serious about heart health may seem like a huge project. Because it means making basic changes in health and living habits, for many it is a major effort. But it doesn't have to be an overwhelming one. Some people find it easier to tackle only one habit at a time. If you smoke cigarettes and also eat a high-fat diet, for example, work on kicking the smoking habit first. Then, once you have gotten used to life without cigarettes, begin skimming the fat from your diet.

And remember: nobody's perfect. Nobody always eats the ideal diet or gets just the right amount of exercise. Few smokers are able to swear off cigarettes without a slip or two along the way. The important thing is to want to make healthful changes, and then to follow a sensible, realistic plan that will gradually lessen your chances of developing cardiovascular diseases.

Women are taking a more active role in their own health care. We are asking more questions and we are seeking more self-help solutions. We are concerned not only about treatment, but about the prevention of a wide range of health problems. Taking steps to prevent cardiovascular diseases is part of this growing movement to promote and protect personal health. The rewards of a healthy heart are well worth the effort.

Resources for a Healthy Heart

If you would like more information on the topics discussed in this chapter, the following organizations may be able to help you.

Federal Government

National Heart, Lung, and Blood Institute (NHLBI)
Information Center
P.O. Box 30105
Bethesda, MD 20824-0105
(301) 951-3260

The NHLBI Information Center is a service of the National Heart, Lung, and Blood Institute (NHLBI). It provides public and patient education materials on high blood pressure, cholesterol, smoking, obesity, and heart disease. Publications include: *Facts About High Blood Pressure; Eating to Lower Your High Blood Cholesterol; Check Your Weight and Heart Disease I.Q.*; and *Check Your Smoking I.Q.: An Important Quiz for Older Smokers.* The NHLBI also offers a number of fact sheets on heart disease-related topics such as *Facts About Coronary Heart Disease.* A directory of publications is available.

Consumer Information Center (CIC)
Pueblo, CO 81009

The Consumer Information Catalog from the CIC lists over 200 free or low-cost booklets on consumer topics. Many are health-related and include booklets on nutrition, foods, exercise, women's health, and smoking. Write for a free copy.

Food and Drug Administration (FDA)
Office of Consumer Affairs, HFE-88
5600 Fishers Lane
Rockville, MD 20857
(301) 443-3170

The FDA offers publications on topics such as general drug information, medical devices, and food-related subjects including fiber, fats, sodium, and cholesterol. The FDA also publishes a monthly journal, *FDA Consumer,* which reports on recent developments in the regulation of foods, drugs, and cosmetics. Recent articles have covered topics such as heart bypass surgery, balloon angioplasty, dieting, and nutrition for women. Subscriptions can be ordered through the Consumer Information Catalog listed above. To order materials, contact the FDA at the address above or contact the consumer affairs office nearest you. Copies are available free of charge.

Food and Nutrition Information Center (FNIC)
National Agricultural Library
10301 Baltimore Avenue, Room 304
Beltsville, MD 20705-2351
(301) 504-5917

The FNIC answers questions concerning food and nutrition and provides database searches, bibliographies, and resource guides on a wide variety of food and nutrition topics.

Human Nutrition Information Service (HNIS)
Department of Agriculture
6505 Belcrest Road
Room 328A
Hyattsville, MD 20782
(301) 436-8617

HNIS reports results of research on food consumption, food composition, and dietary guidance in both technical and popular publications. A list of Department of Agriculture publications is available.

National Cancer Institute (NCI)
Office of Cancer Communications
Bldg. 31, Room 10A24
9000 Rockville Pike
Bethesda, MD 20892
(800) 4-CANCER
(301) 496-5583

The NCI provides information on how to stop smoking. Publications include: *Why Do You Smoke?* (a self-test); *Clearing the Air: A Guide to Quitting Smoking*; and *Guia Para Dejar de Fumar*. Publications are available free of charge.

National Clearinghouse for Alcohol and Drug Abuse Information (NCADI)
P.O. Box 2345
Rockville, MD 20852
(800) 729-6686
(301) 468-2600

NCADI is the central point within the Federal Government for current print and audiovisual information about alcohol and other drugs. Publications for women include: *Alcohol Alert #10; Alcohol and Women; Alcohol, Tobacco, and Other Drugs May Harm the Unborn*; and *Women and Alcohol*. A publications catalog is available.

National Diabetes Information Clearinghouse (NDIC)
Box NDIC
9000 Rockville Pike
Bethesda, MD 20892
(301) 468-2162

The NDIC provides information to diabetic patients and provides materials on topics such as diabetes management and treatment, nutrition, dental care, insulin, and self-blood glucose monitoring. Topical bibliographies are produced on subjects such as diet and nutrition, sports and exercise, and pregnancy. A bimonthly newsletter, *Diabetes Dateline*, is also available. Some mailing fees may apply.

Office of Disease Prevention and Health Promotion
National Health Information Center (ONHIC)
P.O. Box 1133
Washington, DC 20013-1133
(800) 336-4797
(301) 565-4167

The ONHIC helps the public and health professionals locate health information through identification of health information resources, an information and referral system, and publications. The ONHIC provides resource guides on a variety of health-related topics. A publications list is available.

Office on Smoking and Health (OSH)
Center for Chronic Disease Prevention and Health Promotion
Mail Stop K-50
Centers for Disease Control
1600 Clifton Road, N.E.
Atlanta, GA 30333
(404) 488-5705

The Office on Smoking and Health provides information on smoking cessation. Current titles include: *Out of the Ashes: Choosing a Method to Quit Smoking; At A Glance — The Health Benefits of Smoking Cessation: A Report of the Surgeon General; Is Your Baby Smoking?*; and a poster, *Pregnant? That's Two Good Reasons to Quit*. Single copies are available free of charge.

Superintendent of Documents
U.S. Government Printing Office
Washington, DC 20402-9352
(202) 783-3238

The Superintendent of Documents makes available many health-related publications from Government agencies. There are charges for publications. Write for a free copy of *U.S. Government Books and New Books* to receive information on what is available.

Voluntary Health Agencies

American Cancer Society (ACS)
1599 Clifton Road, N.E.
Atlanta, GA 30329
(404) 320-3333
(800) ACS-2345

Contact the local chapters or the national office for information. The ACS provides materials, individual and group support, self-help groups, and a speakers bureau. Publications include: *How Can We Reach You?*, which describes risks specific to women who smoke and tips for quitting without weight gain; *Why Start Life Under a Cloud; Eating Smart*; and *Nutrition, Common Sense, and Cancer*. The Taking Control program provides an introduction to a healthful, enjoyable lifestyle that may reduce one's risk of developing cancer. All publications and services are free.

American Diabetes Association
1660 Duke Street
Alexandria, VA 22314
(800) 232-3472
(703) 549-1500

Contact the local chapters or the national office. The group offers patient and family education activities such as educational meetings, weekend retreats, counseling and discussion, self-help, and support groups. Patient education publications include: *Diabetes in the Family; Diabetes: A to Z*; and the *Family Cookbook* series. *Diabetes Forecast*, a monthly magazine, and *Diabetes*, a quarterly newsletter, are available. There are membership fees and costs for some publications.

American Heart Association (AHA)
National Center
7320 Greenville Avenue
Dallas, TX 75231
(214) 373-6300

The AHA provides fact sheets, brochures, and audiovisuals on topics such as general cardiovascular disease risk reduction, exercise, high blood pressure, smoking, and nutrition. Publications include: *What Every Woman Should Know About High Blood Pressure; About Your Heart and Blood Pressure; American Heart Association Diet: An Eating Plan for Healthy Americans; Now You're Cookin': Healthful Recipes to Help Control High Blood Pressure; Eat Well, But Eat Wisely—To Reduce Your Risk of Heart Attack; Exercise and Your Heart*; and more. Write to the national office or the local AHA affiliate nearest to you. Single copies of most publications are free.

American Lung Association (ALA)
1740 Broadway
New York, NY 10019
(212) 315-8700

The ALA and its local affiliates conduct smoking cessation programs and offer a catalog of publications, including many on smoking. *The Stop Smoking, Stay Trim* booklet explains how stopping smoking affects weight and what you can do to prevent weight gain. *Freedom From Smoking in 20 Days* is a self-help quit smoking program. Other publications include: *Q and A of Smoking and Health; Because You Love Your Baby*; and *Facts About Nicotine, Addiction, and Cigarettes*. Contact your local ALA affiliate or write to the above address. Some fees may apply.

Professional Association

American Dietetic Association (ADA)
216 W. Jackson Blvd., Suite 800
Chicago, IL 60606
(312) 899-0040

The ADA offers cookbooks and other materials for consumers designed to educate about food and nutrition. These include: *Lowfat Living: A Guide to Enjoying a Healthful Diet; Food Facts: What You Should Know About Nutrition and Health*; and *Food 3: Eating the Moderate Fat and Cholesterol Way*. Write or call for price information.

The National Center for Nutrition and Dietetics is the public education initiative of the ADA. It sponsors a consumer nutrition hotline that can be reached at (800) 366-1655 (9:00-4:00, central time). Callers can listen to recorded messages on current issues in nutrition or speak to a registered dietitian.

—by Marian Sandmaier

Chapter 24

Nutritional Health and Weight Management

Chapter Contents

Section 24.1

Methods for Voluntary Weight Loss and Control

Excerpts from NIH Technology Assessment Conference, March 1992.

Introduction

A health paradox exists in modern America. On the one hand, many people who do not need to lose weight are trying to do so. On the other hand, the percentage of Americans whose health is jeopardized by too much weight is growing. Most who need to lose weight are not succeeding. A consideration of voluntary weight loss must encompass a continuum from severe overweight persons with clear adverse medical consequences to persons of normal or low weight who wish to lose weight for cultural, social, or psychological reasons.

Being overweight has serious adverse effects on health and longevity. It is associated with elevated serum cholesterol, elevated blood pressure, and noninsulin-dependent diabetes. Overweight also increases risk for gallbladder disease, gout, coronary heart disease, and some types of cancer and has been implicated in the development of osteoarthritis of the weight-bearing joints.

A widely used means to define overweight is by the body mass index (BMI, weight (kilograms)/height (meters) squared). Agreement has not been established for an exact range of BMI that constitutes a "healthy" weight. This weight varies by factors such as age and gender. Ideally, healthy weight would fall within a range of BMI levels at which adverse health consequences are lowest, and "overweight" is that level of BMI at which adverse health effects begin to increase. A variety of Government and scientific groups have suggested slightly different, desirable ranges of BMI's, ranging from 19 to 27 for adults through middle age. Obese persons have an abnormally high proportion of body fat. Most overweight people are obese.

Approximately one-quarter to one-third of the adult population is classified as overweight, depending on the BMI cut-point used. The prevalence of overweight adults has increased during the last two decades. The problem is disproportionately high in many sub-populations, especially in women, the poor, and members of certain ethnic groups.

The underlying causes of overweight are unknown. The basic mechanism is an imbalance between caloric intake and energy expenditure, but why this imbalance occurs is unclear. Evidence suggests that overweight is multifactorial in origin, reflecting inherited, environmental, cultural, socioeconomic, and psychological conditions. There is increasing physiological, biochemical, and genetic evidence that overweight is not a simple disorder of willpower, as sometimes implied, but is a complex disorder of energy metabolism. For many people, the tendency toward becoming overweight is chronic and needs life-long attention. Many persons attempt to lose weight by employing methods such as caloric restriction, exercise, behavior modification, drugs, or combinations of these methods, with or without medical supervision. Some attempts may be successful in the short term, but most often the weight lost is regained. Repeated weight gain and loss may have adverse psychological and physical effects.

This section will address the following issues:

- How often and in what ways do Americans try to lose weight?

- How successful are various methods for weight loss and control? What are the attributes of and barriers to successful weight loss methods/approaches?

- What are the short- and long-term benefits and adverse effects of weight loss?

- What are the fundamental principles that should be used to select a personal weight loss and control strategy?

- What should be the future directions for research on weight loss and control?

Weight loss and control methods examined here include; diet, exercise, behavioral modification, and drug treatment.

How Often and in What Ways Do Americans Try to Lose Weight?

Who Is Trying to Lose Weight?

The frequency and nature of weight loss efforts in the U.S. population were estimated from participant self-reports in four recent Federal nutrition surveys. Data from these surveys indicate that 33 to 40 percent of adult women and 20 to 24 percent of men are currently trying to lose weight, with an additional 28 percent of each sex trying to maintain weight. Among women and men trying to lose weight, the reported time on a weight loss regimen in the past year averaged 6.4 and 5.8 months, respectively, and the number of attempts to lose weight in the past 2 years averaged 2.5 and 2.0, respectively. Weight loss efforts were not restricted to persons with high BMI. The percent trying to lose weight varied with age (being lower in the youngest and oldest subJects), increased with increasing education and family income, and was positively related to BMI. The percent of men trying to lose weight varied with race (being highest in Hispanic men and lowest in African American men). In women, the percent trying to lose weight did not differ by race even though African-American and Hispanic women have a higher prevalence of overweight compared with white women.

A self-administered questionnaire of a nationally representative sample of high school students showed that 44 percent of female and 15 percent of male students were trying to lose weight; 26 percent of females and 15 percent of males were trying to keep from gaining weight.

Reasons for Weight Loss Efforts

Americans try to lose weight for several reasons. First, a large number of people are seeking to improve their self-images. These people may or may not have physical health problems caused by their weight. Second, some people are severely overweight by current medical standards and are frequently at high risk for weight-related health problems. A third reason involves people who may or may not be classified as being severely overweight; these people attempt weight reduction to improve their perception of their health. A fourth reason involves our society's discrimination against overweight individuals. For these people, weight reduction is attempted to regain greater acceptance.

Future and current health concerns and concerns about fitness and appearance were cited frequently by survey respondents as the most important reasons for trying to lose weight. Health concerns were cited more frequently by persons with higher BMI; appearance/fitness concerns were cited more frequently by persons with lower BMI. Appearance was more important than fitness to women, while the reverse was true for men. Other reasons cited included trying to lose weight gained after smoking cessation or pregnancy.

Methods Used for Weight Loss

Various methods for losing weight were reported, and each of the surveys asked about different methods. Among women trying to lose weight, 84 percent were eating fewer calories, and 60 to 63 percent were increasing their physical activity. Among men trying to lose weight, 76 to 78 percent were eating fewer calories, and 60 to 62 percent were increasing their physical activity. Use of these methods varied with race, education, income, and age.

Another survey of weight loss practices obtained more detail about the methods being used by adults attempting weight loss. Diet and exercise were the most cited methods for both men and women, each at a frequency of more than 80 percent. Vitamins, use of meal replacements, use of over-the-counter products, participation in a weight loss program, and use of diet supplements were cited by both sexes in decreasing order from 28 to 3 percent. The methods used varied with BMI.

In the week preceding the survey, students reported using the following weight loss methods: exercise (51 percent of females and 30 percent of males), skipping meals (49 and 18 percent), using diet pills (4 and 2 percent), and vomiting (3 and 1 percent). The percentage of students who reported ever using these methods was generally much higher: exercise (80 percent of females and 44 percent of males), diet pills (21 and 5 percent), and vomiting (14 and 4 percent).

How Successful Are Various Methods for Weight Loss and Control? What Are the Attributes of and Barriers to Successful Weight Loss Methods/Approaches?

An understanding of the likelihood of successes with the different approaches to weight loss is a key element as individuals or health professionals make informed choices from among the many dietary, exercise, and behavioral options available to the public. In this section, these various weight loss methods will be evaluated with respect to their effectiveness in facilitating weight change.

Strategies for losing weight may or may not work. For most, there are few scientific studies evaluating their safety and efficacy. The available studies indicate that persons participating in such programs tend, over time, to regain whatever weight might have been lost initially. Further, there are examples where weight loss strategies have caused harm. For these reasons, the panel cautions that before individuals adopt any program for the purpose of losing weight, they should examine the scientific data available documenting their safety and efficacy. If no such data exist, the panel recommends that the program not be utilized. The lack of data on the many commercial programs being sold and advertised to effect or enhance weight loss is of special concern. This situation is especially disconcerting in view of the large number of Americans spending an excess of $30 billion yearly in hopes that they will meet their expectations.

Clearly, there is anecdotal information testifying to success in short-term loss for some users; however, there are only very limited data indicating the proportions of individuals initiating programs who actually complete them and on how much weight they lose by program completion and later.

There is considerable diversity within each of the broad categories of weight loss strategies, and their individual success rates can be expected to vary according to initial weight, the length of the treatment period, the magnitude of weight loss desired, and the motivation for wanting to lose weight. The effectiveness of unsupervised efforts to lose weight is difficult to judge due to the limited follow-up data available. Survey data do indicate that many overweight individuals have tried to lose weight on multiple occasions, and because many of these persons presumably are using these strategies, their long-term success rates may be low.

Dietary Change

Dietary change is the most commonly used weight loss strategy. Methods range from caloric restriction, through a variety of methods, to changes in the composition of the diet in terms of proportions of fat, protein, and carbohydrate. There is useful scientific information as to the short-term success for some of these methods and limited information for a few as to their long-term success up to 5 years. Dietary programs can also have other positive health effects.

The weight loss at the end of these relatively short-term programs can exceed 10 percent of initial body weight; however, there is a strong tendency to regain weight, with as much as two-thirds of the weight lost regained within 1 year of completing the program and almost all by 5 years. Importantly, a small percentage of participants do maintain their weight loss over more extended periods.

Key aspects of the evaluation of programs are their duration and dropout rate. The duration of most programs appears to be from several weeks to a few months. Dropout rates can be as high as 80 percent and seem to vary considerably from program to program.

There are two common levels of caloric restriction diets, one being a low-calorie diet (LCD) of about 1,200 to 1,500 calories per day. This comes in a variety of forms, including structured commercial programs often including the use of commercially formulated and calorically defined food products or guidelines in selecting conventional foods. The other is a very low-calorie diet (VLCD) at 800 or fewer calories per day. VLCD's are conducted under physician supervision and monitoring and are restricted to severely overweight persons. VLCD's as well as LCD's may produce side effects, including excessive loss of lean body mass. Attempts to use VLCD's in unsupervised settings have been associated with severe complications. In the short term, the VLCD's tend to produce greater weight loss than do the LCD's; however, for both types of programs, participants tend to return to preprogram weight within 5 years.

There is evidence that the proportion of the calories in the diet from fat, carbohydrate, and protein can have a limited effect on weight loss; however, these effects appear to be quite small in comparison with the direct effect of caloric restriction.

Exercise

The amount of weight loss that can be achieved by exercise programs alone is more limited than that which can be obtained by caloric restriction. However, exercise has beneficial effects independent of weight loss, including increased HDL cholesterol, decreased morbidity, and an increase in lean body mass. Further, exercise can be an important adjunct to other strategies and can, if continued, diminish the tendency for rapid post-program weight gain. The amount of weight lost through exercise can be of the order of 2 to 3 kg over a several-week period. This amount is usually added to that lost through participation in a caloric-restriction program.

Behavior Modification

Behavior modification involves:

1. Identification of the behaviors to be modified
2. The setting of specific behavioral goals
3. The modification of the determinants of the behavior to be changed, and
4. The reinforcement of the desired behavior.

The goal of behavioral treatment is to modify eating and physical activity habits, typically focusing on gradual changes. This can be undertaken through group or individual sessions and through the use of professional or lay personnel. These procedures can be offered alone or in conjunction with other approaches.

When used alone, the typical program takes about 18 weeks and can generate a 1 to 1.5 pound/week weight loss over this period. Typically about one-third of this weight will be regained at the end of 1 year and most regained by 5 years post-program. As with other methods, however, there is a small percentage of participants who have been able to maintain weight loss over an extended period.

Drug Treatment

In carefully controlled research programs, treatment with currently investigational drugs has been effective in producing weight loss. The magnitude of the loss, with some degree of caloric restriction, can be equivalent to VLCD's over comparable periods of treatment. With one drug, prolonging use has resulted in a slowing of weight loss and eventually a weight plateau. Long-term benefits and complications need to be evaluated.

Phenylpropanolamine is a Food and Drug Administration-approved over-the-counter appetite suppressant that has some efficacy in producing weight loss. The long-term benefit of this drug is not well documented. Thus, as with other over-the-counter preparations, there is potential for its misuse.

Combination Therapies

Combination approaches of dietary and exercise changes and dietary and exercise changes reinforced with behavior modification strategies are the most frequently used. In this context, it appears that combining changes in diet and exercise can lead to greater short-term weight loss than changes of either alone. Further, utilizing behavior modification strategies appears to help extend the amount of time it takes to regain lost weight, especially if contact between the program deliverers and participants is continued and maintenance activities are utilized.

Attributes and Barriers

In general, successful programs are those based on realistic goals that involve a caloric deficit leading to a slow and steady weight loss. This requires a diet that can be adhered to for a sufficient period to reach the goal. The development of a new set of dietary practices that can be maintained to enhance the possibility of a lifetime of weight control is also important. Such programs also involve preparing the individual to deal with high-risk emotional and social situations, to self-monitor progress, to solve problems, to reduce stress, and to maintain continual professional contact. Barriers to success include lack of feelings of self-efficacy, failure to lose weight early, early termination of diet and/or exercise modifications, and lack of social and professional support.

It is likely that the effectiveness of the various programs in bringing about weight loss will vary among different cultural groups; however, the data to evaluate this are lacking. As these programs undergo further study, it is important to consider that some of then also may be effective in preventing overweight.

What Are the Short- and Long-Term Benefits and Adverse Effects of Weight Loss?

While there seems to be little doubt that individuals at higher levels of body weight have increased risk of future morbidity and mortality, it does not immediately follow that weight loss reduces that increased risk. Understanding the health consequences of weight loss requires data on what happens to people who have lost weight. Our knowledge of the health effects of weight loss derives from two sources: observational studies of individuals who by self-report or actual measurement have lost weight by whatever means or cause and clinical trial data where we know the circumstances under which weight was lost. Most of the longer term data come from the former studies because follow-up time in trials has generally been short. It is the latter that provides clearer evidence as to the nature of the relationship between weight loss and health.

Benefits of Weight Loss

Both the incidence and severity of diabetes and hypertension are reduced by weight loss among heavy persons. Recent studies have shown that a diet and exercise program leading to weight loss can prevent the onset of hypertension and that the same may be true for diabetes mellitus. Diabetics who can lose weight will improve glycemic control and may eliminate their need for oral agents. Similarly, randomized trial data indicate that weight loss in hypertensive patients also is associated with significant reductions in blood pressure and the need for continued drug therapy. Weight loss also affects other risk factors for cardiovascular disease. In particular, it has well documented positive effects on lipid and lipoprotein levels. Given the high likelihood that weight will be regained, it remains to be determined whether these time-limited improvements confer more permanent health benefits.

Among the very obese individuals, weight loss has been reported to be followed by greater functional status, reduced work absenteeism, less pain, and greater social interaction. The prevalence and severity of sleep apnea also can be substantially reduced by weight loss, but monitoring for weight regain is important.

Adverse Effects of Weight Loss

However, VLCD's and fasting are associated with a variety of short-term adverse effects. Serious complications like cardiac arrhythmias or death, seen in early studies, have largely been eliminated by enriching diets with high quality protein and minerals. Patients on VLCD's frequently report fatigue, hair loss, dizziness, and other symptoms, but these appear to be transitory. More seriously, there appears to be an increased risk of gallstones and acute gall bladder disease during severe calorie restriction.

Because data on health effects come from programs that only include overweight individuals, it is reasonable to posit that some of these complications may be more severe in individuals who are not overweight but are severely restricting calories. Laboratory evidence suggests that weight loss in the lean individual can result in a greater loss of lean body mass than in the severely overweight individual. This may well increase adverse effects such as fatigue.

Weight loss in participants in formal programs may reduce baseline depression and anxiety. These findings, however, apply to those evidencing some success in losing weight. We need to know much more about the emotional impacts of lesser degrees of success. While some argue that failure to lose weight is depressing, confirmation in careful studies is lacking. There also is increasing evidence that mild to moderately overweight women who are dieting may be binge-eating not associated with vomiting and purging. Whether involvement in well-designed dietary modification program increases the risks of bulimia is unknown and in need of careful study.

The evidence that reductions in mortality follow weight loss is meager. In fact, most major epidemiologic studies suggest that losses of weight are, in fact, associated with increased mortality. Most of these studies cannot distinguish purposeful weight loss from that associated with illness, psychosocial distress, or other reasons. We need to know much more about the individuals who have lost weight and why they, unlike participants in programs, appear to keep weight off. Finally the fact that many people who stop smoking gain weight makes comparisons of weight gainers and weight losers more difficult.

Data presented on the health effects of repeated weight gains and losses, or weight cycling, also are inconclusive. Cycling appears to affect energy metabolism and may result in faster regains of weight, but the evidence that weight cycling has longer term negative effects on psychological and physical health needs further confirmation.

While currently used weight-reducing drugs appear to be safe in controlled studies, the studies are short term and examine populations where the potential for abuse may be low. The fact that large numbers of adolescents and young adults report use of over-the-counter preparations urges further examination of their safety in real-world use.

What Are the Fundamental Principles that Should Be Used to Select a Personal Weight Loss and Control Strategy?

A fundamental principle of weight loss and subsequent control is that for almost all people, it requires a life-long commitment to a permanent change in lifestyle, behavioral responses, and dietary practices. Whether one should make this commitment depends partially on the risks and benefits of losing weight versus those of not losing weight. The more one's BMI exceeds the healthy range described in the Introduction, the higher one's risk is for a number of medical conditions, and the need for a weight reduction plan becomes more urgent. In addition, attempts to lower weight are indicated for those persons with current health problems whose symptoms can be lessened by weight loss (such as sleep apnea, hypertension, or diabetes). Finally, for those persons near the upper limit of the healthy weight range, beginning a program of weight control may be appropriate to prevent increases in weight.

Contraindications to non-supervised weight loss exist for severely overweight persons, pregnant or lactating women, children, persons over the age of 65, and those with medical conditions that make such an undertaking dangerous. A trained physician or other health professional can be helpful in making these determinations. This person should also screen the individual for preexisting eating disorders or underlying psychological disorders. If a person is at high medical risk, a properly trained physician should be involved in a multi-disciplinary approach to his or her care throughout the weight loss process. VLCD's (800 or fewer calories per day) should not be undertaken without medical supervision and monitoring because of attendant health risks.

For those who are within the healthy weight range but who desire to lose weight for other reasons, such as improved appearance or sense of well-being, the decision to lose weight should take into account the difficulty of the task as well as the potential adverse physical and psychological effects of weight loss regimens. These include the risk of poor nutrition, the possible development of eating disorders, the effects of weight cycling, and the sometimes serious psychological consequences of repeated failed attempts to lose weight.

Realistic Expectations

No matter how much weight an individual would like to lose, it is generally recognized that modest goals and a slow course of weight loss will maximize the probability of both losing the weight and keeping it off. In setting these goals, it should also be recognized that even in highly structured, medically supervised plans, the dropout rate is often high, and even for those who complete the program, maximum weight loss rarely exceeds 10 percent of the initial body weight. The rate of weight loss in these plans is generally less than 1.5 pounds per week. In addition, if the pattern of eating and activity after the conclusion of the structured portion of such programs is not permanently altered, most participants will regain their lost weight over the next 1 to 5 years. In less structured or self-monitored settings, these results are unknown. These realities should help an individual avoid disappointment by providing guidelines for reasonable goals for how much weight one wants or needs to lose, how fast one wants to lose it, and how long weight loss can be maintained. These facts also should help one recognize that, for most people, achieving body weights and shapes presented to us in the media is not a reasonable, appropriate, or achievable goal, and thus the failure to do so does not represent a weakness of willpower or character.

Setting Weight Loss Goals and Choosing a Program

Characteristics to consider in setting weight loss goals include one's weight history, the weights of biological relatives, the outcomes of past weight loss efforts, and one's emotional profile. When choosing a program, important elements include personal food preferences; the desire for structure in a weight loss program; and the degree of support in the home, workplace, or a chosen group. There may also be a variety of logistical details to consider: time; money (including the costs of programs and special diet foods or supplements); transportation; and the ability to integrate the eating pattern of the dieter with others in the home, particularly if one is a primary food preparer.

In evaluating a weight loss method or program, one should not be distracted by anecdotal "success" stories or by advertising claims. The information that should be obtained about the program includes:

- The percentage of all participants starting the program who complete it.

- The percentage of those completing the program who achieve various degrees of weight loss.

- The proportion of that weight loss that is maintained at 1, 3, and even 5 years.

- The number of participants who experienced negative medical effects as well as their kind and severity.

Valid and reliable statistics of this kind are important but routinely provided by a commercial diet plan or program. This information (preferably in the form of peer-reviewed published studies) should be available for all supervised programs, including those based in hospitals or clinics.

Additional information on program characteristics that should be obtained includes:

- The relative mix of diet, exercise, and behavioral modifications.

- The amount and kind of counseling: individual and/or closed groups (membership does not change except by attrition) are both more successful forms of supervision than open groups in which members may come and go.

- The nature of available multi-disciplinary expertise (including medical, nutritional, psychological, and physiological).

- The training provided for relapse prevention to deal with high-risk emotional and social situations.

- The nature and duration of the maintenance phase.

- The flexibility of food-choices, suitability of food types, and whether weight goals are set unilaterally or cooperatively with the program director.

Weight Maintenance

Maintenance of stable weight, or of a newly lowered weight, is the most important feature of a successful weight loss program. For those who have participated in formal programs to lose weight, continued, regular contact with a supervising professional may be required to maintain that loss. In any case, new eating behaviors must be learned and adopted, and this can be an involved process. These include modifying the quantity and kinds of food consumed and possibly developing a different psychological attitude toward eating and one's self. Therefore, an individual weight loss method should be based not merely on weight loss goals but should be part of a general long-term approach of which the goal is better health. This goal should take into account currently accepted guidelines for healthful eating. Even though total calories must be reduced, the diet must provide all essential nutrients. In addition, a regular exercise regimen, which could be as simple as walking, is essential both to better health as well as long-term weight loss maintenance.

Any program of which the primary goal is short term, rapid or unsupervised weight loss, or which relies on diet aids such as drinks, prepackaged foots, or pharmacologic agents without an education in and eventual transition to a lasting pattern of healthful eating and activity has never been shown to be successful over the long term. It has been fairly said that such programs fail people, not vice versa. A recognition of this by society and individuals and a focus on approaches that can produce health benefits independently of weight loss may be the best way to improve the physical and psychological health of Americans seeking to lose weight.

What Should Be the Future Direction for Research on Weight Loss and Control?

Because voluntary weight loss is associated with important health conditions and because Americans frequently attempt voluntary weight loss, it is imperative that the appropriate scientific base be developed to maximize the chances for all Americans to achieve their healthy weight.

Evidence suggests that the causes of obesity are multifactorial. Thus, an appropriate research base must span the entire spectrum of health research from genetic, biochemical, physiologic, and neurophysiologic to individual, community, and population investigations. Research is needed within and across these areas. Specifically, the biomedical perspective should be incorporated into clinical trials and population studies.

Genetics

Obesity in humans has a substantial genetic basis. Furthermore, numerous animal models of obesity are attributable to defects in as yet unidentified genes. Molecular genetic technology now makes it feasible to identify such genes in both animals and humans. Once identified, characterization of the function of the gene products should facilitate understanding of the biochemical, physiological, and neural basis for regulation of body weight and body fat, the resting metabolic rate, and metabolic efficiency in humans. Genes alone may not explain all of the adiposity in obese humans. Interactions between genetic and environmental effects during early childhood or environmental effects themselves may influence the development of obesity. An understanding of the basic mechanisms elucidated by gene analysis also may provide important new understanding of environmentally induced weight gain.

Therapy

Physiologic research is helping to define weight loss mechanisms that may be useful in therapy. Mechanisms so far identified include appetite suppression, inhibiting gastric emptying, blocking carbohydrate or lipid digestion, stimulating lipid oxidation, and increasing thermogenesis. These mechanisms should be explored with pharmacotherapy research. Further efforts should be made to identify other mechanisms. Because of the association between body fat distribution and health effects, it is important to elucidate the physiologic basis for body fat distribution.

Other Research Areas

There is a paucity of well-designed long-term clinical trials evaluating various methods advocated for voluntary weight loss. This is particularly so for minority populations and for persons who are mildly to moderately overweight. Such trials will provide the most convincing evidence about the longer term health effects of weight loss. Methods to improve participant compliance with the weight loss regimens and methods for long-term maintenance of weight control should receive investigative priority. In this vein, we need to know more about the relationship of binge-eating, diet, and weight loss.

Commercial voluntary weight loss programs should routinely compile operational research data on characteristics, attrition rates, degree and duration of weight loss, and adverse effects for all participants.

Because several observational studies found weight loss was associated with increased mortality, further analysis of existing data sets and survival studies of persons losing weight voluntarily are urgently needed. Better studies are needed to clarify long-term psychological effects of voluntary weight loss. Physical and psychological outcomes of weight cycling deserve additional investigation.

Population studies are needed to determine better the range of healthy weights for individuals at various ages and for the different sexes and different ethnic groups. In addition, the effects of obesity in childhood, obesity treatment in children, and long-term consequences of childhood obesity are important research priorities.

Another research priority is the prevention of unhealthy weights. Voluntary weight loss practices are closely tied to cultural and societal attitudes toward weight and body image. Interdisciplinary research involving all types of behavioral scientists is necessary to develop and evaluate prevention programs that encourage Americans to adopt healthy eating habits and lifestyles that will effect life-long control of weight. Effective methods must be developed to deal with such problems as an unrealistically thin ideal among some women and an uncritical acceptance of dangerously overweight states among certain cultures.

Conclusions

A quarter to a third of Americans are overweight, and many have undertaken a variety of methods to lose weight. Most overweight individuals have had limited success keeping off their excess weight. In controlled settings, weight loss techniques, including diets, behavior modification, exercise, and drugs, produce short-term weight losses with reasonable safety. Unfortunately, most people who achieve weight loss with any of these programs regain their weight. For many overweight persons, overweight is a life-long challenge.

Successful weight loss improves control of diabetes and hypertension, reduces cardiovascular risk factors, and enhances self-image. Long-term health effects are much less clear. Several epidemiologic studies raise the possibility that weight loss is associated with increased mortality. The relevance of these findings to voluntary weight loss programs is not clear.

Survey evidence also confirms that many Americans who are not overweight, particularly young women, are trying to lose weight. This practice may have significant physical and psychological health consequences.

Because of the importance of these issues, research on the biologic and social influences on weight and weight control and the health consequences of weight and weight loss should assume a high-priority position on the nation's health agenda.

Section 24.2

Choosing a Safe and Successful Weight-Loss Program

NIH Publication No. 94-3700, December 1993.

Obesity affects about one four adult Americans, and during any one year, over half of Americans go on a weight-loss diet or are trying to maintain their weight. For many people who try to lose weight it is difficult to lose more than a few pounds and few succeed in remaining at the reduced weight. The difficulty in losing weight and keeping it off leads many people to turn to a professional or commercial weight-loss program for help. These programs are quite popular and are widely advertised in newspapers and on television. What is the evidence that any of these programs is worthwhile, that they will help you lose weight and keep it off, and that they will do it safely.

Almost any of the commercial weight-loss programs can work, but only if they motivate you sufficiently to decrease the amount of calories you eat or increase the amount of calories you burn each day (or both). What elements of a weight-loss program should an intelligent consumer look for in judging its potential for safe and successful weight loss? A responsible and safe weight-loss program should be able to document for you the five following features:

1. The diet should be safe. It should include all of the Recommended Daily Allowances (RDAs) for vitamins, minerals, and protein. The weight-loss diet should be low in *calories* (energy) only, not in essential foodstuffs.

2. The weight-loss program should be directed towards a *slow, steady* weight loss unless your doctor feels your health condition would benefit from more rapid weight loss. Expect to lose only about *a pound a week* after the first week or two. With

506

many calorie-restricted diets there is an initial rapid weight loss during the first 1 to 2 weeks but this loss is largely fluid. The initial rapid loss of fluid also is regained rapidly when you return to a normal-calorie diet. Thus, a reasonable goal of weight loss must be expected.

3. If you plan to lose more than 15 to 20 pounds, have any health problems, or take medication on a regular basis, you should be evaluated by your doctor before beginning your weight-loss program. A doctor can assess your general health and medical conditions that might be affected by dieting and weight loss. Also, a physician should be able to advise you on the need for weight loss, the appropriateness of the weight-loss program, and a sensible goal of weight loss for you. If you plan to use a very-low-calorie diet (a special liquid formula diet that replaces all food intake for 1 to 4 months), you definitely should be examined and monitored by a doctor.

4. Your program should include plans for *weight maintenance* after the weight loss phase is over. It is of little benefit to lose a large amount of weight only to regain it. Weight maintenance is the most difficult part of controlling weight and is not consistently implemented in weight-loss programs. The program you select should include help in permanently changing your dietary habits and level of physical activity, to alter a lifestyle that may have contributed to weight gain in the past. Your program should provide behavior modification help, including education in healthy eating habits and long-term plans to deal with weight problems. One of the most important factors in maintaining weight loss appears to be increasing daily physical activity, often by sensible increases in daily activity, as well as incorporating an individually tailored exercise program.

5. A commercial weight-loss program should provide a detailed statement of fees and costs of additional items such as dietary supplements.

Obesity is a chronic condition. Too often it is viewed as a temporary problem that can be treated for a few months with a strenuous diet. However, as most overweight people know, weight control must be considered a life-long effort. To be safe and effective, any weight-loss program must address the long-term approach or else the program is largely a waste of money and effort.

Section 24.3

Very Low-Calorie Diets

NIH Publication No. 95-3894, March 1995.

Obesity affects up to one-fourth of adult Americans, increasing risk of death from diseases like diabetes, high blood pressure, and heart disease. Traditional weight loss methods include low calorie diets between 800 to 1,500 calories a day and regular exercise. An alternative method sometimes considered for bringing about significant short-term weight loss in moderately to severely obese people is the very low-calorie diet (VLCD).

What Is a Very Low-Calorie Diet (VLCD)?

VLCDs are commercially prepared formulas of 800 calories or less that replace all usual food intake. VLCDs are not the same as over-the-counter meal replacements, which are meant to be substituted for one or two meals a day. VLCDs, when used under proper medical supervision, effectively produce significant short-term weight loss in moderately to severely obese patients.

Who Should Use a VLCD?

VLCDs are generally safe when used under proper medical supervision in patients with a body mass index (BMI) greater than 30. BMI is a mathematical formula that takes into account both a person's height and weight. To calculate BMI, a person's weight in kilograms is divided by height in meters squared. Use of VLCDs in patients with a BMI of 27 to 30 should be reserved for those who have medical complications resulting from their obesity. VLCDs are not recommended for pregnant women or breastfeeding women. VLCDs are not appropriate for children or adolescents, except in specialized treatment programs.

Very little information exists regarding the usage of VLCDs in older individuals. Because individuals over 50 already experience normal depletion of lean body mass, use of a VLCD may not be warranted. Additionally, persons over 50 may not tolerate the side effects associated with VLCDs because of pre-existing medical conditions or need for other medications. Therefore, a physician, on a case by case basis, must evaluate increased risks and potential benefits of drastic weight loss in older individuals. Additionally, people with significant medical problems or who are on medications may be able to use a VLCD, but this too must be determined on an individual basis by a physician.

Health Benefits Associated with a VLCD

A VLCD may allow a severely to moderately obese patient to lose about 3 to 5 pounds per week, for an average total weight loss of 44 pounds over 12 weeks. Such a weight loss can improve obesity-related medical conditions, including diabetes, high blood pressure, and high cholesterol. Combining a VLCD with behavioral therapy and exercise may also increase weight loss and may slow weight regain. However, VLCDs are no more effective than more modest dietary restrictions in the long-term maintenance of reduced weight.

Adverse Effects Associated with a VLCD

Many patients on a VLCD for 4 to 16 weeks report minor side effects such as fatigue, constipation, nausea, and diarrhea, but these conditions usually improve within a few weeks and rarely prevent patients from completing the program. The most common serious side effect seen with VLCDs is gallstone formation. Gallstones, which often develop in obese people, anyway, (especially women), are even more common during rapid weight loss. Some research indicates that rapid weight loss appears to decrease the gallbladder's ability to contract bile. But, it is unclear whether VLCDs directly cause gallstones or whether the amount of weight loss is responsible for the formation of gallstones.

Conclusion

For most obese individuals, obesity is a long-term condition that requires a lifetime of attention even after a formal weight loss treatment ends. Although VLCDs are efficient for short-term weight loss, they are no more effective than other dietary treatments in the long-term maintenance of reduced weight. Therefore, obese patients should be encouraged to commit to a long-term treatment program that includes permanent lifestyle changes of healthier eating, regular physical activity, and an improved outlook about food because without a long-term commitment, their body weights will drift back up the scale.

Section 24.4

Weight Cycling

NIH Publication No. 95-3901, March 1995.

What Is Weight Cycling?

Weight cycling is the repeated loss and regain of body weight. When weight cycling is the result of dieting, it is often called "yo-yo" dieting. A weight cycle can range from small weight losses and gains (5 to 10 lbs. per cycle) to large changes in weight (50 lbs. or more per cycle).

You may have heard stories in the press claiming that weight cycling may be harmful to your health. You also may have heard that staying at one weight is better for you than weight cycling, even if you are obese. However, no convincing evidence supports these claims, and most obesity researchers believe that obese individuals should continue to try to control their body weight.

If I Regain Lost Weight, Won't Losing It Again Be Even Harder?

People who repeatedly lose and regain weight should not experience more difficulty losing weight each time they diet. Most studies have shown that weight cycling does not affect one's metabolic rate. Metabolic rate is the rate at which food is burned for energy. Based on these findings, weight cycling should not affect the success of future weight-loss efforts. However, everyone, whether they have dieted or not, experiences a slowing of the metabolism as they age. In addition, older people are often less physically active than when they were younger. Therefore, people often find it more difficult to lose weight as they get older.

Will Weight Cycling Leave Me with More Fat and Less Lean Tissue than If I Had Not Dieted at All?

Weight cycling has not been proven to increase the amount of fat tissue in people who lose and regain weight. Researchers have found that after a weight cycle people have the same amount of fat and lean tissue as they did prior to weight cycling.

Some people are concerned that weight cycling can cause more fat to collect in the abdominal area. People who tend to carry their excess fat in the abdominal area (apple-shaped), instead of in the hips and buttocks (pear-shaped), are more likely to develop the health problems associated with obesity. However, studies have not found that after a weight cycle people have more abdominal fat than they did before weight cycling.

Is Weight Cycling Harmful to My Health?

A number of studies have suggested that weight cycling (and weight loss) may be associated with an increase in mortality. Unfortunately, these studies were not designed to answer the question of how intentional weight loss by an obese person affects health. Most of the studies did not distinguish between those who lost and regained weight through dieting from those whose change in weight may have been due to other reasons, such as unsuspected illness or stress. In addition, most of the people followed in these studies were not obese. In fact, some evidence shows that if weight cycling does have any negative effects on health, they are seen mostly in people of low or normal weight. Some studies have looked at the relationship between weight cycling and risk factors for illness, such as high blood pressure, high blood cholesterol, or high blood sugar. Most of these studies have not found an association between weight cycling and harmful changes in risk factors.

Is Remaining Overweight Healthier than Weight Cycling?

At this time, no conclusive studies have shown that weight cycling is harmful to the health of an obese person. On the other hand, the health risks of obesity are well known. The costs of obesity-related illnesses are more than $39 billion each year. Obesity is linked to serious medical conditions such as:

- High blood pressure
- Heart disease
- Stroke
- Diabetes
- Certain types of cancer
- Gout, and
- Gallbladder disease.

Not everyone who is obese has the same risk for these conditions— a person's sex, amount of fat, location of fat, and family history of disease all play a role in determining an individual's risk of obesity-related problems. However, experts agree that even a modest weight loss can improve the health of an obese person.

Conclusions

Further research on the effects of weight cycling is needed. In the meantime, if you are obese, don't let fear of weight cycling stop you from achieving a modest weight loss. Although health problems associated with weight cycling have not been proven, the health-related problems of obesity are well known.

If you are not obese and have no risk factors for obesity-related illness, focus on preventing further weight gain by increasing your exercise and eating healthy foods, rather than trying to lose weight. If you do need to lose weight, you should be ready to commit to lifelong changes in your eating behaviors, diet, and physical activity.

Section 24.5

Dieting and Gallstones

NIH Publication No. 94-3677, November 1993.

As most people know, there are significant health benefits to be gained from losing excess pounds. For example, many people can reduce high blood pressure and cholesterol levels through weight loss. Overweight people are at a greater risk of developing gallstones than people of average weight. However, people considering a diet program, requiring very low intake of calories each day should be aware that during rapid or substantial weight loss, a person's risk of developing gallstones is increased.

What Are Gallstones?

Gallstones are clumps of solid material that form in the gallbladder. They may occur as a single, large stone or many small ones. Gallstones are a mixture of compounds, but typically they are mostly cholesterol.

One in ten Americans has gallstones. However, most people with gallstones don't know they have them and experience no symptoms. Painless gallstones are called *silent gallstones*. For an unfortunate minority, however, gallstones can cause painful attacks. Painful gallstones are called *symptomatic gallstones,* because they cause symptoms. In rare cases gallstones can cause life-threatening complications. Symptomatic gallstones result in 600,000 hospitalizations and more than 500,000 operations each year in the United States.

What Causes Gallstones?

Gallstones develop in the *gallbladder,* a pear-shaped organ beneath the liver on the right side of the abdomen. It's about 3 inches long

513

and an inch wide at its thickest part. The gallbladder stores and releases *bile* into the intestine to aid digestion.

Bile is a fluid made by the liver that helps in digestion. Bile contains substances called bile salts that act like natural detergents to break down fats in the food we eat. As food passes from the stomach into the small intestine, the gallbladder releases bile into the bile ducts. These ducts, or tubes, run from the liver to the intestine. Bile also helps eliminate excess cholesterol from the body. The liver secretes cholesterol into the bile, which is then eliminated from the body via the digestive system.

Most researchers believe three conditions are necessary to form gallstones. First, the bile becomes supersaturated with cholesterol, which means the bile contains more cholesterol than the bile salts can dissolve. Second, an imbalance of proteins or other substances in the bile causes the cholesterol to start to crystallize. Third, the gallbladder does not contract enough to empty its bile regularly.

Are Obese People More Likely to Develop Gallstones?

Yes. Obesity is a strong risk factor for gallstones.

Scientists often use a mathematical formula called *body mass index* (BMI) to define obesity. (BMI = weight in kilograms divided by height in meters squared. The accompanying table shows BMI in pounds and inches.) For example, an obese woman who is 5 ft. 4 in. tall (64 in.) and weighs 174 pounds has a BMI of 30. The more obese a person is, the greater his or her risk is of developing gallstones. Several studies have shown that women with a BMI of 30 or higher have at least double the risk of developing gallstones than women with a BMI of less than 25.

Why obesity is a risk factor for gallstones is unclear. But researchers believe that in obese people, the liver produces too much cholesterol. The excess cholesterol leads to supersaturation in the gallbladder.

Are People on a Diet to Lose Weight More at Risk for Developing Gallstones?

Yes. People who lose a lot of weight rapidly are at greater risk for developing gallstones. *Gallstones are one of the most medically important complications of voluntary weight loss.* The relationship of dieting to gallstones has only recently received attention.

Body Mass Index (kg/m²)

Height (in.)	19	20	21	22	23	24	25	26	27	28	29	30	35	40
	Body Weight (lb.)													
58	91	96	100	105	110	115	119	124	129	134	138	143	167	191
59	94	99	104	109	114	119	124	128	133	138	143	148	173	198
60	97	102	107	112	118	123	128	133	138	143	148	153	179	204
61	100	106	111	116	122	127	132	137	143	148	153	158	185	211
62	104	109	115	120	126	131	136	142	147	153	158	164	191	218
63	107	113	118	124	130	135	141	146	152	158	163	169	197	225
64	110	116	122	128	134	140	145	151	157	163	169	174	204	232
65	114	120	126	132	138	144	150	156	162	168	174	180	210	240
66	118	124	130	136	142	148	155	161	167	173	179	186	216	247
67	121	127	134	140	146	153	159	166	172	178	185	191	223	255
68	125	131	138	144	151	158	164	171	177	184	190	197	230	262
69	128	135	142	149	155	162	169	176	182	189	196	203	236	270
70	132	139	146	153	160	167	174	181	188	195	202	207	243	278
71	136	143	150	157	165	172	179	186	193	200	208	215	250	286
72	140	147	154	162	169	177	184	191	199	206	213	221	258	294
73	144	151	159	166	174	182	189	197	204	212	219	227	265	302
74	148	155	163	171	179	186	194	202	210	218	225	233	272	311
75	152	160	168	176	184	192	200	208	216	224	232	240	279	319
76	156	164	172	180	189	197	205	213	221	230	238	246	287	328

Figure 24.1. *Body Weight in Pounds According to Height and Body Mass Index. Each entry gives the body weight in pounds (lb.) for a person of a given height and body mass index. Pounds have been rounded off. To use the table, find the appropriate height in the left-hand column. Move across the row to a given weight. The number at the top of the column is the body mass index for the height and weight. Adapted with permission from Bray, G.A., Gray, D.S. Obesity. Part 1. Pathogenesis. West J Med 1988; 149:429-41.*

One major study found that women who lost from 9 to 22 pounds (over a 2-year period) were 44 percent more likely to develop gallstones than women who did not lose weight. Women who lost more than 22 pounds were almost twice as likely to develop gallstones.

Other studies have shown that 10 to 25 percent of obese people develop gallstones while on a *very-low-calorie diet.* (Very-low-calorie diets are usually defined as diets containing 800 calories a day or less. The food is often in liquid form and taken for a prolonged period, typically 12 to 16 weeks.) The gallstones that developed in people on very-low-calorie diets were usually silent and did not produce any symptoms. However, about a third of the dieters who developed gallstones did have symptoms, and a proportion of these required gallbladder surgery.

In short, the likelihood of a person developing symptomatic gallstones during or shortly after rapid weight loss is about 4 to 6 percent. This estimate is based on reviewing just a few clinical studies, however and is not conclusive.

Why Does Weight Loss Cause Gallstones?

Researchers believe dieting may cause a shift in the balance of bile salts and cholesterol in the gallbladder. The cholesterol level is increased and the amount of bile salts is decreased. Going for long periods without eating (skipping breakfast, for example), a common practice among dieters, also may decrease gallbladder contractions. If the gallbladder does not contract often enough to empty out the bile, gallstones may form.

Are Some Weight Loss Methods Better than Others in Preventing Gallstones?

Possibly. If substantial or rapid weight loss increases the risk of developing gallstones, more gradual weight loss would seem to lessen the risk of getting gallstones. However, studies are needed to test this theory.

Some very-low-calorie diets may not contain enough fat to cause the gallbladder to contract enough to empty its bile. A meal or snack containing approximately 10 grams (one-third of an ounce) of fat is necessary for the gallbladder to contract normally. But again, no studies have directly linked a diet's nutrient composition to the risk of gallstones.

516

Also, no studies have been conducted on the effects of repeated dieting on gallstone formation.

Are People Who Have Surgery to Lose Weight Also at Risk for Gallstones?

You bet. Gallstones are common among obese patients who lose weight rapidly after gastric bypass surgery. (In gastric bypass surgery, the size of the stomach is reduced, preventing the person from overeating.)

One study found that more than a third (38 percent) of patients who had gastric bypass surgery developed gallstones afterward. Gallstones are most likely to occur within the first few months after surgery.

Should People Who Already Have Gallstones Try to Lose Weight?

Scientists know that weight loss increases the risk of gallstone formation. However, they don't know whether weight loss increases the risk of silent gallstones becoming symptomatic gallstones or of other complications developing. In addition to painful gallstone attacks, complications include inflammation of the gallbladder, liver, or pancreas. These are usually caused by a gallstone getting lodged in a bile duct.

Although excluding people with pre-existing gallstones from a weight-loss program seems prudent, there is no evidence to support this action. If people have had their gallbladders removed, there is little risk of them having gallstones or bile problems while participating in a weight-loss program. Shedding excess pounds can bring significant health benefits. Weight loss can lessen the severity of high blood pressure and diabetes, sometimes eliminating the need to take medications for these conditions.

What Is the Treatment for Gallstones?

Silent gallstones are usually left alone and occasionally disappear on their own. Usually only patients with symptomatic gallstones are treated.

The most common treatment for gallstones is surgery to remove the gallbladder. This operation is called a *cholecystectomy*. In rare cases, drugs are used to dissolve the gallstones. Other nonsurgical methods are still considered experimental.

The drug *ursodeoxycholic acid* prevented gallstones from forming in one clinical trial of patients on very-low-calorie diets. However, the drug is costly. Given the small proportion of patients who develop symptomatic gallstones on very-low-calorie diets, it is not known if ursodeoxycholic acid would be a cost-effective drug to recommend for all patients undergoing such diets, though people with pre-existing gallstones may benefit from this drug.

Are the Benefits of Weight Loss Greater Than the Risk of Getting Gallstones?

There's no question that obesity poses serious health risks. Obesity has been linked to heart disease, stroke, high blood pressure, high cholesterol levels, and diabetes. Obesity has also been associated with higher rates of certain types of cancer, such as gallbladder, colon, prostate, breast, cervical, and ovarian cancers.

Weight loss also reduces the risk of heart disease by lowering cholesterol levels. Even a modest weight loss of 10 to 20 pounds can bring positive changes. And the psychological boost from losing weight, such as improved self-image and greater social interaction, should not be ignored.

Patients who are thinking about beginning a commercial diet program to lose a significant amount of weight should talk with their doctors. A physician can evaluate a patient's medical history, individual circumstances, and the proposed weight-loss program. Doctor and patient can then discuss the potential benefits and risks of dieting, including the risks of developing gallstones.

Additional Reading

Clayman CB, ed. *The American Medical Association Encyclopedia of Medicine*. New York: Random House. 1989. This authoritative reference guide for patients has entries on the gallbladder, gallstones, and the biliary system. It is widely available in libraries and bookstores.

Everhart, J.E. Contributions of Obesity and Weight-Loss to Gallstone Disease. *Annals of Internal Medicine* 1993, Vol. 119, pp 1029-35. This article, written for physicians, shows how obesity as well as weight loss and low calorie diets increase the risk of gallstones.

Gallstones. NIH Publication No. 93-2897. This fact sheet provides basic information about gallstones and treatment options. It is published by the National Institute of Diabetes and Digestive and Kidney Diseases and is available through the National Digestive Diseases Information Clearinghouse, Box NDDIC, 9000 Rockville Pike, Bethesda, MD 20892, Tel: 301-654-3810.

Weinsier RL, et. al. Gallstone Formation and Weight Loss. *Obesity Research,* 1993; 1 (1):51 -56. This review article, written for physicians, examines gallstone formation rates in patients on very-low-calorie diets, including the role that fasting and diet composition may play.

Yang H., et. al. Risk Factors for Gallstone Formation during Rapid Loss of Weight. *Digestive Diseases and Sciences,* Vol. 37, No. 6 (June 1992), pp 912-18. This article, written for physicians, discusses gallstone formation in patients on very-low-calorie diets.

Section 24.6

Exercise and Weight Control

The President's Council on Physical Fitness and Sports

Just about everybody seems to be interested in weight control. Some of us weigh just the right amount, others need to gain a few pounds. Most of us "battle the bulge" at some time in our life. Whatever our goals, we should understand and take advantage of the important role of exercise in keeping our weight under control.

Carrying around too much body fat is a major nuisance. Yet excess body fat is common in modern-day living. Few of today's occupations require vigorous physical activity, and much of our leisure time is spent in sedentary pursuits.

Recent estimates indicate that 34 million adults are considered obese (20 percent above desirable weight). Also, there has been an increase in body fat levels in children and youth over the past 20 years. After infancy and early childhood, the earlier the onset of obesity, the greater the likelihood of remaining obese.

Excess body fat has been linked to such health problems as coronary heart disease, high blood pressure, osteoporosis, diabetes, arthritis and certain forms of cancer. Some evidence now exists showing that obesity has a negative effect on both health and longevity.

Exercise is associated with the loss of body fat in both obese and normal weight persons. A regular program of exercise is an important component of any plan to help individuals lose, gain or maintain their weight.

Overweight or Overfat?

Overweight and overfat do not always mean the same thing. Some people are quite muscular and weigh more than the average for their age and height. However, their body composition, the amount of fat versus lean body mass (muscle, bone, organs and tissue), is within a desirable range. This is true for many athletes. Others weigh an average amount yet carry around too much fat. In our society, however, overweight often implies overfat because excess weight is commonly distributed as excess fat. The addition of exercise to a weight control program helps control both body weight and body fat levels.

A certain amount of body fat is necessary for everyone. Experts say that percent body fat for women should be about 20 percent, 15 percent for men. Women with more than 30 percent fat and men with more than 25 percent fat are considered obese.

How much of your weight is fat can be assessed by a variety of methods including underwater (hydrostatic) weighing, skinfold thickness measurements and circumference measurements. Each requires a specially trained person to administer the test and perform the correct calculations. From the numbers obtained, a body fat percentage is determined. Assessing body composition has an advantage over the standard height-weight tables because it can help distinguish between "overweight" and "overfat."

An easy self-test you can do is to pinch the thickness of the fat folds at your waist and abdomen. If you can pinch an inch or more of fat (make sure no muscle is included) chances are you have too much body fat.

People who exercise appropriately increase lean body mass while decreasing their overall fat level. Depending on the amount of fat loss, this can result in a loss of inches without a loss of weight, since muscle weighs more than fat. However, with the proper combination of diet and exercise, both body fat and overall weight can be reduced.

Energy Balance: A Weighty Concept

Losing weight, gaining weight or maintaining your weight depends on the amount of calories you take in and use up during the day, otherwise referred to as energy balance. Learning how to balance energy intake (calories in food) with energy output (calories expended through physical activity) will help you achieve your desired weight.

Although the underlying causes and the treatments of obesity are complex, the concept of energy balance is relatively simple. If you eat more calories than your body needs to perform your day's activities, the extra calories are stored as fat. If you do not take in enough calories to meet your body's energy needs, your body will go to the stored fat to make up the difference. (Exercise helps ensure that stored fat, rather than muscle tissue, is used to meet your energy needs.) If you eat just about the same amount of calories to meet your body's energy needs, your weight will stay the same.

On the average, a person consumes between 800,000 and 900,000 calories each year! An active person needs more calories than a sedentary person, as physically active people require energy above and beyond the day's basic needs. All too often, people who want to lose weight concentrate on counting calorie intake while neglecting calorie output. The most powerful formula is the combination of dietary modification with exercise. By increasing your daily physical activity and decreasing your caloric input you can lose excess weight in the most efficient and healthful way.

Counting Calories

Each pound of fat your body stores represents 3,500 calories of unused energy. In order to lose one pound, you would have to create a calorie deficit of 3,500 calories by either taking in 3,500 less calories over a period of time than you need or doing 3,500 calories worth of exercise. It is recommended that no more than two pounds (7,000 calories) be lost per week for lasting weight loss.

Adding 15 minutes of moderate exercise, say walking one mile, to your daily schedule will use up 100 extra calories per day. (Your body uses approximately 100 calories of energy to walk one mile, depending on your body weight.) Maintaining this schedule would result in an extra 700 calories per week used up, or a loss of about 10 pounds in one year, assuming your food intake stays the same.

To look at energy balance another way, just one extra slice of bread or one extra soft drink a day—or any other food that contains approximately 100 calories—can add up to ten extra pounds in a year if the amount of physical activity you do does not increase.

If you already have a lean figure and want to keep it you should exercise regularly and eat a balanced diet that provides enough calories to make up for the energy you expend. If you wish to gain weight you should exercise regularly and increase the number of calories you consume until you reach your desired weight. Exercise will help ensure that the weight you gain will be lean muscle mass, not extra fat.

The Diet Connection

A balanced diet should be part of any weight control plan. A diet high in complex carbohydrates and moderate in protein and fat will complement an exercise program. It should include enough calories to satisfy your daily nutrient requirements and include the proper number of servings per day from the "basic four food groups": vegetables and fruits (4 servings), breads and cereals (4 servings), milk and milk products (2-4 depending on age) and meats and fish (2).

Experts recommend that your daily intake not fall below 1200 calories unless you are under a doctor's supervision. Also, weekly weight loss should not exceed two pounds.

Remarkable claims have been made for a variety of "crash" diets and diet pills. And some of these very restricted diets do result in noticeable weight loss in a short time. Much of this loss is water and such a loss is quickly regained when normal food and liquid intake is resumed. These diet plans are often expensive and may be dangerous. Moreover, they do not emphasize lifestyle changes that will help you maintain your desired weight. Dieting alone will result in a loss of valuable body tissue such as muscle mass in addition to a loss in fat.

How Many Calories?

The estimates for number of calories (energy) used during a physical activity are based on experiments that measure the amount of oxygen consumed during a specific bout of exercise for a certain body weight.

The energy costs of activities that require you to move your own body weight, such as walking or jogging, are greater for heavier people since they have more weight to move. For example, a person weighing 150 pounds would use more calories jogging one mile than a person jogging alongside who weighs 115 pounds. Always check to see what body weight is referred to in caloric expenditure charts you use.

Exercise and Modern Living

One thing is certain. Most people do not get enough exercise in their ordinary routines. All of the advances of modern technology—from electric can openers to power steering —have made life easier, more comfortable and much less physically demanding. Yet our bodies need activity, especially if they are carrying around too much fat. Satisfying this need requires a definite plan, and a commitment. There are two main ways to increase the number of calories you expend:

1. Start a regular exercise program if you do not have one already.

2. Increase the amount of physical activity in your daily routine.

The best way to control your weight is a combination of the above. The sum total of calories used over time will help regulate your weight as well as keep you physically fit.

Active Lifestyles

Before looking at what kind of regular exercise program is best, let's look at how you can increase the amount of physical activity in your daily routine to supplement your exercise program.

- Recreational pursuits such as gardening on weekends, bowling in the office league, family outings, an evening of social dancing, and many other activities provide added exercise. They are fun and can be considered an extra bonus in your weight control campaign.

- Add more "action" to your day. Walk to the neighborhood grocery store instead of using the car. Park several blocks from the office and walk the rest of the way. Walk up the stairs instead of using the elevator; start with one flight of steps and gradually increase.

Energy Expenditure Chart

	Energy Costs Cals/Hour*
A. Sedentary Activities	
Lying down or sleeping	90
Sitting quietly	84
Sitting and writing, card playing, etc.	114
B. Moderate Activities	**(150-350)**
Bicycling (5 mph)	174
Canoeing (2.5 mph)	174
Dancing (Ballroom)	210
Golf (2-some, carrying clubs)	324
Horseback riding (sitting to trot)	246
Light housework. cleaning, etc.	246
Swimming (crawl, 20 yards/min)	288
Tennis (recreational doubles)	312
Volleyball (recreational)	264
Walking (2 mph)	198
C. Vigorous Activities	**(More than 350)**
Aerobic Dancing	546
Basketball (recreational)	450
Bicycling (13 mph)	612
Circuit weight training	756
Football (touch, vigorous)	498
Ice Skating (9 mph)	384
Racquetball	588
Roller Skating (9 mph)	384
Jogging (10 minute mile, 6 mph)	654
Scrubbing Floors	440
Swimming (crawl, 45 yards/min)	522
Tennis (recreational singles)	450
X-country Skiing (5 mph)	690

*Hourly estimates based on values calculated for calories burned per minute for a 150 pound (68 kg) person.

(Sources: William D McArdle. Frank I. Katch. Victor L Katch. "Exercise Physiology: Energy, Nutrition and Human Performance" (2nd edition). Lea & Febiger, Philadelphia, 1986; Melvin H. Williams, *"Nutrition for Fitness and Sport,"* William C. Brown Company Publishers. Dubuque. 1983.)

- Change your attitude toward movement. Instead of considering an extra little walk or trip to the files an annoyance, look upon it as an added fitness boost. Look for opportunities to use your body. Bend, stretch, reach, move, lift and carry. Time-saving devices and gadgets eliminate drudgery and are a bonus to mankind, but when they substitute too often for physical activity they can demand a high cost in health, vigor and fitness.

These little bits of action are cumulative in their effects. Alone, each does not burn a huge amount of calories. But when added together they can result in a sizable amount of energy used over the course of the day. And they will help improve your muscle tone and flexibility at the same time.

What Kind Of Exercise?

Although any kind of physical movement requires energy (calories), the type of exercise that uses the most energy is "aerobic" exercise. The term "aerobic" is derived from the Greek word meaning "with oxygen." Jogging, brisk walking, swimming. biking, cross-country skiing and aerobic dancing are some popular forms of aerobic exercise.

Aerobic exercises use the body's large muscle groups in continuous, rhythmic, sustained movement and require oxygen for the production of energy. When oxygen is combined with food (which can come from stored fat) energy is produced to power the body's musculature. The longer you move aerobically, the more energy needed and the more calories used. Regular aerobic exercise will improve your cardiorespiratory endurance, the ability of your heart, lungs, blood vessels and associated tissues to use oxygen to produce energy needed for activity. You'll build a healthier body while getting rid of excess body fat.

In addition to the aerobic exercise. supplement your program with muscle strengthening and stretching exercises. The stronger your muscles, the longer you will be able to keep going during aerobic activity, and the less chance of injury.

How Much? How Often?

Experts recommend that you do some form of aerobic exercise at least three times a week for a minimum of 20 continuous minutes. Of course, if that is too much, start with a shorter time span and gradually build up to the minimum. Then gradually progress until you are able to work aerobically for 20-40 minutes. If you need to lose a large amount of weight, you may want to do your aerobic workout five times a week.

It is important to exercise at an intensity vigorous enough to cause your heart rate and breathing to increase. How hard you should exercise depends to a certain degree on your age, and is determined by measuring your heart rate in beats per minute.

The heart rate you should maintain is called your target heart rate, and there are several ways you can arrive at this figure. The simplest is to subtract your age from 220 and then calculate 60 to 80 percent of that figure. Beginners should maintain the 60 percent level, more advanced can work up to the 80 percent level. This is just a guide however, and people with any medical limitations should discuss this formula with their physician.

You can do different types of aerobic activities, say walking one day, riding a bike the next. Make sure you choose an activity that can be done regularly, and is enjoyable for you. The important thing to remember is not to skip too many days between workouts or fitness benefits will be lost. If you must lose a few days, gradually work back into your routine.

The Benefits of Exercise in a Weight Control Program

The benefits of exercise are many, from producing physically fit bodies to providing an outlet for fun and socialization. When added to a weight control program these benefits take on increased significance.

We already have noted that proper exercise can help control weight by burning excess body fat. It also has two other body-trimming advantages: 1) exercise builds muscle tissue and muscle uses calories up at a faster rate than body fat; and 2) exercise helps reduce inches and a firm, lean body looks slimmer even if your weight remains the same.

Remember, fat does not "turn into" muscle, as is often believed. Fat and muscle are two entirely different substances and one cannot become the other. However, muscle does use calories at a faster rate than fat which directly affects your body's metabolic rate or energy requirement. Your basal metabolic rate (BMR) is the amount of energy required to sustain the body's functions at rest and it depends on your age, sex, body size, genes and body composition. People with high levels of muscle tend to have higher BMRs and use more calories in the resting stage.

Some studies have even shown that your metabolic rate stays elevated for some time after vigorous exercise, causing you to use even more calories throughout your day.

Additional benefits may be seen in how exercise affects appetite. A lean person in good shape may eat more following increased activity, but the regular exercise will burn up the extra calories consumed. On the other hand, vigorous exercise has been reported to suppress appetite. And, physical activity can be used as a positive substitute for between meal snacking.

Better Mental Health

The psychological benefits of exercise are equally important to the weight conscious person. Exercise decreases stress and relieves tensions that might otherwise lead to overeating. Exercise builds physical fitness which in turn builds self-confidence, enhanced self-image, and a positive outlook. When you start to feel good about yourself, you are more likely to want to make other positive changes in your lifestyle that will help keep your weight under control.

In addition, exercise can be fun, provide recreation and offer opportunities for companionship. The exhilaration and emotional release of participating in sports or other activities are a boost to mental and physical health. Pent-up anxieties and frustrations seem to disappear when you're concentrating on returning a serve, sinking a putt or going that extra mile.

Tips to Get You Started

Hopefully, you are now convinced that in order to successfully manage your weight you must include exercise in your daily routine. Here are some tips to get you started:

1. Check with your doctor first. Since you are carrying around some extra "baggage," it is wise to get your doctor's "OK" before embarking on an exercise program.

2. Choose activities that you think you'll enjoy. Most people will stick to their exercise program if they are having fun, even though they are working hard.

3. Set aside a regular exercise time. Whether this means joining an exercise class or getting up a little earlier every day, make

time for this addition to your routine and don't let anything get in your way. Planning ahead will help you get around interruptions in your workout schedule, such as bad weather and vacations.

4. Set short term goals. Don't expect to lose 20 pounds in two weeks. It's taken awhile for you to gain the weight, it will take time to lose it. Keep a record of your progress and tell your friends and family about your achievements.

5. Vary your exercise program. Change exercises or invite friends to join you to make your workout more enjoyable. There is no "best" exercise—just the one that works best for you.

It won't be easy, especially at the start. But as you begin to feel better, look better and enjoy a new zest for life, you will be rewarded many times over for your efforts.

Tips to Keep You Going

1. Adopt a specific plan and write it down.
2. Keep setting realistic goals as you go along, and remind yourself of them often.
3. Keep a log to record your progress and make sure to keep it up-to-date.
4. Include weight and/or percent body fat measures in your log. Extra pounds can easily creep back.
5. Upgrade your fitness program as you progress.
6. Enlist the support and company of your family and friends.
7. Update others on your successes.
8. Avoid injuries by pacing yourself and including a warmup and cooldown period as part of every workout.
9. Reward yourself periodically for a job well done!

Chapter 25

Health Benefits of Smoking Cessation

Preface to the Executive Summary

This Report of the Surgeon General is the twenty-first report of the U.S. Public Health Service on the health consequences of smoking and the first issued during my tenure as Surgeon General. Whereas previous reports have focused on the health effects of smoking, this Report is devoted to the benefits of smoking cessation.

The public health impact of smoking is enormous. As documented in the 1989 Surgeon General's Report, an estimated 390,000 Americans die each year from diseases caused by smoking. This toll includes 115,000 deaths from heart disease; 106,000 from lung cancer; 31,600 from other cancers; 57,000 from chronic obstructive pulmonary disease; 27,500 from stroke; and 52,900 from other conditions related to smoking. More than one of every six deaths in the United States are caused by smoking. For more than a decade the Public Health Service has identified cigarette smoking as the most important preventable cause of death in our society.

It is clear, then, that the elimination of smoking would yield substantial benefits for public health. What are the benefits, however, for the individual smoker who quits? A large body of evidence has accumulated to address that question and derives from cohort and case-control studies, cross-sectional surveys, and clinical trials. In studies of the health effects of smoking cessation, persons classified as former

---

A Report of the Surgeon General, 1990. U.S. DHHS Pub. No. 90-8416, 1990.

smokers may include some current smokers; this misclassification is likely to cause an underestimation of the health benefits of quitting. Taken together, the evidence clearly indicates that smoking cessation has major and immediate health benefits for men and women of all ages.

Overall Benefits of Smoking Cessation

People who quit smoking live longer than those who continue to smoke. To what extent is a smoker's risk of premature death reduced after quitting smoking? The answer depends on several factors, including the number of years of smoking, the number of cigarettes smoked per day, and the presence or absence of disease at the time of quitting. Data from the American Cancer Society's Cancer Prevention Study II (CPS-II) were analyzed in this Report to estimate the risk of premature death in ex-smokers versus current smokers. These data show, for example, that persons who quit smoking before age 50 have one-half the risk of dying in the next 15 years compared with continuing smokers.

Smoking cessation increases life expectancy because it reduces the risk of dying from specific smoking-related diseases. One such disease is lung cancer, the most common cause of cancer death in both men and women. The risk of dying from lung cancer is 22 times higher among male smokers and 12 times higher among female smokers compared with people who have never smoked. The risk of lung cancer declines steadily in people who quit smoking; after 10 years of abstinence, the risk of lung cancer is about 30 to 50 percent of the risk for continuing smokers. Smoking cessation also reduces the risk of cancers of the larynx, oral cavity, esophagus, pancreas, and urinary bladder.

Coronary heart disease (CHD) is the leading cause of death in the United States. Smokers have about twice the risk of dying from CHD compared with lifetime nonsmokers. This excess risk is reduced by about half among ex-smokers after only 1 year of smoking abstinence and declines gradually thereafter. After 15 years of abstinence the risk of CHD is similar to that of persons who have never smoked.

Compared with lifetime nonsmokers, smokers have about twice the risk of dying from stroke, the third leading cause of death in the United States. After quitting smoking, the risk of stroke returns to the level of people who have never smoked; in some studies this reduction in risk has occurred within 5 years, but in others as long as 15 years of abstinence were required.

Cigarette smoking is the major cause of chronic obstructive pulmonary disease (COPD), the fifth leading cause of death in the United States. Smoking increases the risk of COPD by accelerating the age-related decline in lung function. With sustained abstinence from smoking, the rate of decline of lung function among former smokers returns to that of never smokers, thus reducing the risk of developing COPD.

Influenza and pneumonia represent the sixth leading cause of death in the United States. Cigarette smoking increases the risk of respiratory infections such as influenza, pneumonia, and bronchitis, and smoking cessation reduces the risk.

Cigarette smoking is a major cause of peripheral artery occlusive disease. This condition causes substantial mortality and morbidity; complications may include intermittent claudication, tissue ischemia and gangrene, and ultimately, loss of limb. Smoking cessation substantially reduces the risk of peripheral artery occlusive disease compared with continued smoking.

The mortality rate from abdominal aortic aneurysm is two to five times higher in current smokers than in never smokers. Former smokers have half the excess risk of dying from this condition relative to current smokers.

About 90 million Americans currently have, or have had, an ulcer of the stomach or duodenum. Smokers have an increased risk of developing gastric or duodenal ulcers, and this increased risk is reduced by quitting smoking.

Benefits at All Ages

According to a 1989 Gallup survey, the proportion of smokers who say they would like to give up smoking is lower for smokers aged 50 and older (57 percent) than for smokers aged 18-29 (68 percent) and 30-49 (67 percent). Older smokers may be less motivated to quit smoking because the highly motivated may have quit already at younger ages, leaving a relatively "hard-core" group of older smokers. But many long-term smokers may lack motivation to quit for other reasons. Some may believe they are no longer at risk of smoking-related diseases because they have already survived smoking for many years. Others may believe that any damage that may have been caused by smoking is irreversible after decades of smoking. For similar reasons, many physicians may be less likely to counsel their older patients to quit.

CPS-II data were used to estimate the effects of quitting smoking at various ages on the cumulative risk of death during a fixed interval after cessation. The results show the benefits of cessation extend to quitting at older ages. For example, a healthy man aged 60-64 who smokes 1 pack of cigarettes or more per day reduces his risk of dying during the next 15 years by 10 percent if he quits smoking.

These findings support the recommendations of the Surgeon General's 1988 Workshop on Health Promotion and Aging for the development and dissemination of smoking cessation messages and interventions to older persons. I am pleased that a coalition of organizations and agencies is now working toward implementation of those recommendations, including the Centers for Disease Control; the National Cancer Institute; the National Heart, Lung, and Blood Institute; the Administration on Aging; the Department of Veterans Affairs; the Office of Disease Prevention and Health Promotion; the American Association of Retired Persons; and the Fox Chase Cancer Center. The major message of this campaign will be that it is never too late to quit smoking.

Two facts point to the urgent need for a strong smoking cessation campaign targeting older Americans:

1. Seven million smokers are aged 60 or older; and

2. Smoking is a major risk factor for 6 of the 14 leading causes of death among those aged 60 and older, and is a complicating factor for 3 others.

Benefits for Smokers with Existing Disease

Many smokers who have already developed smoking-related disease or symptoms may be less motivated to quit because of a belief that the damage is already done. For the same reason, physicians may be less motivated to advise these patients to quit. However, the evidence reviewed in this report shows that smoking cessation yields important health benefits to those who already suffer from smoking-related illness.

Among persons with diagnosed CHD, smoking cessation markedly reduces the risk of recurrent heart attack and cardiovascular death. In many studies, this reduction in risk has been 50 percent or more. Smoking cessation is the most important intervention in the management of peripheral artery occlusive disease; for patients with this condition, quitting smoking improves exercise tolerance, reduces the risk of amputation after peripheral artery surgery, and increases overall survival. Patients with gastric and duodenal ulcers who stop smoking improve their clinical course relative to smokers who continue to smoke. Although the benefits of smoking cessation among stroke patients have not been studied, it is reasonable to assume that quitting smoking reduces the risk of recurrent stroke just as it reduces the risk of recurrence of other cardiovascular events.

Even smokers who have already developed cancer may benefit from smoking cessation. A few studies have shown that persons who stopped smoking after diagnosis of cancer had a reduced risk of acquiring a second primary cancer compared with persons who continued to smoke. Although relevant data are sparse, longer survival might be expected among smokers with cancer or other serious illnesses if they stop smoking. Smoking cessation reduces the risk of respiratory infections such as pneumonia, which are often the immediate causes of death in patients with an underlying chronic disease.

The important role of health care providers in counseling patients to quit smoking is well recognized. Health care providers should give smoking cessation advice and assistance to all patients who smoke, including those with existing illness.

Benefits for the Fetus

Maternal smoking is associated with several complications of pregnancy including abruptio placentae, placenta previa, bleeding during pregnancy, premature and prolonged rupture of the membranes, and preterm delivery. Maternal smoking retards fetal growth, causes an average reduction in birth-weight of 200 g, and doubles the risk of having a low birth-weight baby. Studies have shown a 25- to 50-percent higher rate of fetal and infant deaths among women who smoke during pregnancy compared with those who do not.

Women who stop smoking before becoming pregnant have infants of the same birth-weight as those born to women who have never smoked. The same benefit accrues to women who quit smoking in the first 3 to 4 months of pregnancy and who remain abstinent throughout the remainder of pregnancy. Women who quit smoking at later stages of pregnancy, up to the 30th week of gestation, have infants with higher birth-weight than do women who smoke throughout pregnancy.

Smoking is probably the most important modifiable cause of poor pregnancy outcome among women in the United States. Recent estimates suggest that the elimination of smoking during pregnancy could prevent about 5 percent of perinatal deaths, about 20 percent of low birth-weight births, and about 8 percent of preterm deliveries in the United States. In groups with a high prevalence of smoking (e.g., women who have not completed high school), the elimination of smoking during pregnancy could prevent about 10 percent of perinatal deaths, about 35 percent of low birth-weight births, and about 15 percent of preterm deliveries.

The prevalence of smoking during pregnancy has declined over time but remains unacceptably high. Approximately 30 percent of U.S. women who are cigarette smokers quit after recognition of pregnancy, and others quit later in pregnancy. However, about 25 percent of pregnant women in the United States smoke throughout pregnancy. A shocking statistic is that half of pregnant women who have not completed high school smoke throughout pregnancy. Many women who do not quit smoking during pregnancy reduce their daily cigarette consumption; however, reduced consumption without quitting may have little or no benefit for birth-weight. Of the women who quit smoking during pregnancy, 70 percent resume smoking within 1 year of delivery.

Initiatives have been launched in the public and private sectors to reduce smoking during pregnancy. These programs should be expanded, and less educated pregnant women should be a special target of these efforts. Strategies need to be developed to address the problem of relapse after delivery.

Benefits for Infants and Children

As a pediatrician, I am particularly concerned about the effects of parental smoking on infants and children. Evidence reviewed in the 1986 Surgeon General's Report, *The Health Consequences of Involuntary Smoking*, indicates that the children of parents who smoke, compared with the children of non-smoking parents, have an increased frequency of respiratory infections such as pneumonia and bronchitis. Many studies have found a dose-response relationship between respiratory illness in children and their level of tobacco smoke exposure.

Several studies have shown that children exposed to tobacco smoke in the home are more likely to develop acute otitis media and persistent middle ear effusions. Middle ear disease imposes a substantial burden on the health care system. Otitis media is the most frequent diagnosis made by physicians who care for children. The myringotomy-and-tube procedure, used to treat otitis media in more than 1 million American children each year, is the most common minor surgical operation performed under general anesthesia.

The impact of smoking cessation during or after pregnancy on these associations has not been studied. However, the dose-response relationship between parental smoking and frequency of childhood respiratory infections suggests that smoking cessation during pregnancy and abstinence after delivery would eliminate most or all of the excess risk by eliminating most or all of the exposure.

If parents are unwilling to quit smoking for their own sake, I would urge them to quit for the sake of their children.

Passive-smoking-induced infections in infants and young children can cause serious and even fatal illness. Moreover, children whose parents smoke are much more likely to become smokers themselves.

Smoking Cessation and Weight Gain

The fear of post-cessation weight gain may discourage many smokers from trying to quit. The fear or occurrence of weight gain may precipitate relapse among many of those who already have quit. In the 1986 Adult Use of Tobacco Survey, current smokers who had tried to quit were asked to judge the importance of several possible reasons for their return to smoking. Twenty-seven percent responded that "actual weight gain" was a "very important" or "somewhat important" reason why they resumed smoking; 22 percent said that "the possibility of gaining weight" was an important reason for their relapse. Forty-seven percent of current smokers and 48 percent of former smokers agreed with the statement that "smoking helps control weight."

Fifteen studies involving a total of 20,000 persons were reviewed in this report to determine the likelihood of gaining weight and the average weight gain after quitting. Although four-fifths of smokers who quit gained weight alter cessation, the average weight gain was only 5 pounds (2.3 kg). The average weight gain among subjects who continued to smoke was 1 pound. Thus, smoking cessation produces a 4-pound greater weight gain than that associated with continued smoking. This weight gain poses a minimal health risk. Moreover, evidence suggests that this small weight gain is accompanied by favorable changes in lipid profiles and in body fat distribution. Smoking cessation programs and messages should emphasize that weight gain after quitting is small on average.

Not only is the average post-cessation weight gain small, but the risk of large weight gain after quitting is extremely low. Less than 4 percent of those who quit smoking gain more than 20 pounds. Nevertheless, special advice and assistance should be available to the rare person who does gain considerable weight after quitting. For these individuals, the health benefits of cessation still occur, and weight control programs rather than smoking relapse should be implemented.

Increase in food intake and decreases in resting energy expenditure are largely responsible for post-cessation weight gain. Thus, dietary advice and exercise should be helpful in preventing or reducing post-cessation weight gain. Unfortunately, minor weight control modification to smoking cessation programs do not generally yield beneficial effects in terms of reducing weight gain or increasing cessation rates. A few studies have investigated pharmacologic approaches to post-cessation weight control; preliminary results are encouraging but more research is needed. High priority should be given to the development and evaluation of effective weight control programs that can be targeted in a cost-effective manner to those at greatest need of assistance.

Psychological and Behavioral Consequences of Smoking Cessation

Nicotine withdrawal symptoms include anxiety, irritability, frustration, anger, difficulty concentrating, increased appetite, and urges to smoke. With the possible exception of urges to smoke and increased appetite, these effects soon disappear. Nicotine withdrawal peaks in first 1 to 2 days following cessation and subsides rapidly during the following weeks. With long-term abstinence, former smokers are likely to enjoy favorable psychological changes such as enhanced self-esteem and increased sense of self-control.

Although most nicotine withdrawal symptoms are short-lived, they often exert a strong influence on smokers' ability to quit and maintain abstinence. Nicotine withdrawal may discourage many smokers from trying to quit and may precipitate relapse among those who have recently quit. In the 1986 Adult Use of Tobacco Survey, 39 percent of current smokers reported that irritability was a "very important" or "somewhat important" reason why they resumed smoking after a previous quit attempt.

Smokers and ex-smokers should be counseled that adverse psychological effects of smoking subside rapidly over time. Smoking cessation materials and programs, nicotine replacement, exercise, stress management, and dietary counseling can help smokers cope with these symptoms until they abate, after which favorable psychological changes are likely to occur.

Support for a Causal Association Between Smoking and Disease

Tens of thousands of studies have documented the associations between cigarette smoking and a large number of serious diseases. It is safe to say that smoking represents the most extensively documented cause of disease ever investigated in the history of biomedical research. Previous Surgeon General's reports, in particular the landmark 1964 Report of the Surgeon General's Advisory Committee on Smoking and Health and the 1982 Surgeon General's Report on smoking and cancer, examined these associations with respect to epidemiologic criteria for causality. These criteria include the consistency, strength, specificity, coherence, and temporal relationship of the association. Based on these criteria, previous reports have recognized a causal association between smoking and cancers of the lung, larynx, esophagus, and oral cavity; heart disease; stroke; peripheral artery occlusive disease; chronic obstructive pulmonary disease; and intrauterine growth retardation. This Surgeon General's Report is the first to conclude that the evidence is now sufficient to identify cigarette smoking as a cause of cancer of the urinary bladder; the 1982 report concluded that cigarette smoking is a contributing factor in the development of bladder cancer.

The causal nature of most of these associations was well established long before publication of this report. Nevertheless, it is worth noting that the findings of this report add even more weight to the evidence that these associations are causal. The criterion of coherence requires that descriptive epidemiologic findings on disease occurrence correlate with measures of exposure to the suspected agent. Coherence would predict that the increased risk of disease associated with an exposure would diminish or disappear after cessation of exposure. As this report shows in great detail, the risks of most smoking-related diseases decrease after cessation and with increasing duration or abstinence.

Evidence on the risk of disease after smoking cessation is especially important for the understanding of smoking-and-disease associations of unclear causality. For example cigarette smoking is associated with cancer of the uterine cervix, but this association is potentially confounded by unidentified factors (in particular by a sexually transmitted etiologic agent). The evidence reviewed in this report indicates that former smokers experience a lower risk of cervical cancer than current smokers even after adjusting for the social correlates of smoking and risk of sexually acquired infections. This diminution of risk after smoking cessation supports the hypothesis that smoking is a contributing cause of cervical cancer.

Conclusion

The Comprehensive Smoking Education Act of 1984 (Public Law 98-474) requires the rotation of four health warnings on cigarette packages and advertisements. One of those warnings reads "SURGEON GENERAL'S WARNING: Quitting Smoking Now Greatly Reduces Serious Risks to Your Health." The evidence reviewed in this report confirms and expands that advice.

The health benefits of quitting smoking are immediate and substantial. They far exceed any risks from the average 5-pound weight gain or any adverse psychological affects that may follow quitting. The benefits extend to men and women to the young and the old, to those who are sick and to those who are well. Smoking cessation represents the single most important step that smokers can take to enhance the length and quality of their lives.

Public opinion polls tell us that most smokers want to quit. This report provides smokers with new and more powerful motivation to give up this self-destructive behavior.

Summary

1. Smoking cessation reduces rates of respiratory symptoms such as cough, sputum production, and wheezing, and respiratory infections such as bronchitis and pneumonia, compared with continued smoking.

2. For persons without overt chronic obstructive pulmonary disease (COPD), smoking cessation improves pulmonary function about 5 percent within a few months after cessation.

3. Cigarette smoking accelerates the age-related decline in lung function that occurs among never smokers. With sustained

abstinence from smoking, the rate of decline in pulmonary function among former smokers returns to that of never smokers.

4. With sustained abstinence, the COPD mortality rates among former smokers decline in comparison with continuing smokers.

—Antonia C. Novello, M.D.. M.P.H.,
Surgeon General of the United States, 1990

Index

Index

Page numbers in *italics* refer to tables and illustrations; the letter "n" following a page number refers to a note.

A

abortion 150, 247–61
Abortion: Commonly Asked Questions 247n
About Your Heart and Blood Pressure 487
abruptio placentae 533
abstinence failure rate 175
acetaminophen 10–11, 16
ACR *see* American College of Radiology (ACR)
ACS *see* American Cancer Society (ACS)
ACTG *see* AIDS Clinical Trials Groups (ACTG)
active lifestyles 523, 525
Acute Renal Infection in Women 282
ADA *see* American Dietetic Association (ADA)
adenomyosis 72
ADFR complex 319
Administration on Aging 532

Adolescent psychopathology 450
adoption 235
adrenal glands 31, 58–59
Adult and Pediatric Urology 382
Adult Use of Tobacco Survey (1986) 535, 536
Advanced Care Products 123
Advil 10
aerobic exercise 309, 312, 495, 525–26
Agency for Health Care Policy and Research (AHCPR) 155, 399n, 406n, 406–7
Age Pages: Preventing Falls and Fractures 360, 361–64
AHA *see* American Heart Association (AHA)
AHCPR *see* Agency for Health Care Policy and Research (AHCPR)
AIDS (Acquired Immune Deficiency Syndrome) 116, 125, 146, 153–54, 233
  Pap smear tests 134
  perinatal transmission 160–61
  pregnancy 142, 146
  protection 166, 169
  sexually transmitted diseases (STDs) 142, 144, 156
  see also HIV (human immunodeficiency virus)